Lung Cancer: Clinical Diagnosis and Treatment

Lung Cancer: Clinical Diagnosis and Treatment

Editor: Marley Barnes

MURPHY & MOORE
www.murphy-moorepublishing.com

www.murphy-moorepublishing.com

MURPHY & MOORE

Cataloging-in-Publication Data

Lung cancer : clinical diagnosis and treatment / edited by Marley Barnes.
p. cm.
Includes bibliographical references and index.
ISBN 978-1-63987-347-0
1. Lungs--Cancer. 2. Lungs--Cancer--Diagnosis. 3. Lungs--Cancer--Treatment. I. Barnes, Marley.
RC280.L8 L86 2022
616.994 36--dc23

Murphy & Moore Publishing,
1 Rockefeller Plaza,
New York City, NY 10020, USA

ISBN 978-1-63987-347-0 (Hardback)

Contents

Preface

Lung cancer is the uncontrolled growth of cells in the lung tissues. This uncontrolled growth can spread beyond the tissues of lungs to other parts of the body through a process known as metastasis. There are two main types of lung cancer, namely, small-cell lung carcinoma and non-small-cell lung carcinoma. Its symptoms are shortness of breath, coughing up blood, weight loss and chest pain. In most cases, the main cause of cancer is prolonged use of tobacco. Other risk factors can be a combination of genetic factors and exposure to radon gas, second-hand smoke, asbestos, and air pollution. There are various diagnostic techniques which can be used to diagnose lung cancer such as computed tomography scans, chest radiographs and biopsy. This book includes some of the vital pieces of work being conducted across the world, on various topics related to the clinical diagnosis and management of lung cancer. It will also provide interesting topics for research which interested readers can take up. This book is a complete source of knowledge on the present status of this important field.

This book unites the global concepts and researches in an organized manner for a comprehensive understanding of the subject. It is a ripe text for all researchers, students, scientists or anyone else who is interested in acquiring a better knowledge of this dynamic field.

I extend my sincere thanks to the contributors for such eloquent research chapters. Finally, I thank my family for being a source of support and help.

Editor

1

Radiotherapy in Lung Cancer

Fiona Lim Mei Ying

Abstract

Lung cancer remains one of the top five cancers worldwide. Around 85% are nonsmall cell lung cancer (NSCLC) and only one-third present with early stage diseases. Radiotherapy had an important role both in radical and palliative treatment. With advancement in technology, newer techniques of stereotactic body radiotherapy allow delivery of much higher biologically effective dose to tumor achieving similar outcomes to radical surgery in early stage diseases. However, the usually large tumor volume together with preexiting poor lung condition makes radiotherapy challenging to deliver a radical dose to tumor while maintaining normal tissue constrains. In this chapter, different indications and techniques used in treating NSCLC will be discussed and reviewed.

Keywords: nonsmall cell lung cancer, external beam radiotherapy, stereotactic body radiotherapy

1. Introduction

According to the World Cancer Report 2014, lung cancer remains the top five most common cancers among both men and women worldwide. And it is also the leading cause of cancer deaths. Majority (around 85%) are nonsmall cell lung carcinomas [1, 2]. Incidence of adenocarcinoma had been rising and now became the most common histological subtypes in both men and women. About one-third of them are presented with early stage localized disease (stage I–II), another one-third with locally advanced disease (stage III), and remaining one-third with metastatic disease (stage IV) at diagnosis [3, 4].

2. Anatomy

Lungs are a paired structure that is separated into left and right by the mediastinum, which contains the tracheal, heart, esophagus, and lymph nodes. The left lung is divided into upper and lower lobe by oblique fissure, while the right lung is divided into three lobes (upper, middle, and lower) by oblique and horizontal fissures.

Lung cancers can arise from mucosa of the tracheobronchial tree or the alveolar lining cells of peripheral lung parenchyma. Tumor can spread locally within lung parenchyma or invading surrounding structures including mediastinum, major vessels, or chest wall (**Figure 1**). They can also spread along major airways causing obstruction, distal collapse, or atelectasis (**Figure 2**).

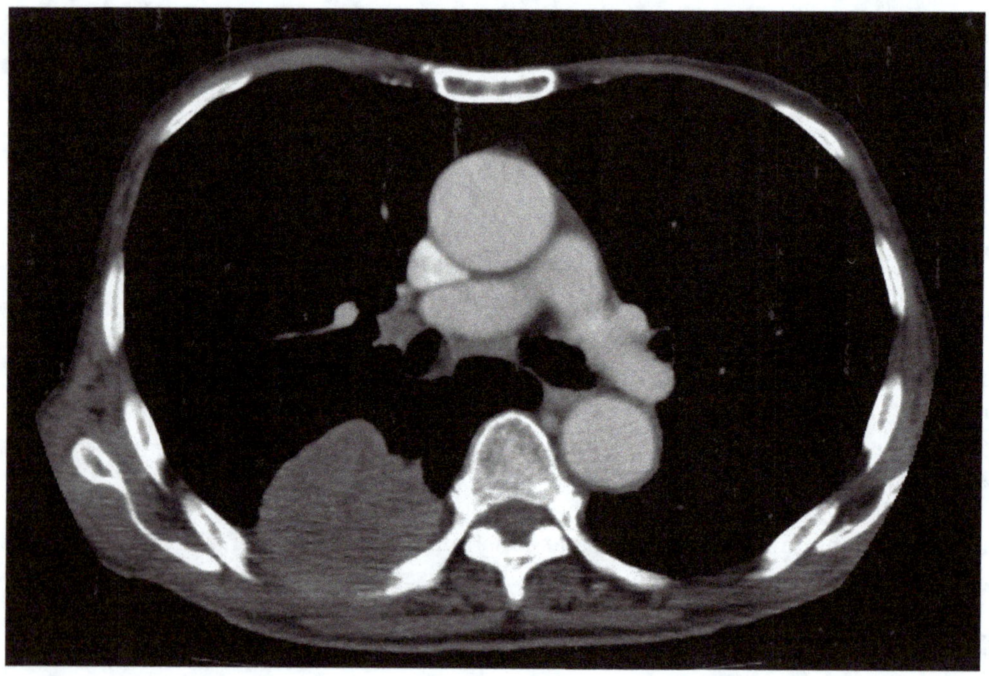

Figure 1. Tumor invasion to chest wall.

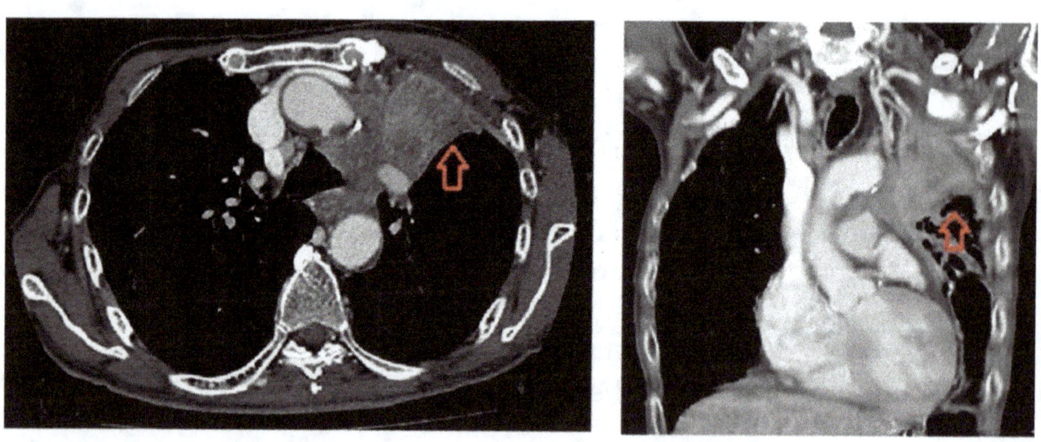

Figure 2. Tumor over left main bronchus causing collapse of left upper lobe (red arrow).

There is rich lymphatic within the respiratory system that accounts for the high rate of nodal metastasis. The lymph node map proposed by the International Association for the Study of Lung Cancer (ISALC) in 2009 divides the lymph nodes into 14 stations and sever zones [5]. It is adopted by the latest seventh edition of AJCC and UICC Manual for N staging, with involvement of ipsilateral hila node as N1, ipsilateral mediastinal nodes as N2, and contralateral mediastinal or supraclavicular nodes as N3. Lymph nodes drainage depends on the location of tumors, with those in left upper lobe drain predominantly into subaortic node and those in right upper lobe drain predominantly into right upper paratracheal node. Middle and lower lobe tumors drain more commonly into subcarinal and lower paratracheal nodes. However, skip metastasis to mediastinal nodes bypassing hilar nodes occur in around 10–25% tumors [6]. Lymph nodes with short axis diameter ≥10 mm is considered suspicious of nodal metastasis (**Figure 3**).

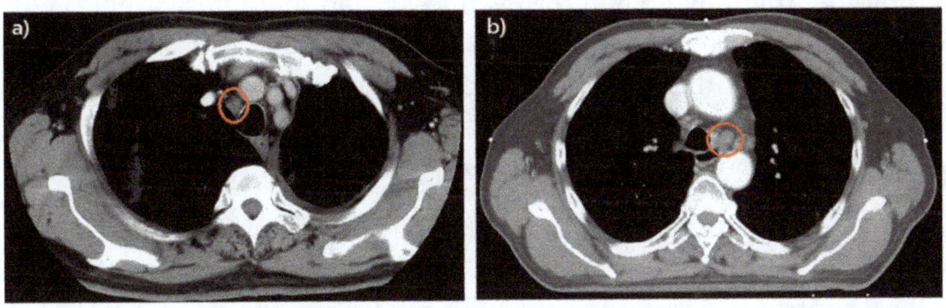

Figure 3. Enlarged mediastinal lymph node over (a) right upper paratracheal node (station 2R) and (b) subaortic node (station 5).

3. Staging and assessment

All patients with suspected lung cancer should have computer tomography (CT) of thorax with intravenous contrast for proper staging. Histological proof from primary tumors can be obtained by bronchoscopy if centrally located or by image-guided approach if peripherally located. For those patients planned for radical treatment, positron emission tomography (PET) scan is recommended to exclude any distant metastasis. Unanticipated metastasis may be detected in up to 10–20% cases. It is also more useful than CT in differentiating collapse or atelectasis from primary tumors (**Figure 4**). Any suspicious lymph nodes based on enlargement on CT or uptake in PET should be confirmed by needle technique (e.g., endoscopic ultrasound) or mediastinoscopy.

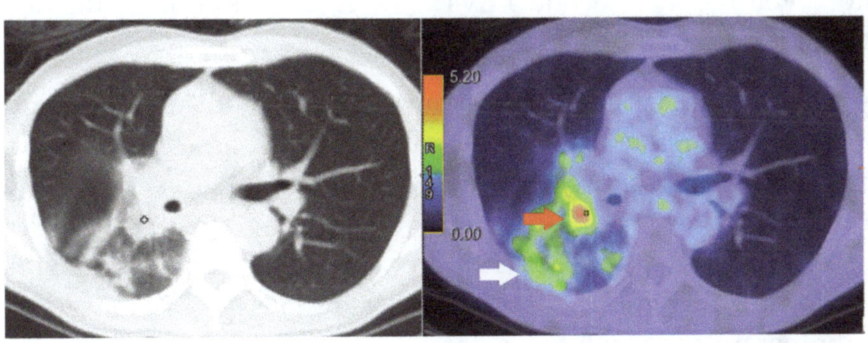

Figure 4. Use of PET in differentiating primary tumor with intense uptake (red arrow) from surrounding collapse or atetactasis (white arrow).

4. Indications of radiotherapy

4.1. Nonsmall cell lung cancer

4.1.1. Early stage I–II disease: curative treatment

Radical surgery remained the preferred treatment in early stage I–II lung cancer with 5-year overall survival rate of around 60–80%. Radical radiotherapy can be an alternative to patients who are medically unfit for surgery due to medical comorbidities or who declined surgery. Currently, there are no phase III trials to directly compare the outcomes after surgery with radiotherapy. Retrospective and historical databases showed that the long-term survival after conventional radiotherapy may be half (or even less) than that after surgery, with 5-year survival of around 20–30% in most series. But this indirect comparison is difficult due to the different population groups with more elderly, comorbidities, or poor lung function in those nonsurgical series. For elderly patients, hypofractionated scheme using 55 Gray (Gy) in 20 daily fractions is as effective as conventional radiotherapy in 2Gy per fraction.

Stereotactic body radiotherapy (SBRT) is now a newly emerging treatment option that allows delivery of a much higher radiation dose to a precise area than conventional radiotherapy. The reported local control rate in early stage lung cancer can be up to 80–90% in 2 years and is well tolerated. Therefore, it becomes the preferred radiotherapy modality for stage I lung cancer patients who are not fit for surgery. But extra care should be given when treating tumors that are centrally located around the major airways due to the potential higher complications with the hypofractionated regime.

4.1.2. Locally advanced stage III disease: curative treatment

This stage of disease was considered locally advanced either due to extensive primary tumor extension to extrathoracic structures nearby (T3 or T4) or mediastinal lymph nodes involvement (N2 or N3). It is a heterogeneous population that requires multimodality treatments. The reported 5-year survival was around 10–30%. A multidisciplinary discussion involving cardiothoracic surgeons, radiologists, and oncologists is needed to individualize and optimize the treatment plan for each patient. Patients with good performance status 0–1, no significant weight loss of >10% in the preceding 3 months and good pulmonary function (forced expiratory volume in 1 second FEV1 > 1.0 L) are candidates for radical combined modality treatment.

For potentially operable N2 disease, induction treatment with either chemotherapy alone or chemoirradiation is recommended over surgery alone. There is no solid evidence to support the superiority of either approach. Addition of preoperative radiotherapy may have the potential effect in downstaging the tumor and achieving a higher pathological complete remission rate of mediastinal disease. Special precaution should be given with its use in candidates before a planned pneumonectomy due to the higher perioperative mortalities. When preoperative radiotherapy is considered, a dose higher than 45–54 Gy in 1.8–2 Gy per fraction had not been shown to give addition survival benefit.

For infiltrative N2 or N3 (contralateral mediastinum) disease, risk of systemic micrometastases is high. Definitive chemoirradation is the commonly used approach. Addition of chemotherapy to radical radiotherapy led to a survival benefit of 5–10% at 5 years. Concomitant use of chemotherapy had a further improvement in survival by 4.5% at 5 years when compared with sequential approach, but with the expense of higher toxicities (mainly esophagitis and/or pneumonitis). Platinum-based doublet chemotherapy is the preferred regime and usually 2–4 cycles are given [7, 8]. Thus, concurrent chemoirradiation is the preferred strategy for fit patients, while sequential approach can be used for less fit patients with disease still within a treatable radical radiotherapy volume. A dose higher than 70 Gy in conventional fractionation is not recommended due to the associated higher toxicities but no added survival benefit. A continuous, hyperfractionated, accelerated radiotherapy (CHART) using 54 Gy in 36 fractions of 1.5 Gy three times per day can be considered for selected patients opting for radiotherapy alone. It had around 20% relative risk reduction in 2-year local progression rate and survival compared with conventional radiotherapy, but implementation can be challenging.

For patients with performance status 3–4, significant comorbidities and poor lung function that preclude a radical treatment approach, palliative radiotherapy may be considered for local symptoms control.

4.1.3. Metastatic stage IV disease: palliative treatment

Early radiotherapy to thorax in patients with incurable disease but no or minimal symptoms had not been shown to improve symptom control, survival, or quality of life. Hence, palliative thoracic radiotherapy can be deferred till symptoms emerged. Common indications are cough, hemoptysis, chest pain, and airway obstruction [9]. The optimal radiotherapy dose and fractionation schedule remained unclear. While there is no significant difference in symptom control with different dose schedules, a small survival improvement may be seen with higher dose radiotherapy.

For malignancy-related superior vena cava obstruction, external beam radiotherapy is effective in 60% patients with nonsmall cell lung cancers and 80% patients with small cell lung cancers [10]. Chemotherapy is another treatment option for patients with chemosensitive tumors like lymphoma, germ cell tumors, or small cell tumors. Intravascular stent insertion may be considered for patients that require rapid relief of symptoms, those who fail to response or relapse after radiotherapy.

Palliative radiotherapy can also be given to distant metastatic sites (e.g., bone, skin). Single fraction radiotherapy is as effective as longer course radiotherapy in pain and local symptom control.

4.1.4. Postoperative treatment

Adjuvant postoperative radiotherapy (PORT) helps to improve local control in patients with high risk of local recurrence after surgery, including those with pathological N2 disease and incomplete resection either microscopically or macroscopically. A careful evaluation of general conditions and remaining lung reserves is required before the start of treatment. It is not routinely given to early stage I–II disease with clear resection due to the potential detrimental effect on overall survival from previous meta-analyses that include trials using large radiation fields and nonconformal radiation techniques. However, its role with the use of modern radiotherapy machine and conformal radiotherapy are unclear and further research is warranted.

5. Radiotherapy data acquisition

5.1. External beam radiotherapy

5.1.1. Immobilization

Patient will lie supine with arms above head holding a T-bar device and elbow supported laterally (**Figure 5**) to facilitate different beam angle entry for treatment. Knee support can be given to allow a more comfortable position when needed. Vacuum bag can be added to reduce movement if treatment time is long. For palliative setting using AP beams only, patients usually lie supine with arms beside body.

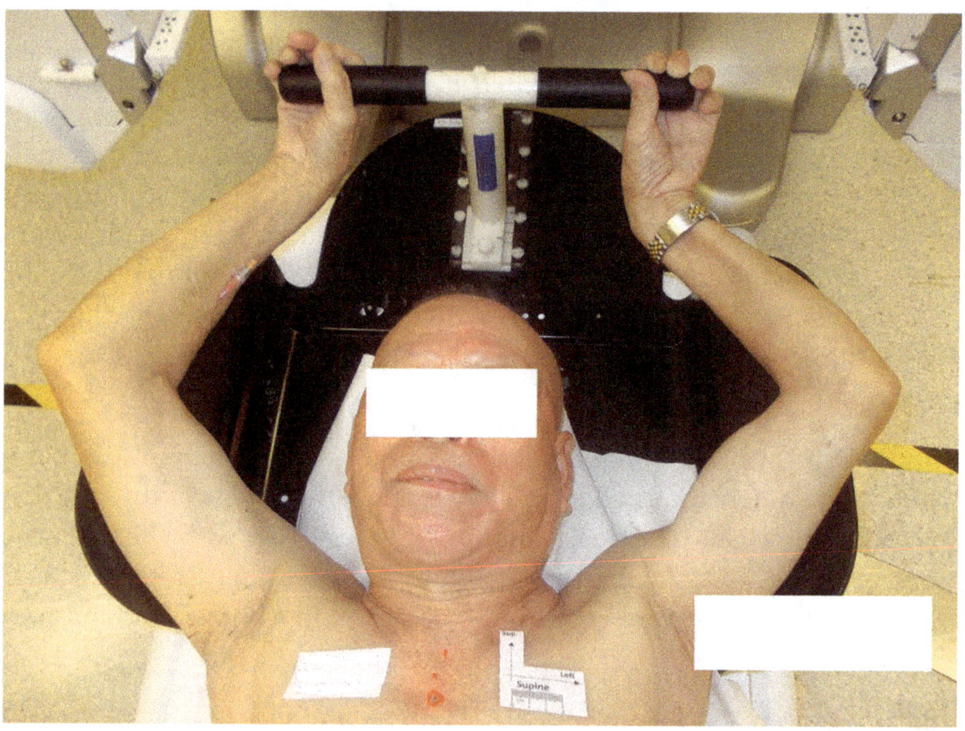

Figure 5. Immobilization for thoracic radiotherapy with T-bar and elbow support.

5.1.2. Simulation

For treatment with radical intent, computer-tomography from cricoid to lower border of L1 is needed to cover the whole lung for calculation of lung dose. Slice thickness of 3–5 mm allows better quality of images for target volume delineation. Intravenous contrast is not essential but is preferred when mediastinal disease is present so as to allow better visualization of the extent.

For treatment of palliative intent, radiation field border can be defined by simple X-ray simulation. Radio-opaque markers (e.g. lead wire) can be used to mark any clinically palpable diseases that are going to be included for radiotherapy (e.g., chest wall mass, supraclavicular lymph nodes).

To aid set-up, tattoos will be marked on beam center or isocenter, together with lateral reference points over left and right side of the body.

5.2. Stereotactic body radiotherapy (SBRT)

5.2.1. Immobilization

Patient should be immobilized in a comfortable position to avoid movement during the longer treatment length of each fraction. In this way, a supine position with arms above head immobilized by wing board and vacuum bag is commonly used (**Figure 6**).

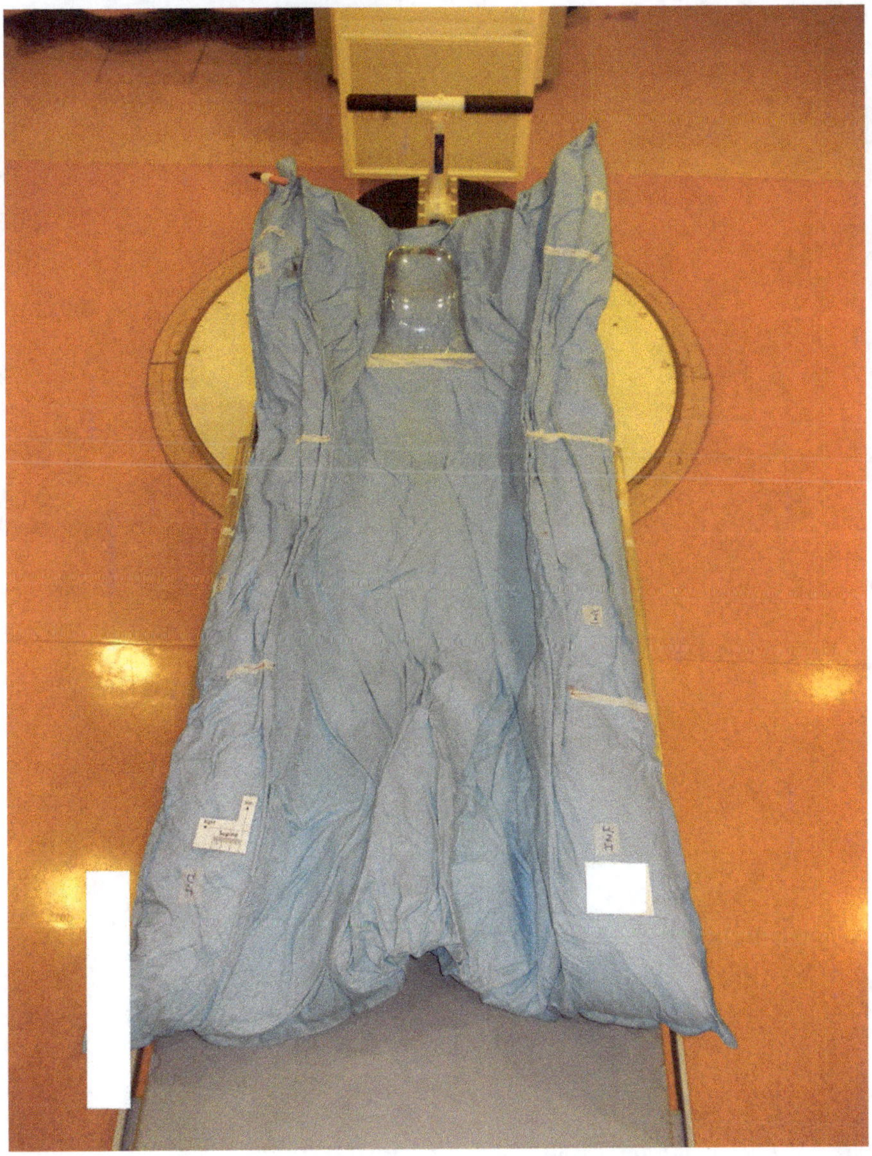

Figure 6. Immobilization with wing board and vacuum bag for SBRT of lung cancer.

5.2.2. Breathing motion assessment and correction

Fluoroscopy can be used to visualize tumor motion. But it only allows tumor motion assessment in two dimensions and can be difficult if with indistinct border of tumors. Noncontrast four-dimensional CT (4D CT) is a better option, which is a fast scanner that acquires multiset of CT images over consecutive phases of breathing cycle. Information about patients' breathing cycle and amplitude can be recorded by infrared reflecting marker and a coupled camera (**Figure 7**). And different CT images set will be sorted according to different phases in the respiratory cycle (**Figure 8**).

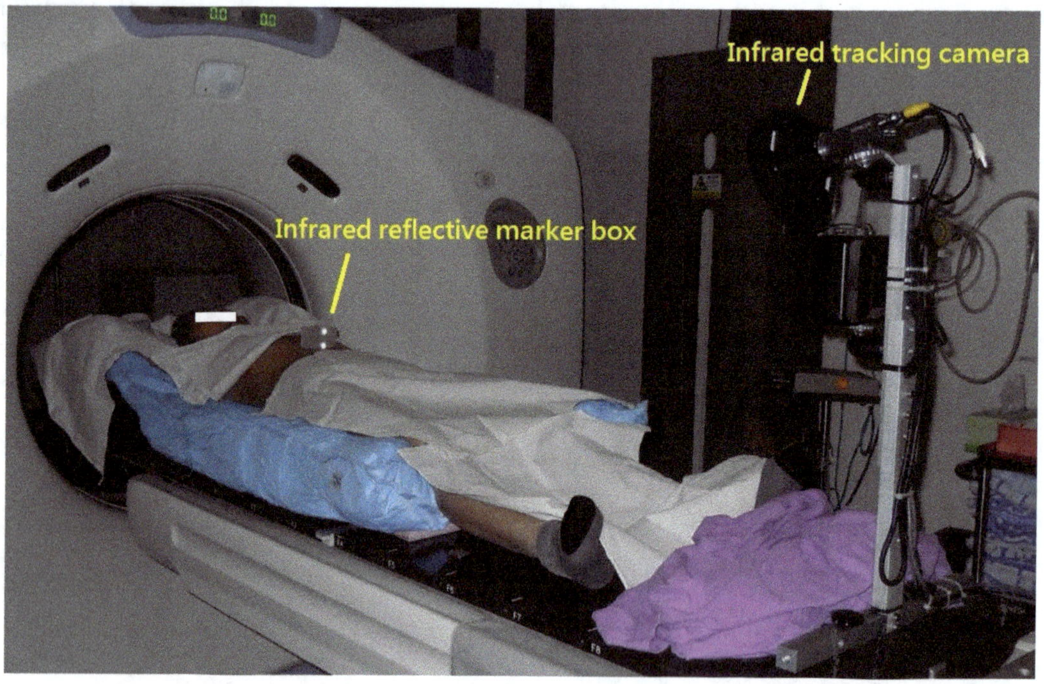

Figure 7. Infrared system including reflecting marker on patient's xiphsternum and coupled camera for tracking breathing cycle.

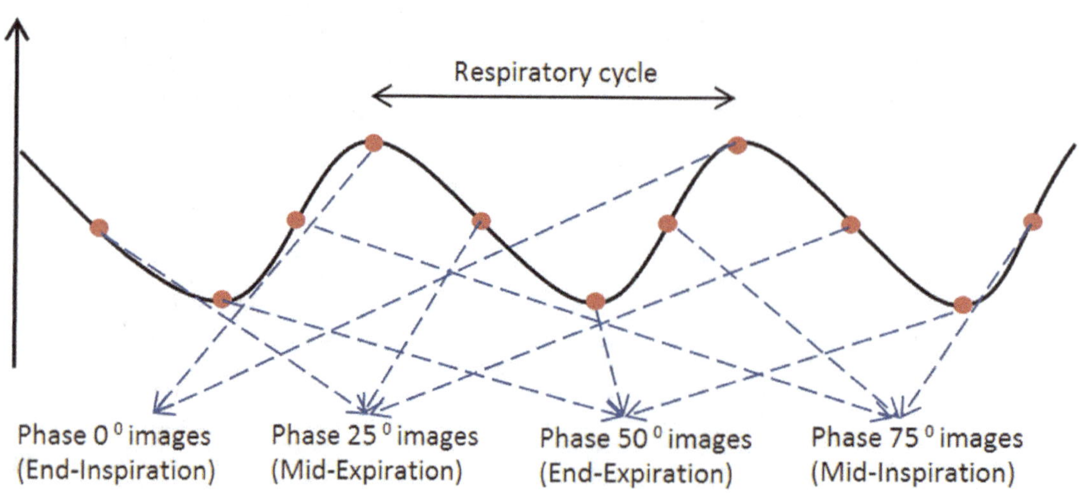

Figure 8. Sorting of 4D CT images by different phases in respiratory cycle.

Additional methods should be considered to reduce the tumor movement when it is ≥1cm, including abdominal compression, breath-hold, respiratory gating, or active breathing control. Both breath-hold and active breathing control require sufficient lung reserve to allow holding each breath for at least 20 seconds, which may be difficult for most of patients with lung cancers. Respiratory gating allows free breathing and beam on in certain phase of respiration. But it requires the use of fiducial markers to track internal tumor motion and is time consuming. Abdominal compression is the most commonly used method but reproducibility can be difficult (**Figure 9**). So the best method to be used depends on the patient's condition, tolerance, and corporation.

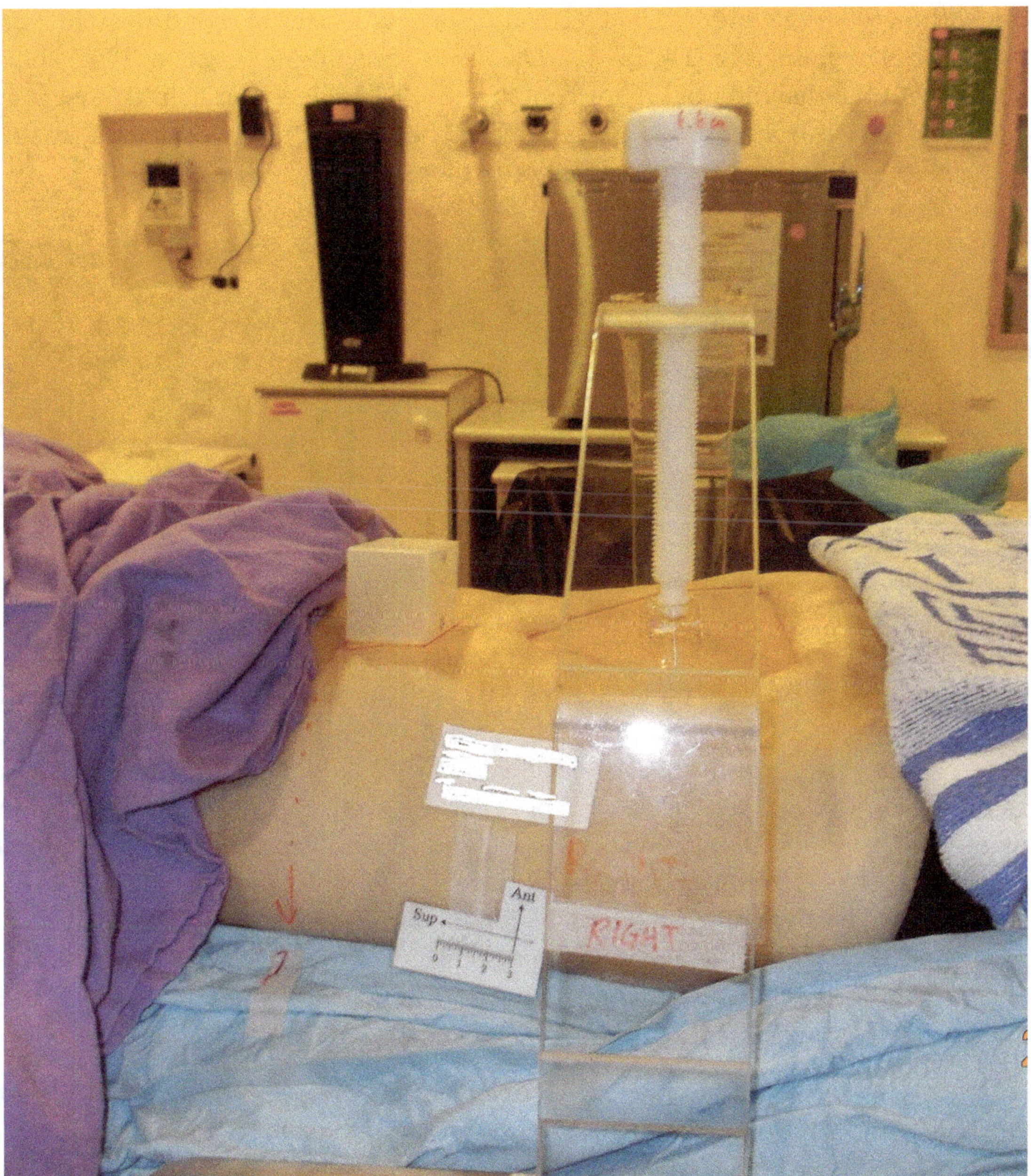

Figure 9. Abdominal compressor on patient's belly to reduce respiratory motion.

6. Target volume delineation

6.1. Conventional radiotherapy

Any clinical information and findings from bronchoscopy and mediastinoscopy should be gathered and correlated with diagnostic images. For postoperative cases, surgical records and pathology reports should be reviewed. And in case with doubt, discussions with surgeons and pathologists are encouraged to identify sites at risk of recurrence. Clips that are placed intraoperatively at sites with incomplete resection are useful for target identification.

An appropriate window setting should be used to delineate different targets on planning CT. Extent of primary lung tumor and mediastinal disease is best visualized by lung setting (window width 1600 and window level -600) and soft tissue setting (window width 400 and window level 20), respectively (**Figure 10**). Diagnostic imaging (e.g., CT or PET) should be coregistered with the planning of CT for contouring. PET images can help delineate area of collapse and atelectasis from tumors, but care should be taken when matching the images due to poor spatial resolution and breathing motion artifact.

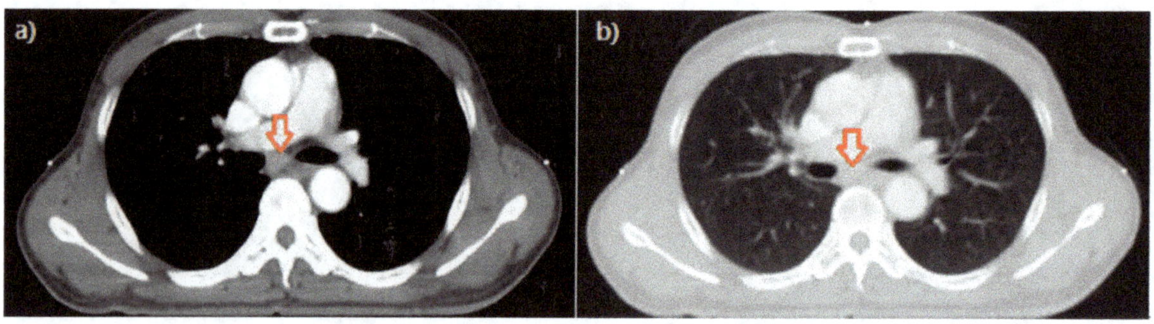

Figure 10. Soft tissue window setting (a) in planning CT to define the mediastinal lymph node (red arrow), which cannot be easily seen in lung window (b).

Gross tumor volume of primary tumor (GTV-P) is best contoured on lung window setting to include any visible tumor within lung parenchyma and the speculated border. Any local invasion to surrounding structures (e.g., chest wall, vertebra) should be included as well based on soft tissue window setting. Areas of collapse or atelectasis were excluded but can be difficult to differentiate. Input from radiologists and PET may be useful. Elective nodal irradiation is not recommended as isolated nodal recurrences are rare. So GTV of lymph node (GTV-N) will only include any pathologically confirmed lymph nodes (fine needle cytology or core biopsy) and any suspicious lymph nodes based on imaging characteristics (including short axis diameter ≥1 cm, necrotic center or PET uptake). If chemotherapy had been used before radiotherapy, all initial sites of tumor involvement should be contoured unless it exceeds a tolerable radiotherapy portal.

An isotropic margin is then added to GTV-P to cover microscopic tumor spread to form the clinical target volume (CTV-P). Usually, a 6 mm margin for adenocarcinoma and an 8 mm margin for squamous cell carcinoma are used as it had been shown to cover around 95% of microscopic tumor extension on pathological specimens [11]. Subsequent CTV-P is edited according to the presence of natural barriers (e.g., great vessels, bone). For GTV-N, usually no additional margin is needed for CTV.

A margin from CTV to PTV (planning target volume) depends on tumor motion and daily set-up errors (**Figure 11**). Tumor motion can be quite variable from zero in cases using implanted fiducial markers in image-guided radiotherapy to certain centimeters in cases without any breathing motion control. Set-up errors are regularly measured in each department and usually within 5 mm in all directions. In common practice with free breathing treatment, a 1 cm isotropic margin is usually given to form the PTV. But a larger superior-inferior margin of 1.5 cm may be used for tumors with greater movement as long as the lung dose is within the tolerance limit.

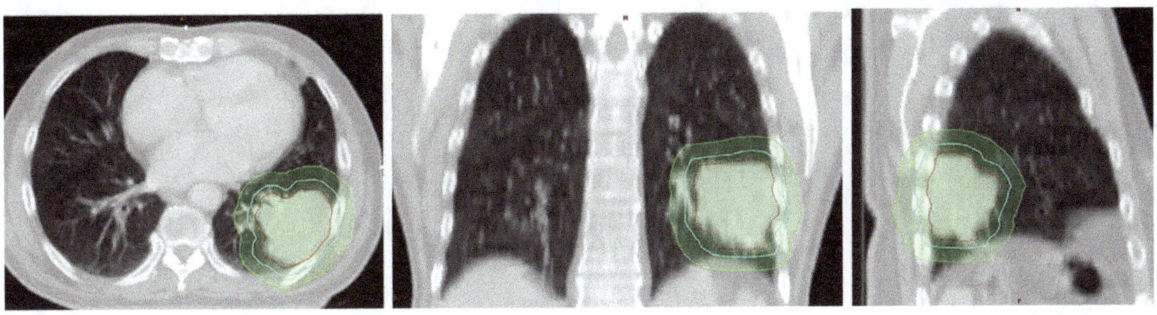

Figure 11. Target volume delineation: primary lung tumor (T) is contoured on lung window as gross tumor volume (GTV; red line); an additional 6 mm is added to form clinical target volume (CTV; blue line) to cover microscopic spread; further 1 cm margin is added to form the planning target volume (PTV; green line) to account for tumor motion and set-up error.

For palliative radiotherapy using AP beams, information about tumor extent from diagnostic imaging can be superimposed on those visible on simulator to form the GTV. And a further 1.5 cm margin from GTV can be used to define the radiotherapy field border.

6.2. Stereotactic body radiotherapy

Internal target volume (ITV) takes into account both GTV and internal tumor motion. It can be generated from the 4D CT using the maximum intensity projection (MIP) scan, maximum inspiratory, and expiratory scans, or all 10 phases of respiratory cycles (**Figure 12**). No CTV is needed. The usual CTV to PTV margin is 3–5mm, but it depends on methods of immobilization, tumor motion assessments, and treatment verification.

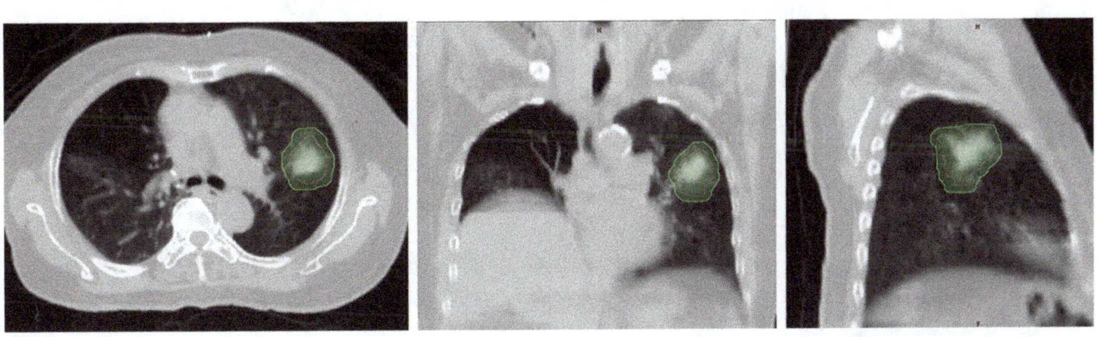

Figure 12. Target delineation on 4D CT: tumor is contoured on MIP images to form the internal target volume (ITV; red line); addition 5 mm margin was used to generate the planning target volume (PTV; green line).

7. Organs at risk delineation

Organs at risk including heart, esophagus, and spinal cord will be contoured using soft tissue window. The heart includes the whole structure within pericardial sac starting from the pulmonary artery to the apex. All layers of esophagus will be included and contoured from the cricoid cartilage to the esophagogastric junction. Spinal cord will be contoured at least 10 cm above and below PTV. For tumors over upper chest, the ipsilateral brachial plexus should also be contoured. Both left and right lungs are also contoured and then used to form a new structure called lung minus PTV after subtraction.

For SBRT, the tracheal and proximal bronchial tree should be contoured as well. Trachea will start from the level of cricoid cartilage to 2 cm above the carina, where it then continuous with the proximal bronchial tree (PBT, **Figure 13**) including the distal 2 cm trachea, main carina, bilateral main bronchi, bilateral upper lobe bronchi, lingular bronchus, intermedia bronchus, right middle lobe bronchus, and bilateral lower lobe bronchi. A 2 cm margin applied around the PTB will then be used to form a PRV (planning organ at risk volume).

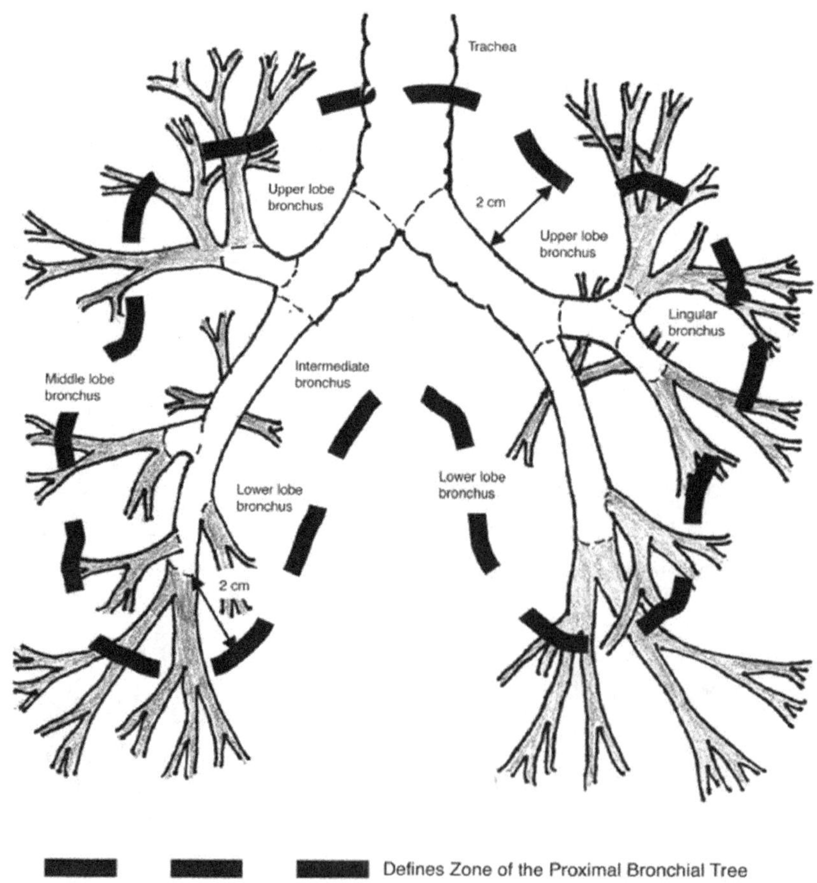

Figure 13. Definition of proximal bronchial tree.

8. Radiotherapy planning

For radical treatment, three-field conformal radiotherapy is most commonly used. The choices of beam numbers and beam angles depend on the location of the tumor and proximity to OARs. For early stage I–II tumors with lateralized target volume, a lateral, anterior, and posterior oblique beams are usually chosen to reduce irradiate contralateral lung (**Figure 14**).

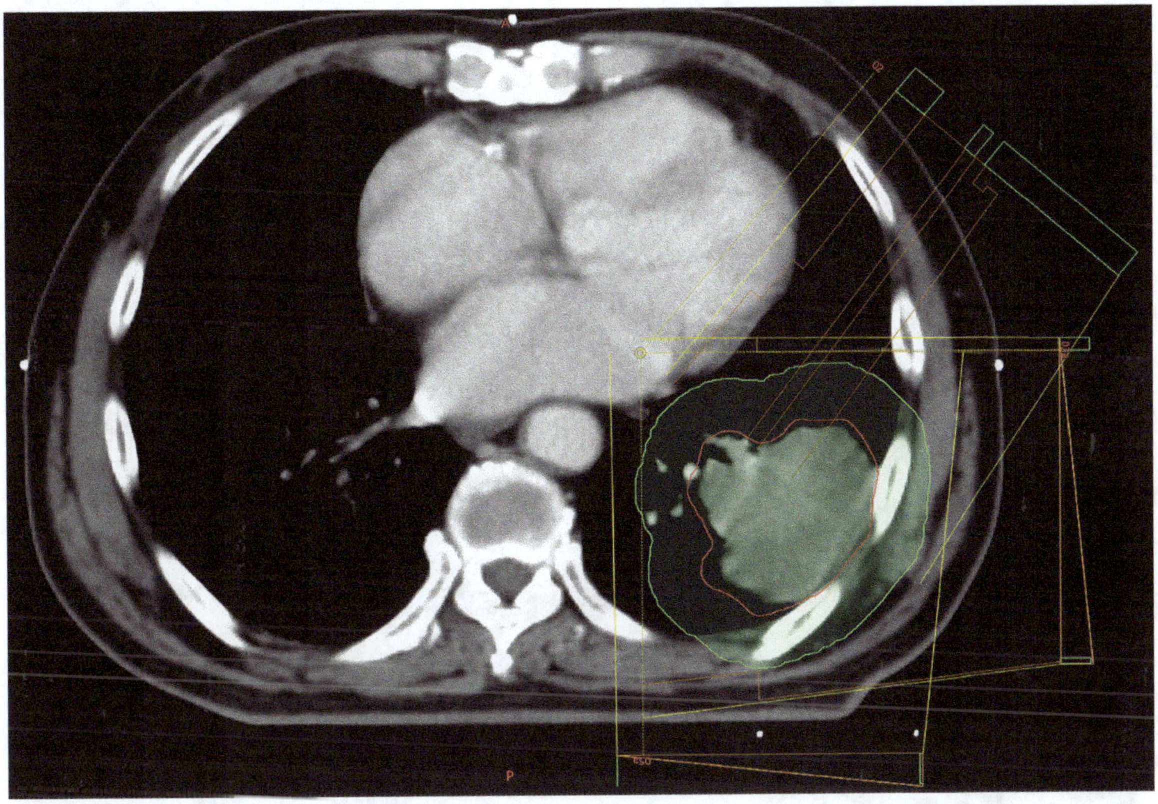

Figure 14. Beam arrangement in a three-field conformal radiotherapy for early stage lung cancer (red line = GTV; green line = PTV).

For more advanced stage disease with tumor involvement to mediastinum or across midline, the above three-field technique using ipsilateral beams only may not give good dose coverage to target, and addition of contralateral beam will increase total lung dose. In such case, two phases treatment should be considered. First phase will treat the mediastinum using AP beams shaped by multileaf collimator (MLC), while the second phase will use conformal technique to give adequate coverage to all the target volume. With this approach, total lung dose can be reduced but OARs near midline (e.g., esophagus, spinal cord) will receive higher dose.

For palliative radiotherapy, anterior and posterior fields modified by MLC are usually used with dose prescribed to midplane. Energy of photon beam used will depend on separation at the center of the field.

Radiotherapy plans should be carefully evaluated using dose-volume histogram (DVH). Optimal plan should aim at 95% PTV receiving at least 100% of the prescribed dose and 99% PTV receiving a minimum of 90% of the prescribed dose. For OARs, commonly used dose constrains for lung minus PTV is V20 (volume receiving >20 Gy) below 35%, preferably below 30%. However, a tighter constrain to reduce the risk of radiation pneumonitis should be considered when there is presence of other risk factors including preexiting lung disease and concurrent use of chemotherapy. Another frequently used limit is the mean lung dose below 20 Gy. The dose constrains for other OARs are maximum dose to spinal cord less than 45 Gy and heart V20 less than 40 Gy. Care should be given to avoid irradiation of more than 10 cm length of the esophagus due to higher long-term risk of stricture.

For SBRT, either intensity-modulated radiotherapy using 6–8 fields (IMRT) or rapidarc therapy is recommended to deliver a high and conformal dose to a precise area (**Figure 15**). Dose to skin should be minimized to avoid cutaneous and subcutaneous toxicities. Recommendations to other OARs can be made reference to that published by ROSEL study and RTOG 0813 study.

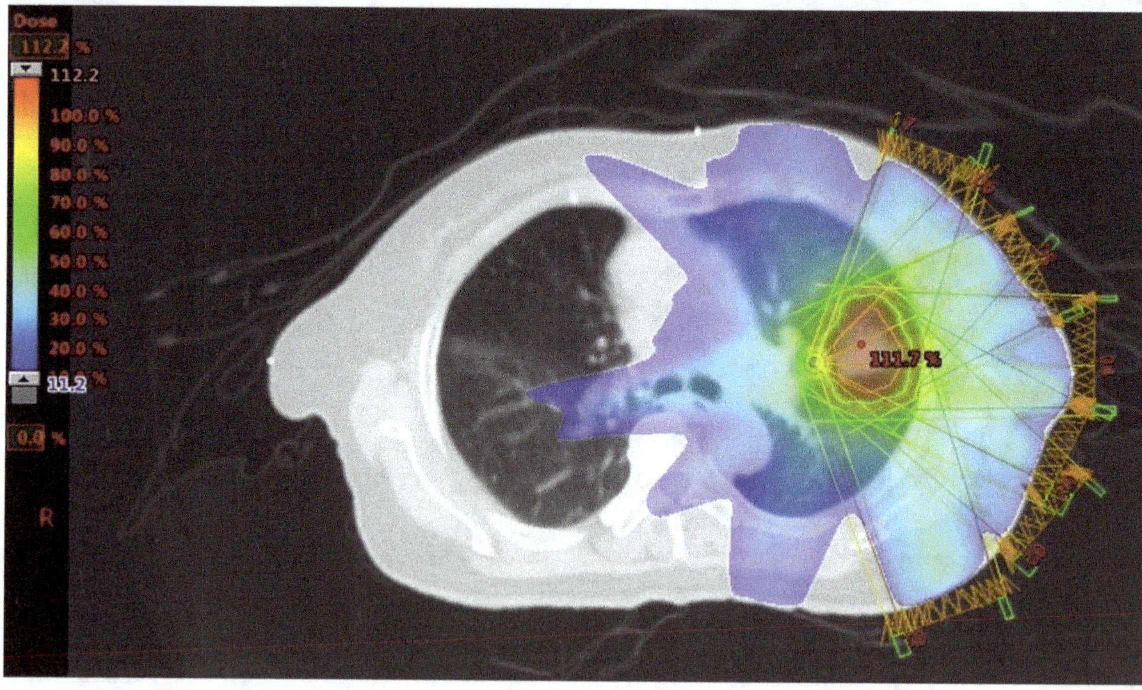

Figure 15. Beam arrangement and dose color wash from SBRT for lung cancer using IMRT technique.

9. Radiotherapy dose and fractionation

9.1. Radical treatment

9.1.1. Early stage T1-3N0 disease and fit patients: use SBRT

- For peripherally located tumor: 54 Gy in three fractions or 60 Gy in five fractions, alternate day treatment over 1–2 weeks (more conservative schedule is recommended if PTV is in contact with chest wall to avoid rib toxicities).

- For centrally located tumor (defined as GTV within 2 cm from proximal bronchial tree): 50 Gy in 10 fractions, alternate day treatment over 2 weeks.

9.1.2. Other early stage I–II disease: use conventional radiotherapy

- 60–70 Gy in 30–35 daily fractions over 6–6.5 weeks.
- Consider hypofractionated regime of 55 Gy in 20 daily fractions over 4 weeks if elderly.

9.1.3. Locally advanced stage III disease: use conventional radiotherapy

- For preoperative treatment (with or without chemotherapy): 45–54 Gy in 1.8–2 Gy per fraction over 5–6 weeks.
- For definitive treatment with concurrent chemotherapy: 60–66 Gy in 30–33 daily fractions over 6–6.5 weeks (consider treat up to 70 Gy in 35 daily fractions over 7 weeks if no chemotherapy given and within lung dose tolerance).

9.2. Adjuvant treatment

- For complete resection: 50 Gy in 25 daily fractions over 5 weeks.
- For incomplete resection: 60 Gy in 30 daily fractions over 6 weeks (consider boost up to 66 Gy in 33 daily fractions if gross residual disease).

9.3. Palliative treatment

- For PS 0–1 and life expectancy >6 months: 30 Gy in 10 daily fractions over 2 weeks (consider 39 Gy in 13 daily fractions over 2.5 weeks if spinal cord not within treated volume).
- For PS ≥ 2: 20 Gy in five daily fractions over 1 week or 10 Gy single fraction.

10. Treatment verification and delivery

Portal images by electronic portal imaging device on treatment machines are taken on first 3 days on treatment and then weekly afterwards. These are compared and registered with digitally reconstructed radiography (DRR) from CT simulations to allow offline corrections. For SBRT, cone beam CT by onboard imaging on treatment machine is done daily to allow online correction before delivery of each fraction of treatment.

During treatment period, patients should be reviewed at least once by radiation oncologists for assessment of any acute radiation side effects. Mild chest symptoms like cough or dyspnea are common but concomitant chest infection should be excluded if symptoms worsened. Dysphagia can occur due to esophagitis which usually start at around third week. Adequate analgesics and diet advice should be given to minimize severity and the impact on nutrition or weight loss.

11. Follow-up

After radical treatment, CT of thorax and upper abdomen should be done 3 monthly in the first 2 years, then half yearly till 5 years, and then annually to evaluate disease status. Long-term toxicities especially on lung function and esophageal stricture should be regularly reviewed and managed accordingly.

Author details

Fiona Lim Mei Ying

Address all correspondence to: fionalimmy@gmail.com

Department of Oncology, Princess Margaret Hospital, Hong Kong

References

[1] International Agency for Research on Cancer. 2014. Available from: http://publications.iarc.fr/Non-Series-Publications/World-Cancer-Reports/World-Cancer-Report-2014

[2] Lortet-Tieulent J, Soerjomataram I, Ferlay J, Rutherford M, Weiderpass E, Bray F. International trends in lung cancer incidence by histological subtype: Adenocarcinoma stabilizing in men but still increasing in women. Lung Cancer. 2014;**84**(1):13–22. DOI: http://dx.doi.org/10.1016/j.lungcan.2014.01.009

[3] Govindan R, Page N, Morgensztern D, et al. Changing epidemiology of small-cell lung cancer in the United States over the last 30 years: Analysis of the surveillance, epidemiologic, and end results database. Journal of Clinical Oncology. 2006;**24**:4539–4544.

[4] Morgensztern D, Ng SH, Gao F, Govindan R. Trends in stage distribution for patients with non-small cell lung cancer. A National Cancer Database Survey. Journal of Thoracic Oncology. 2010;**5**:29–33.

[5] Rusch VW, Asamura H, Watanabe H, Giroux DJ, Rami-Porta R, Goldstraw P. The IASLC Lung Cancer Staging Project. A proposal for a new international lymph node map in the forthcoming seventh edition of the TNM classification for lung cancer. Journal of Thoracic Oncology. 2009;**4**:568–577.

[6] Riquet M, Hidden G, Debesse B. Direct lymphatic drainage of lung segments to the mediastinal nodes. An anatomic study on 260 adults. The Journal of Thoracic and Cardiovascular Surgery. 1989;**97**:623–632.

[7] O'Rourke N, Roque i Figuls M, Farre Bernado N, Macbeth F. Concurrent chemoradiotherapy in non-small cell lung cancer. Cochrane Database of Systematic Reviews. 2010;6:CD002140. DOI: 10.1022/14651858.CD002140.pub3.

[8] Auperin A, Pechoux CL, Rolland E, Curran WJ, Furuse K et al. Meta-analysis of concomitant versus sequential radiochemotherapy in locally advanced non-small-cell lung cancer. Journal of Clinical Oncology. 2010;**28**:2181–2190. DOI: 10.1200/JCO.2009.26.2543

[9] Fairchild A, Harris K, Barnes E, Wong R, Lutz S, Bezjak A, et al. Palliative thoracic radiotherapy for lung cancer: a systematic review. Journal of Clinical Oncology. 2008;**26**:4001–4011. DOI: 10,1200/JCO.2007,15,3312

[10] Rowell NP, Gleeson FV. Steroids, radiotherapy, chemotherapy and stents for superior vena caval obstruction in carcinoma of the bronchus. Cochrane Database Systemic Review. 2001;**4**(4):CD001316.

[11] Giraud P, Antoine M, Larrouy A, Milleron B, Callard P, De Rycke Y, et al. Evaluation of microscopic tumor extension in non-small-cell lung cancer for three-dimensional conformal radiotherapy planning. International Journal of Radiation Oncology Biology Physics. 2000;**48**(4):1015–1024.

2

Chemoresistance of Lung Cancer Cells: 2D and 3D *In Vitro* Models for Anticancer Drug Screening

Vivek Kaushik, Juan Sebastian Yakisich,
Yogesh Kulkarni, Neelam Azad and
Anand Krishnan V. Iyer

Abstract

Chemoresistance of lung cancer cells is a key factor that limits the treatment of lung cancer patients. Patients may initially respond to standard chemotherapy, but this is often followed by rapid development of drug resistance and disease progression. Tumor heterogeneity and the presence of putative cancer stem-like cells (CS-LCs) provide a viable explanation for the chemoresistance of several types of tumors. In this book chapter, we will first describe the current knowledge of the role of both tumor heterogeneity and CS-LCs in lung cancer chemoresistance, tumor progression and metastasis. Next, we will discuss ongoing strategies at the *in vitro* level to screen for more effective anticancer drugs. We will specifically focus in three-dimensional (3D) culture systems (Spheroids and tumorspheres) and their application in anticancer drug discovery for lung cancer.

Keywords: chemoresistance, tumor heterogeneity, cancer stem cells, spheroids tumorspheres, 3D systems

1. Introduction

Lung cancer is the leading cause of cancer death among men and the second leading cause of cancer death among women worldwide [1]. Despite important advances in our knowledge of cancer cell biology and anti-cancer therapies such as chemotherapy, radiotherapy and targeted therapies, the five-year survival rates remain poor (<15%). Lung tumors are broadly classified into small cell lung cancer (SCLC) and non-small lung cancer (NSCLC). SCLCs are defined by neuroendocrine differentiation and small cell morphology of the tumor cells and account for

15–20% of newly diagnosed lung malignancies. Interestingly, SCLC tumors tend to recur as chemoresistant variants and occasionally show progression to a NSCLC phenotype [2]. Regardless of the type, chemoresistance appears in most lung tumors, presenting a challenge to the development of new therapeutic regimes. The failure of the management of lung cancer is largely attributed to the inherent and/or acquired resistance that limits the efficacy of current therapies. Several characteristics of lung tumors have been identified for long time as key driving factors that lead to increased chemoresistance. Among them, mutations, amplifications and overexpression of multidrug-resistant proteins have been investigated *in vitro* using cell lines growing as adherent monolayers (2D systems). Intratumoral heterogeneity was also recognized long time ago as a key factor contributing to chemoresistance and soon tumor spheroids were developed with the aim to replicate *in vitro* "mini-tumor" with more complex and heterogeneous 3D architecture mimicking primary tumors. These tumor spheroids were routinely obtained by culturing cancer cells in serum-containing media under anchorage-independent conditions. The isolation of putative cancer stem cells from solid tumors was done by culturing cancer cells under anchorage-independent condition but in serum-free media (initially with few supplements). Under these conditions, cancer cells grow as "floating tumorspheres" and form complex 3D structures similar to spheroids. It is widely accepted that "floating tumorspheres" are enriched with cancer stem-like cells that are inherently chemoresistant. For clarity and consistency, we will call "spheroids" and "tumorspheres" to masses of cancer cells growing as floating spheres in serum-containing and serum-free media, respectively. The aim of this chapter is to (1) briefly describe the main factors—relevant to 3D *in vitro* models contributing to chemoresistance (intratumoral heterogeneity and the presence of CS-LCs) and (2) discuss the application of spheroids and tumorspheres as tools for screening anticancer drugs targeting chemoresistant cancer cells.

1.1. Intratumoral heterogeneity

Intratumoral heterogeneity is a term that refers to the presence of cells within a tumor with varying degrees of morphology, proliferation rate, ability to metastasize, sensitivity to drugs, dependence on growth signals and tumor initiation/repopulation capacity. It has long been recognized as a salient feature of most cancers and largely associated with tumor relapse. Both genotypic and phenotypic diversity exist within tumors that arise driven by genetic mutations, epigenetic alterations or microenvironmental influence. As a consequence, expansion of selected clones as well as establishment of differentiation hierarchies of cancer stem cells (CSCs) and non-CSCs creates a wide diversity of cells [3]. The basis for the genotypic heterogeneity is the inherent genetic instability of cancer cells and the clonal evolution theory that proposes that a tumor of monoclonal origin may become heterogeneous due to advantageous tumorigenic growth of clonal subpopulations. Over time, as the tumor progresses, cancer cells accumulate different mutations and different clones may compete or evolve in parallel generating a tumor composed of cells with varied genetic imprints. The latter is called branched evolution, and this process has been confirmed by genetic analysis in a variety of tumors [3]. Non-genetic heterogeneity (phenotypic heterogeneity) is the result of microenvironmental pressures due to, for instance, alterations in oxygen, pH and nutrient availability based on their regional location within the primary tumor largely influenced by their relative distance to blood vessels. Both genotypic and phenotypic heterogeneity are associated with chemoresistance that have a profound impact on the clinical outcome of lung cancer patients. For instance, at the clinical level, it has been recently suggested that increased metabolic heterogeneity should be considered as a high-risk subpopulation for early EGFR TKI failure [4].

1.2. Presence of cancer stem-like cells in lung tumors

The cancer stem cell hypothesis (CSCH) suggests that most cancers contain a rare subpopulation of cancer cells with properties such as indefinite self-renewal, slow replication and ability to give rise to differentiated progeny. These cells possess intrinsic resistance to chemotherapy and radiotherapy and are thought to be responsible for tumor initiation and growth and tumor relapse [5, 6]. The CSCH is a hierarchical model in which cancer stem cells (CSCs) can differentiate into non-cancer stem cells (non-CSCs) but not the other way around. According to this model, eliminating the CSC subpopulation would eventually lead to a cure. This concept has been recently challenged by several alternative models of cancer stem cell biology [7, 8] since experimental evidence demonstrated that cancer cells are extremely plastic [9, 10] and evidence of interconversion between CSCs and non-CSCs was found in a variety of cancer types including lung [11], breast [12] and colon [13] cancers. Contrary to the CSCH, all the alternative models propose that to cure cancer all cancer cells should be eliminated at once. At present, it is safe to assume that tumors may consist of a heterogeneous population of cancer cells with different "stemness" properties ranging from a pure non-CSC phenotype (typically sensitive to conventional anticancer drugs) to a pure CSC phenotype (usually highly resistant to conventional anticancer drugs). *In vitro*, CS-LCs are able to grow in the absence of serum as 3D spheres under anchorage-independent conditions as floating "tumorspheres" (FTs) and it is thought that the ability to form clonal spheres is a unique characteristic of CSCs [14, 15]. Because of its 3D architecture, and the notion that FTs consist of mostly CSCs with inherent chemoresistant properties, they have widely adopted as system models for drug screening (see Section 2.2.2.).

2. *In vitro* models for anticancer drug screening

Several *in vitro* models of lung cancer have been widely used for testing new anticancer drugs. Historically, 2D cultures were introduced first and chemoresistant cells lines were isolated and widely used to screen for more effective anticancer drugs. However, since 2D cultures typically consist of a more homogenous population of cells, 2D systems may not be able to account for intratumoral heterogeneity. As a result that 3D systems would recapitulate more faithfully, the heterogeneous nature of cancer cells existing *in vivo* were soon developed. Before describing these 3D systems, we will briefly discuss 2D systems.

2.1. 2D systems

Some cell lines were found to be inherently resistant to one or more drugs. In addition, several drug-resistant cancer cell lines have been generated in the laboratory to investigate either the underlying mechanism of resistance to a particular drug and/or to screen for alternative drug able to circumvent the acquired resistant. The next three sections will focus in the development and characterization of cancer-resistant cell lines and their application to identify mechanism of resistance and identification of new targets.

2.1.1. *Development of drug-resistant cellular models of lung cancer*

Developing models of chemoresistant cancer cells is a well-utilized approach to investigate mechanisms of acquired drug resistance, anticancer drug screening and developing novel drugs to resensitize resistant cancers to apoptotic stimuli. Developing a stable clinically relevant drug-resistant model involves using doses and exposure times consistent with the clinical setting [16]. In order to mimic clinical conditions, developing *in vitro* models of cancer resistance involves chronic exposure to lower concentration of drug with a pulsed treatment strategy that involves cycles of exposure to drug followed by recovery in drug-free medium [17]. Alternatively, continuous selection strategy with increasing doses or acute exposure to high concentration of gefitinib and erlotinib has been used to develop resistant models of NSCLC [18–20].

2.1.2. *Characterization of drug-resistant models*

Several assays have been used to characterize chemoresistance by comparing the resistant phenotype with the parental cell line. Measurement of drug sensitivity using viability assays such as the MTT assay, flow cytometry analysis to determine cell cycle arrest, clonogenic survival assay, characterization of stemness markers, determination of ALDH activity, expression of EMT markers, characterization of MDR modulators and quantification of cellular uptake of drug used to induce drug resistance are commonly used assays to characterize drug resistance. A dose and time-response curve of cell viability is used to calculate IC_{50}. The fold resistance is calculated by comparing the ratios of IC_{50} of the resistant cells with parental cells [17]. A marked feature of drug-resistant cell lines is enrichment of cancer stem cells, a subpopulation of tumor cells with capacity for self-renewal and tumorigenicity potential. Aldehyde dehydrogenase (ALDH) is involved in differentiation of cancer stem cells and promoting resistance and survival mechanisms [21]. Aberration in regular cell cycle can circumvent or potentiate apoptosis, and drug-resistant cells undergo cell cycle arrest to prevent apoptotic cell death [22]. Epithelial mesenchymal transition has been associated with resistance to gefitinib and erlotinib in NSCLC [23, 24]. Quantifying decreased cellular drug accumulation in the resistant phenotype using inductively coupled plasma mass spectrometry (ICP-MS) due to overexpression of transporter proteins is another novel method of characterizing acquired drug resistance [25, 26].

2.1.3. *Identifying mechanisms of resistance and novel drug targets for resistant lung cancer*

Epidermal growth factor receptor (EGFR), a transmembrane receptor tyrosine kinase (RTK), involved in cellular proliferation is overexpressed in NSCLC and SCLC. Targeting EGFR signaling using tyrosine kinase inhibitors (TKI) such as gefitinib and erlotinib was a reasonable clinical success, particularly in patients with EGFR mutations [27, 28]. Acquisition of resistance due to a secondary mutation of EGFR (T790M) is a major therapeutic problem necessitating discovery of novel drugs that can inhibit TKI-resistant NSCLC after developing T790 M mutation [29]. A panel of 12 NSCLC cell lines comprising wild-type EGFR (TKI-resistant), EGFR mutation with an additional TKI-resistance inducing mutation and EGFR mutation yet sensitive to TKI-inhibitor was used to screen 10 anticancer compounds. All 12 NSCLC cell lines showed inhibition of proliferation with 17-DMAG, an Hsp90 inhibitor and belinostat, a histone-deacetylase inhibitor (HDACi). 17-DMAG and belinostat inhibited EGFR and p-Akt expression in one cell line of each group. Combination of 17-DMAG and belinostat showed synergistic antiproliferative activity and inhibited the growth of TKI-resistant cell lines. These drugs were effective in mice xenografts and completely suppressed tumor growth with the combination being more effective than either drug alone. Immunoblotting of mice tumors showed decreased expression of p-EGFR, total EGFR and p-Akt substantiating a need to validate a combination therapy of 17-DMAG and belinostat in patients with EGFR-TKI-resistant NSCLC [30].

Some mechanisms shown to confer resistance to gefitinib and erlotinib in EGFR-mutated patients in addition to T790 M mutation, stemness and EMT have been shown to be MET amplification, FGFR1 overexpression and IGF1R overexpression [30–32]. These multiple resistance mechanisms can exist in parallel giving rise to heterogeneous resistant cell population. NSCLC grown resistant to erlotinib identified subclones that underwent MET amplification or induced EMT phenotype. MET subclones, while maintaining erlotinib resistance, showed increased sensitivity to MET inhibitors, crizotinib and capmatinib. EMT subclones overexpressed FGFR1 and showed increased sensitivity to FGFR1 inhibitor AZD4547. Inhibitors of MET and FGFR1 showed reduced sensitivity to mixed NSCLC cell line as compared to the individual subclones. This study highlights the coexistence of parallel resistance mechanisms giving rise to heterogeneous resistant population [33]. Anaplastic lymphoma kinase (ALK) gene rearrangements act as oncogenic drivers and are present in a small subset of NSCLC, which are responsive to ALK kinase inhibitors such as ceritinib (LDK378) [34]. Ceritinib-resistant cells were grown by chronic exposure to the drug and assayed for resistance using cell proliferation and viability assays. Ceritinib treatment upregulated Src, an oncogene involved in tumorigenesis and metastatic progression. Knockdown of Src with siRNA in resistant phenotype resensitized cells to ALK inhibition with ceritinib. Resistant ALK-positive cell lines showed sensitivity to Src inhibitor ADZ0530, which has promising therapeutic potential to be explored in patients with ALK-TKI-resistant tumors [35]. In another study, combinatorial treatment of ALK and IGF1R inhibitor was used to overcome crizotinib resistance in ALK-positive lung cancer, positing IGF1R to be an independent drug target in this subset of lung cancer [36]. Interleukin-8 is upregulated in gefitinib-resistant cells and is associated with shorter progression-free survival in EGFR-TKI-treated lung cancer patients. IL-8 expressing EGFR-mutant cell line showed increased phosphorylation of Akt and NF-κB translocation and decreased sensitivity to gefitinib-induced apoptosis. Knocking down IL-8 increased the apoptotic sensitivity to gefitinib. IL-8 expressing cells showed stemness as characterized by ALDH activity, increased expression of Nanog, Oct4 and Sox2 and forming more and larger colonies than controls. This acquisition of stemness was IL-8 dependent, as knocking down IL-8 reversed the stem cell-like properties in EGFR-TKI- resistant cells [37]. Gefitinib-resistant cells were developed to investigate the induction of EMT phenotype associated with EGFR-TKI resistance in NSCLC. While these resistant phenotypes were negative for T790 M mutation or MET-amplification, they had acquired the EMT phenotype with increased migratory and invasive phenotype. The acquisition of EMT phenotype was mediated via the activation of IGF1R/NF-κB signaling pathway. Inhibition of IGF1R/NF-κB signaling restored the sensitivity to gefitinib and suppressed the migration and invasion capability, suggesting that this pathway could be a novel target for gefitinib-resistant EGFR-mutant NSCLC therapy [38].

To summarize, despite the wide variety of cancer drugs available to treat lung cancer, acquired resistance to therapy is still a frequently encountered problem. It is important to identify the resistance conferring mechanisms, so that the resistance can be circumvented or reversed with novel anticancer drugs. Although drug-resistant cell lines provide robust preclinical models to interrogate underlying mechanisms of resistance and anticancer drug screening, they lack key features present *in vivo* in primary tumors that may provide additional mechanism associated with chemoresistance.

2.2. 3D systems

Although a plethora of 3D systems have been developed for anticancer drug screening at present, despite some technical traits, none of these systems showed a clear advantage over other regarding the ability to select successful clinically useful anticancer drugs. For space limitations, only floating spheroids and floating tumorspheres will be addressed in this chapter. **Figure 1** shows representative microscopy image of spheroids and tumorspheres.

2.2.1. *Floating spheroids*

The 3D multicellular aggregates formed from single cell suspensions in FBS containing media under anchorage-dependent or independent conditions are commonly known as "Spheroids." It is an excellent 3D model for drug screening as it can closely mimic tumor heterogeneity, tumor microenvironment niches (normoxic, hypoxic, pH gradient zones) and tumor structural as well as functional intricacies. Spheroids with constant size and consistent structural features are necessary to generate consistent and reproducible results.

Researchers have developed various techniques to develop spheroids to achieve these targets. The commonly used 3D cell culture methods can be divided into two main categories—(i) scaffold

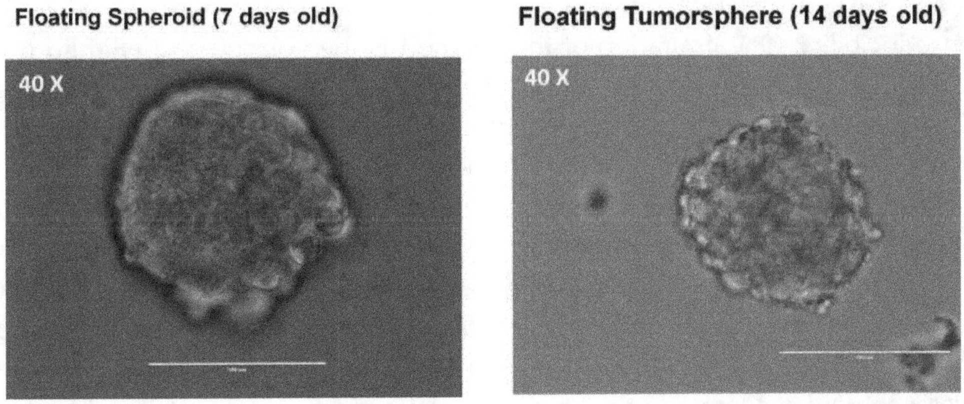

Figure 1. Representative images of H460 lung cancer cells growing as floating spheroids in serum-containing media (A) or as floating tumorspheres in serum-free media (B). Image in B was reprinted with permission from [39]. Bar = 100 μm.

based (hydrogel and inserts) and (ii) non-scaffold based. Scaffold-based methods involve collagen-, chitosan- and polycaprolactone-based biomaterials, which serve as extracellular matrix and provide a 3D architecture for the growth of cells in anchorage-dependent manner in 3D cellular entities. Non-scaffold-based approaches employ techniques such as forced floating, rotary devices, hanging drop arrays, microfluidics, etc. to generate spheroids. Forced floating is the simplest and most commonly used method for the spheroids in a laboratory setting. As the name suggests, forced floating of cells is achieved by culturing them in vessels that have been coated with poly-HEMA or agarose suspensions, which prevents attachment of cells to the substratum. This method has been successfully used to generate spheroids of various types of cancers. It is a simple, inexpensive and convenient method for generating spheroids; however, it produces spheroids of variable sizes and shapes. In a recent study, Ivascu et al. reported the use of centrifugation to generate spheroids of fixed size using forced suspension method [40]. They added cell suspensions containing a fixed number of cells in each well of poly-HEMA-coated 96-well plates and subsequently centrifuged the plates to colocalize them. They reported formation of uniform single spheroids per well as early as 24 hours. Rotary 3D culture techniques work on agitation principle, which prevents cells from attaching to the container and instead cells interact with each other and develop 3D spheroids. Rotary culture methods can be sub divided into two main categories: (i) spinner flask and (ii) rotational culture systems. In spinner flask method, cell suspensions are constantly agitated by magnetic stirrer, while in rotational culture system cell suspension media is moved by rotating the culture vessel itself. Both these methods can produce large amount of spheroids and can be used for long-term production of spheroids. As culture is constant, agitated cells receive constant supply of nutrients and oxygen. However, size and structure of the spheroids cannot be controlled in these 3D culture methods. As these methods rely on constant moving of culture media, it exerts extensive force on cells which can either damage or affect cellular physiology of the cells. Rotational culture system is a superior technique than spinner flask method as it exerts far less force on the cells [41]. Kelm et al. developed hanging drop method for the generation of multicellular spheroids [42]. This method employs gravity as a force to bring the cells together to generate spheroids. Small aliquots of cell suspension media (usually 20 μL) carrying fixed number of cells are placed in wells of microtiter plate. These plates are then inverted and suspension media forms a drop and cells migrate to the tip of the drop due to gravity. These cells are then allowed to proliferate and generate a single spheroid per well. This method is good for high throughput, and spheroids with consistent size can be generated with excellent reproducibility. One limitation of this method is the volume of the liquid (up to 50 μL) that can be used to generate drop as surface tension can keep only small volumes of media together. Since small volumes of media are used for drop generation, this method requires constant media replacement making maintenance of culture challenging [43]. Tan et al. used a microfluidic platform to generate spheres [44]. This platform consists of a main channel and an array of coated microwells. Media containing single cell suspension flows through the channel and the cells get trapped into the wells where they grow in close contact and generate a single spheroid per well. Size and shape of the spheroids can be controlled by this method. It is a very good platform for high throughput drug screening and compatible with multidimensional imaging. However, spheroids generated in microfluidic platform cannot be retrieved for further study and structural analysis. In addition, several coculture methods have been developed to mimic complex cancer cell and microenvironment interactions. Tumor microenvironment is a complex system that involves interactions between tumor cells and adjacent stroma cells (fibroblasts, endothelial and inflammatory cells) embedded in extracellular matrix (ECM). Spheroids generation using a coculture model by coculturing cancer cells and fibroblasts and/or immune cells has been reported and studied for their unique interaction and subsequent effect on carcinogenesis [45, 46]. Spheroids perfectly mimic an avascular tumor microenvironment and cellular heterogeneity. Similar to tumor a nutrient, oxygen and pH gradient exist in spheroids leading to three distinct cellular zones in the spheroids [47]. The central necrotic zone, which mostly constituted by dead cells, is devoid of oxygen and nutrients. This is followed by middle dormant (senescent) zone consisted of quiescent cells. The peripheral layer, which has sufficient supply of nutrients and oxygen, has proliferative cells. Microelectrodes and proton magnetic resonance with pH-sensitive indicators are commonly used techniques to study oxygen flow and pH inside the spheroids [48, 49]. **Figure 2** illustrates the complex 3 architecture of spheroids.

In general, 3D spheroids show less chemosensitivity towards various drugs compared to 2D *in vitro* cell culture models [50, 51]. This differential response can be attributed to structural and functional complexity of 3D model vs. a 2D model. Drug penetration is one of the reasons of this resistance as the structural and microenvironmental barriers prevent effective convection of drug in 3D spheroids. As a result, drug fails to achieve an effective concentration inside the tumor to deliver a strong anticancer response. Kerr et al. demonstrated that reduced penetration of anthracycline-based drugs was responsible for a mild cytotoxic effect of these drugs in lung spheroids and a more lipophilic analogue partitioned better hence can be a better therapeutic option against 3D spheroids [52]. A recent study by Gupta et al. showed improved efficacy of paclitaxel when coadministered with tumor penetrating peptide iRGD due to increased availability of the drug in the interior of A549 spheroids [53]. Similarly, tumor

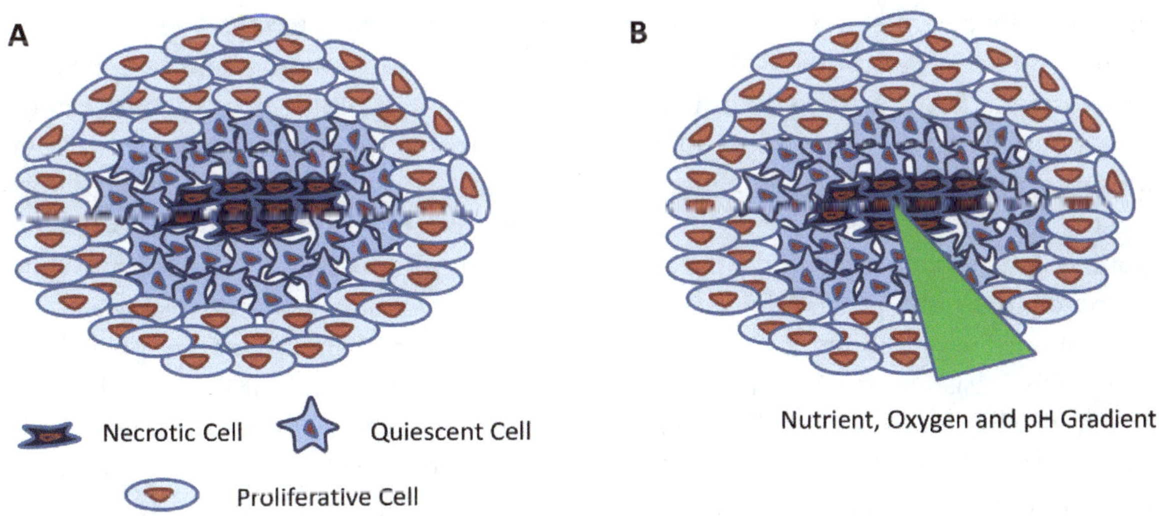

Figure 2. Structural organization of spheroids. (A) Cells are organized in three distinct zones based on viability and proliferative status of the contributing cells. The innermost necrotic layer is mostly composed of dead cells, which is followed by middle senescent layer consisting of slowly growing quiescent cells. The outermost layer is proliferative and contains rapid dividing cells. (B) A gradient of nutrients, oxygen and pH is responsible for this structural organization of cells in spheroids. Since the interior section of the spheroids receives least amount of nutrients and oxygen, the survival of cells in this part of the spheroid is compromised. As supply of nutrients and oxygen improve from moderate to high in the middle and outer section of spheroids, cells change from quiescent to highly proliferative in these zones.

heterogeneity arising from the distinct arrangement of cells in different proliferative zones in spheroids can promote resistance to certain drugs. For example, antiproliferative drugs such as paclitaxel, which confers most activity towards rapidly dividing cells, showed a reduced activity towards interior region of spheroid as it consists of quiescent cells [54]. Drugs like doxorubicin which induce anticancer effect by producing reactive oxygen species show limited response under hypoxic conditions [55]. However, drugs which get activated under hypoxic conditions can potentially treat hypoxic tumors. In 2012, Meng et al. observed that a hypoxia-selective drug TH-302 showed 650-fold greater activity in hypoxic H460 lung cancer cell spheroids than in monolayer cells [56]. Cancer cells switch their metabolism to glycolysis and produce lactic acid in the process. A lack of effective clearing of this excess lactic acid results in accumulation of lactic acid and subsequent reduction of pH in the interior of the tumor. A reduced pH of the tumor microenvironment can adversely affect the cytotoxicity of weak basic drugs such as doxorubicin, mitoxantrone, vincristine, etc. These drugs get protonated under acidic conditions resulting in decreased cellular uptake, hence lose their activity [57]. Activations of mechanisms related to drug efflux in spheroid can be responsible for increased resistance to the drugs. In 2015, Rodriguez et al. showed an increased expression of MDR-1 and P-glycoprotein in spheroids of INER-37 human NSCLC cell line compared to 2D culture likely responsible for increased drug resistance [58]. Several studies have indicated CSC enrichment in spheroids as possible explanation for drug resistance and metastasis [59, 60]. A 3D spheroid platform is a more relevant model for anti-cancer drug screening, and represents a much better approach to achieving therapeutic outcomes for cancer patients as compared to current therapeutic practices. There is need to develop drugs with better penetrating ability to improve its availability to the most interior sections of tumors. Improved drug delivery techniques employing vehicles, such as nanoparticles, liposomes, nanospheres, etc., can (i) improve drug delivery and (ii) protect drug decomposition under harsh tumor microenvironment. Tumor heterogeneity arising from cells of different metabolic, proliferative, chemosensitivity, metastatic and stemness profile calls for a more complex and versatile therapy approach for cancer treatment. For example—a cotherapy approach using multiple drugs which can target different populations of cancer cells will have better outcome for patients than a simple single therapy approach. Development of better drugs with single drugs targeting multiple pathways can remove the need to use multiple drugs simultaneously. So, an effective and improved drug development, drug delivery and drug testing programme are the need of hour to make significant inroads in a fight against cancer. It is important to mention that Steadman et al. raised concerns about the possibility that the chemoresistance mechanisms found in spheroids may differ from the resistance found in intractable solid tumors in patients [61]. If this is the case, drugs selected by this system will be ineffective in primary tumors. Future studies should be aimed to attempt to recapitulate *in vitro,* the complex architecture of lung tumors should take in consideration several factors known to simultaneously contribute to chemoresistance.

2.2.2. Floating tumorspheres

Cancer is a complex disease with several preventive mechanisms put in place to escape elimination by immune response, drug efflux or expulsion mechanisms to mitigate drug activity and a microenvironment uniquely suitable for cancer cells. The matter is further complicated by tumor heterogeneity resulting in mixed population of cells with varying degree of chemoresistance, invasive and migratory potential. Several cancer models have been proposed to explain tumor heterogeneity and related tumor characteristics. Clonal evolution model (CEM) and cancer stem cell model (CSCM) are two of the most popular and widely accepted models. CEM postulates clonal evolution of tumor and suggests existence of several clones with varying genetic and epigenetic modifications as the contributor for tumor heterogeneity. Lately, CSCM has become most commonly used model for tumor biology. According to CSCM, a rare but fixed population of cells known as cancer stem cells (CSCs) with indefinite self-renewal potential and pluripotency are responsible for tumor origin, heterogeneity, metastasis, resistance and relapse. CSCs are rare cells and most of the times only constitute 1% of tumor volume. Over the period, various methods and techniques have been developed to enrich and study the CSC. Fluorescence-activated cell sorting (FACS) using surface markers, culture of cells in suspension for generating tumorspheres with increased stemness, sorting of cells based on the activity of intracellular enzymes such as aldehyde dehydrogenase (ALDH) and 26S proteosome and sorting of side population cells due to their ability to exclude Hoechst 33342 are some of the most commonly used methods for CSC sorting and subsequent enrichment. Generation of tumorspheres is most convenient and cost-effective way for enriching CSCs as it does not require previous knowledge of surface marker or enzyme expression and costly cell sorting FACS set up. For this chapter, we will focus on generation of floating tumorspheres and their use as a model for studying chemoresistance. In 1996, Reynolds et al. described the generation of normal neural stem cells as "neurospheres" upon culture of brain cells in floating conditions in serum-free medium supplemented with epidermal growth factor (EGF) and fibroblast growth factor (FGF) [62]. Following the same culture protocol, Singh et al. generated tumorspheres from the brain tumor cells [63]. Soon after, the method was widely accepted and researcher all over the world used this protocol to generate tumorspheres from a wide variety of cancers [64–68]. Over the course of time, researchers have tried to improve upon the existing protocol of sphere formation in order to make it more efficient, consistent, reliable and physiologically relevant. Various types of scaffolds consisting of chitosan-alginate, collagen, alginate and agarose have been used as 3D matrices to substitute low attachment plates [69–72]. In 2014, Cao et al. generated tumorspheres from primary neuroblastoma cells driven from MYCN transgenic mice using a medium supplemented with fetal bovine serum (FBS) and β-mercaptoethanol. These spheres exhibited indefinite renewal as they could be passaged more than 20 times and also demonstrated enhanced metastatic potential [73]. More recently, in one of our studies, we described culture of lung tumorspheres (LTs) from H460 cells solely in serum-free media without supplementation of growth factors [39]. This method was further extended to mammospheres (MSs) generation in MCF-7 cells [74].

Over a period, several targeted therapies have been developed towards various oncogenic drivers (EGFR, ALK, ROS1, RET, etc.) in lung cancer [75]. However, most of these drugs have shown a transient effect on cancer as initial remission of disease is followed by outbreak of more aggressive and resistant cancer resulting in modest overall survival. Therapy resistance is a leading hurdle in cancer treatment and mostly responsible for poor outcome for the patients. Several researchers have identified acquired mutations during the prolonged treatment with a single drug as the leading cause for the therapy resistance. As discussed in more detail in the previous section (Section 2.1.3.), secondary mutations, bypass pathways such as MET, amplification of HER2, overexpression of AXL kinase, etc. have been shown to induce therapy resistance in lung cancer [75–78]. With the advent of concept of CSCs and subsequent discovery of CSCs in several types of cancers, researchers started to explore a possible link between therapy resistance and possible changes in the CSCs population. In 2008, Levina et al. were the first researchers to report the enrichment of cancer stem-like cells (CSLCs) in response to therapy treatment in lung tumor. They observed that the surviving cancer cell expressed stemness-related markers such as CD133, CD117, SSEA-3, TRA1-81, Oct4 and nuclear β-catenin. These cells retained a higher capability to form spheres, self-renewal, differentiation and showed high metastatic and tumorigenic potential [79]. Several studies have pointed towards enrichment of CSLCs as a contributing factor for acquired resistance in lung cancer in response to Cisplatin therapy [25, 80]. Similar findings have been reported for other commonly used anticancer therapies in lung cancer [81]. Normally, a 2D *in vitro* model is used for the screening of potential anticancer agents and more often they fail to translate *in vitro* antiproliferative efficacy of a drug in *in vivo* settings. This is due to an inherently flawed 2D model which does not replicate a real tumor at structural, physicochemical, mechanical and biochemical levels. A tumor is a 3D entity composed of cells exhibiting varying degree of resistance, proliferative and metastatic tendencies. Tumor microenvironmental conditions which play a critical role in determining tumor heterogeneity, resistance and metastasis cannot be replicated by an *in vitro* model, and hence it often fails to impress upon aforementioned attributes of tumor. Therefore, a more physiologically relevant drug screening tool is a real necessity to improve upon often failing *in vitro* cytotoxicity model. Tumorspheres with their 3D structure and often increased stemness can serve as more resistant and invasive model with closely relatable microenvironmental conditions as that of a real tumor. It can serve as a more realistic approach for drug screening with better chances of replication of drug efficacy in *in vivo* system. Tumorspheres assay can serve as a quick and more economical intermediary testing platform for *in vivo* tumor xenograft studies in a high-throughput setting while *in vivo* studies can be reserved for validating findings observed in the tumorsphere assays.

In recent years, researchers have successfully employed tumorsphere model for effective screening of potential anticancer drugs. A number of studies exploring anticancer efficacy of different classes of compounds such as inorganic [82], natural ingredients [83], antibiotics [84], Chinese medicine [85], cardiac glycosides [86], etc. against LTs have been published. *In vivo* studies have been performed to explore and extend observed drug efficacy against LTs in a more physiological setting [87, 88]. Several studies have tried combination therapy approaches in LTs setting to develop effective drug combinations to alleviate therapy resistance-related concerns and improve efficacy of existing cancer drugs [68, 89–92]. The promising anticancer drugs selected using tumorspheres described above need to pass the test of more relevant animal models and later on successful clinical trials to validate the applicability of this 3D system for anticancer drug screening.

2.2.3. 3D systems as models to test drug delivery and efficacy

Drug delivery refers to approaches, formulations, technologies and systems for transporting and administering *in vivo* an active pharmaceutical ingredient (API) to achieve a therapeutic effect in the patient. In tumors, there are gradients of drug concentrations, oxygen and nutrients created by the distance from blood vessels. These similarities make 3D systems the more physiological models for drug delivery testing and therefore better predictors of chemosensitivity. Metha et al. [93] described in detail six characteristics of spheroids, which are absent in conventional culture formats, that mimic how drug delivery might occur *in vivo*: (1) spheroids model the 3D architecture of tissues, including multicellular arrangement and extracellular matrix deposition, found *in vivo*. (2) Spheroids have sizeable cell-cell interactions, including tight junctions that are known to influence response of cells to drugs, (3) spheroids have diffusional limits to mass transport of drugs, nutrients and other factors, (4) spheroids are formed with two or more cell types in varying ratios representing intercellular signaling and architecture that can help to understand how multiple cell types might impact drug delivery, (5) rare cells such as cancer stem cells or primary stem cells may be present or incorporated and maintained in spheroids which can facilitate targeting these specific cells with drugs and (6) larger spheroids develop central necrosis and regions of hypoxia present in many cancers. These specific microenvironments have been shown to contain cancer cells with increased chemoresistance. Tumorspheres share most of these characteristics with few differences: (1) they are considered to be enriched with CS-LCs that are inherently more resistant than non-CS-LCs and (2) tumorspheres can be generated in complete absence of external mitogenic stimulation that makes ideal system to study how specific factors (sometimes present in serum-containing media) may alter the response of cancer cells to anticancer drugs. For instance, lung tumorspheres grown in the absence of external mitogenic stimuli when exposed to exogenously added EGF demonstrated increased sensitivity to Erlotinib and Gefitinib [10]. In summary, despite their limitations, both spheroids and tumorspheres are useful and complementary systems for drug delivery testing.

3. Implications for translational oncology

The *in vitro* identification of effective anticancer is a crucial part of the anticancer drug screening program. Drug development is a long and expensive business, and billions of dollars are invested for a single successful drug release in market. It starts at identification of potential drug candidate with subsequent testing *in vitro* and *in vivo* setting followed by testing in various phases of clinical trials. Upon successful completion of clinical trial, drug is approved by FDA for marketing. Therefore, development of realistic models of drug screening is extremely important for vetting of drug candidates in earlier preclinical stages for them to have better chances to be successful in later clinical trials. Traditionally, 2D *in vitro* culture model is used for cancer drug screening. However, it completely fails to recapture finer intricacies of 3D tumor. It does not have any semblance with a 3D tumor at microenvironmental, biological and physiological levels and hence in most instances miserably fails in therapy translation from an *in vitro* to an *in vivo* setting. In order to address these issues, researchers have developed various drug screening 3D models, which align well, mimic essence of natural tumors and carry more significance as drug screening platforms. Despite these important technical advances, few drugs have been translated into clinical practice and the prognosis of lung cancer patients remains poor, suggesting that current *in vitro* 3D models are still not good models of primary tumors.

4. Conclusions

At present, current *in vitro* 3D models offer significant advantages over 2D systems in terms of recapitulating intratumoral heterogeneity and enrichment of cancer stem cells and have been extremely useful for understanding cancer cell biology. However, for anticancer drugs discovery, this success has not been translated into the clinic because the prognosis of lung cancer patients still remains poor. Future development in the field should concentrate on (i) efforts to better mimic *in vivo* conditions and (ii) identifying the underlying mechanism of chemoresistance of *in vitro* system in correlation with *in vivo* conditions. Otherwise, drugs selected with the current method will only target a subpopulation of chemoresistant cells or as suggested by Steadman et al. will be ineffective due to differences in the underlying mechanism of chemoresistance between *in vitro* 3D system and *in vivo* conditions.

Acknowledgements

Research in Dr. Iyer and Dr. Azad's lab is supported by grants CA173069 from National Cancer Institute (NIH/NCI) and HL112630, respectively. The content is solely the responsibility of the authors and does not represent the official views of the National Institutes of Health. We apologize to authors whose important work has not been cited due to limited space.

Conflict of interest

The author declares no conflict of interest, financial or otherwise.

Author details

Vivek Kaushik, Juan Sebastian Yakisich, Yogesh Kulkarni, Neelam Azad and Anand Krishnan V. Iyer*

*Address all correspondence to: anand.iyer@hamptonu.edu

Department of Pharmaceutical Sciences, School of Pharmacy, Hampton University, Hampton, VA, USA

References

[1] Torre LA, Siegel RL, Jemal A. Lung cancer statistics. Advances in Experimental Medicine and Biology. 2016;**893**:1-19. DOI: 10.1007/978-3-319-24223-1_1

[2] Abeloff MD, Eggleston JC, Mendelsohn G, Ettinger DS, Baylin SB. Changes in morphologic and biochemical characteristics of small cell carcinoma of the lung. A clinicopathologic study. The American Journal of Medicine. 1979;**66**(5):757-764

[3] Neelakantan D, Drasin DJ, Ford HL. Intratumoral heterogeneity: Clonal cooperation in epithelial-to-mesenchymal transition and metastasis. Cell Adhesion & Migration. 2015; **9**(4):265-276. DOI: 10.4161/19336918.2014.972761

[4] Park S, Ha S, Lee SH, Paeng JC, Keam B, Kim TM, et al. Intratumoral heterogeneity characterized by pretreatment PET in non-small cell lung cancer patients predicts progression-free survival on EGFR tyrosine kinase inhibitor. PLoS One. 2018;**13**(1):e0189766. DOI: 10.1371/journal.pone.0189766

[5] MacDonagh L, Gray SG, Breen E, Cuffe S, Finn SP, O'Byrne KJ, et al. Lung cancer stem cells: The root of resistance. Cancer Letters. 2016;**372**(2):147-156. DOI: 10.1016/j.canlet.2016.01.012

[6] O'Flaherty JD, Barr M, Fennell D, Richard D, Reynolds J, O'Leary J, et al. The cancer stem-cell hypothesis: Its emerging role in lung cancer biology and its relevance for future therapy. Journal of Thoracic Oncology. 2012;**7**(12):1880-1890. DOI: 10.1097/JTO.0b013e31826bfbc6

[7] Cruz MH, Siden A, Calaf GM, Delwar ZM, Yakisich JS. The stemness phenotype model. ISRN Oncology. 2012;**2012**:392647. DOI: 10.5402/2012/392647

[8] Vermeulen L, de Sousa e Melo F, Richel DJ, Medema JP. The developing cancer stem-cell model: Clinical challenges and opportunities. The Lancet Oncology. 2012;**13**(2):e83-e89. DOI: 10.1016/S1470-2045(11)70257-1

[9] Marjanovic ND, Weinberg RA, Chaffer CL. Cell plasticity and heterogeneity in cancer. Clinical Chemistry. 2013;**59**(1):168-179. DOI: 10.1373/clinchem.2012.184655

[10] Yakisich JS, Azad N, Kaushik V, Iyer AK. Cancer cell plasticity: Rapid reversal of chemosensitivity and expression of stemness markers in lung and breast cancer tumorspheres. Journal of Cellular Physiology. 2016;**232**(9):2280-2286. DOI: 10.1002/jcp.25725

[11] Akunuru S, Zhai QJ, Zheng Y. Non-small cell lung cancer stem/progenitor cells are enriched in multiple distinct phenotypic subpopulations and exhibit plasticity. Cell Death & Disease. 2012;**3**(7):e352. DOI: 10.1038/cddis.2012.93

[12] Gupta PB, Fillmore CM, Jiang G, Shapira SD, Tao K, Kuperwasser C, et al. Stochastic state transitions give rise to phenotypic equilibrium in populations of cancer cells. Cell. 2011; **146**(4):633-644. Erratum in: Cell. 2011; 147(5):1197. Cell. 2011;**146**(6):1042. DOI: 10.1016/j.cell.2011.07.026

[13] Yang G, Quan Y, Wang W, Fu Q, Wu J, Mei T, et al. Dynamic equilibrium between cancer stem cells and non-stem cancer cells in human SW620 and MCF-7 cancer cell populations. British Journal of Cancer. 2012;**106**(9):1512-1519. DOI: 10.1038/bjc.2012.126

[14] Pastrana E, Silva-Vargas V, Doetsch F. Eyes wide open: A critical review of sphere-formation as an assay for stem cells. Cell Stem Cell. 2011;**8**(5):486-498. DOI: 10.1016/j.stem.2011.04.007

[15] Tirino V, Desiderio V, Paino F, De Rosa A, Papaccio F, La Noce M, et al. Cancer stem cells in solid tumors: An overview and new approaches for their isolation and characterization. The FASEB Journal. 2013;**27**(1):13-24. DOI: 10.1096/fj.12-218222

[16] Stordal BK, Davey MW, Davey RA. Oxaliplatin induces drug resistance more rapidly than cisplatin in H69 small cell lung cancer cells. Cancer Chemotherapy and Pharmacology. 2006;**58**(2):256-265. DOI: 10.1007/s00280-005-0148-7

[17] McDermott M, Eustace AJ, Busschots S, Breen L, Crown J, Clynes M, et al. In vitro development of chemotherapy and targeted therapy drug-resistant cancer cell lines: A practical guide with case studies. Frontiers in Oncology. 2014;**4**:40. DOI: 10.3389/fonc.2014.00040

[18] Ghosh G, Lian X, Kron SJ, Palecek SP. Properties of resistant cells generated from lung cancer cell lines treated with EGFR inhibitors. BMC Cancer. 2012;**12**:95. DOI: 10.1186/1471-2407-12-95

[19] Kurokawa M, Ise N, Omi K, Goishi K, Higashiyama S. Cisplatin influences acquisition of resistance to molecular-targeted agents through epithelial-mesenchymal transition-like changes. Cancer Science. 2013;**104**(7):904-911. DOI: 10.1111/cas.12171

[20] Shien K, Toyooka S, Yamamoto H, Soh J, Jida M, Thu KL, et al. Acquired resistance to EGFR inhibitors is associated with a manifestation of stem cell-like properties in cancer cells. Cancer Research. 2013;**73**(10):3051-3061. DOI: 10.1158/0008-5472.can-12-4136

[21] Januchowski R, Wojtowicz K, Zabel M. The role of aldehyde dehydrogenase (ALDH) in cancer drug resistance. Biomedicine & Pharmacotherapy. 2013;**67**(7):669-680. DOI: 10.1016/j.biopha.2013.04.005

[22] Shah MA, Schwartz GK. Cell cycle-mediated drug resistance: An emerging concept in cancer therapy. Clinical Cancer Research. 2001;**7**(8):2168-2181

[23] Nurwidya F, Takahashi F, Murakami A, Takahashi K. Epithelial mesenchymal transition in drug resistance and metastasis of lung cancer. Cancer Research and Treatment. 2012;**44**(3):151-156. DOI: 10.4143/crt.2012.44.3.151

[24] Yauch RL, Januario T, Eberhard DA, Cavet G, Zhu W, Fu L, et al. Epithelial versus mesenchymal phenotype determines in vitro sensitivity and predicts clinical activity of erlotinib in lung cancer patients. Clinical Cancer Research. 2005;**11**(24 Pt 1):8686-8698. DOI: 10.1158/1078-0432.ccr-05-1492

[25] Barr MP, Gray SG, Hoffmann AC, Hilger RA, Thomale J, O'Flaherty JD, et al. Generation and characterisation of cisplatin-resistant non-small cell lung cancer cell lines displaying a stem-like signature. PLoS One. 2013;**8**(1):e54193. DOI: 10.1371/journal.pone.0054193

[26] Krishna R, Mayer LD. Multidrug resistance (MDR) in cancer. Mechanisms, reversal using modulators of MDR and the role of MDR modulators in influencing the pharmacokinetics of anticancer drugs. European Journal of Pharmaceutical Sciences. 2000;**11**(4):265-283

[27] Kris MG, Natale RB, Herbst RS, Lynch TJ, Prager D, Belani CP, et al. Efficacy of gefitinib, an inhibitor of the epidermal growth factor receptor tyrosine kinase, in symptomatic

patients with non-small cell lung cancer: A randomized trial. Journal of the American Medical Association. 2003;**290**(16):2149-2158. DOI: 10.1001/jama.290.16.2149

[28] Marchetti A, Martella C, Felicioni L, Barassi F, Salvatore S, Chella A, et al. EGFR mutations in non-small-cell lung cancer: Analysis of a large series of cases and development of a rapid and sensitive method for diagnostic screening with potential implications on pharmacologic treatment. Journal of Clinical Oncology. 2005;**23**(4):857-865. DOI: 10.1200/jco.2005.08.043

[29] Yun CH, Mengwasser KE, Toms AV, Woo MS, Greulich H, Wong KK, et al. The T790M mutation in EGFR kinase causes drug resistance by increasing the affinity for ATP. Proceedings of the National Academy of Sciences of the United States of America. 2008; **105**(6):2070-2075. DOI: 10.1073/pnas.0709662105

[30] Sudo M, Chin TM, Mori S, Doan NB, Said JW, Akashi M, et al. Inhibiting proliferation of gefitinib-resistant, non-small cell lung cancer. Cancer Chemotherapy and Pharmacology. 2013;**71**(5):1325-1334. DOI: 10.1007/s00280-013-2132-y

[31] Engelman JA, Zejnullahu K, Mitsudomi T, Song Y, Hyland C, Park JO, et al. MET amplification leads to gefitinib resistance in lung cancer by activating ERBB3 signaling. Science (New York, NY). 2007;**316**(5827):1039-1043. DOI: 10.1126/science.1141478

[32] Terai H, Soejima K, Yasuda H, Nakayama S, Hamamoto J, Arai D, et al. Activation of the FGF2-FGFR1 autocrine pathway: A novel mechanism of acquired resistance to gefitinib in NSCLC. Molecular Cancer Research. 2013;**11**(7):759-767. DOI: 10.1158/1541-7786.mcr-12-0652

[33] Jakobsen KR, Demuth C, Madsen AT, Hussmann D, Vad-Nielsen J, Nielsen AL, et al. MET amplification and epithelial-to-mesenchymal transition exist as parallel resistance mechanisms in erlotinib-resistant, EGFR-mutated, NSCLC HCC827 cells. Oncogenesis. 2017; **6**(4):e307. DOI: 10.1038/oncsis.2017.17

[34] Shaw AT, Engelman JA. ALK in lung cancer: Past, present, and future. Journal of Clinical Oncology. 2013;**31**(8):1105-1111. DOI: 10.1200/jco.2012.44.5353

[35] Zhao Y, Yang Y, Xu Y, Lu S, Jian H. AZD0530 sensitizes drug-resistant ALK-positive lung cancer cells by inhibiting SRC signaling. FEBS Open Bio. 2017;**7**(4):472-476. DOI: 10.1002/2211-5463.12162

[36] Wilson C, Nimick M, Nehoff H, Ashton JC. ALK and IGF-1R as independent targets in crizotinib resistant lung cancer. Scientific Reports. 2017;**7**(1):13955. DOI: 10.1038/s41598-017-14289-w

[37] Liu YN, Chang TH, Tsai MF, Wu SG, Tsai TH, Chen HY, et al. IL-8 confers resistance to EGFR inhibitors by inducing stem cell properties in lung cancer. Oncotarget. 2015;**6**(12): 10415-10431. DOI: 10.18632/oncotarget.3389

[38] Li L, Gu X, Yue J, Zhao Q, Lv D, Chen H, et al. Acquisition of EGFR TKI resistance and EMT phenotype is linked with activation of IGF1R/NF-kappaB pathway in EGFR-mutant NSCLC. Oncotarget. 2017;**8**(54):92240-92253. DOI: 10.18632/oncotarget.21170

[39] Yakisich JS, Azad N, Venkatadri R, Kulkarni Y, Wright C, Kaushik V, et al. Formation of tumorspheres with increased stemness without external mitogens in a lung cancer model. Stem Cells International. 2016;**2016**:5603135. DOI: 10.1155/2016/5603135

[40] Ivascu A, Kubbies M. Rapid generation of single-tumor spheroids for high-throughput cell function and toxicity analysis. Journal of Biomolecular Screening. 2006;**11**(8):922-932. DOI: 10.1177/1087057106292763

[41] Goodwin TJ, Prewett TL, Wolf DA, Spaulding GF. Reduced shear stress: A major component in the ability of mammalian tissues to form three-dimensional assemblies in simulated microgravity. Journal of Cellular Biochemistry. 1993;**51**(3):301-311. DOI: 10.1002/jcb.240510309

[42] Kelm JM, Timmins NE, Brown CJ, Fussenegger M, Nielsen LK. Method for generation of homogeneous multicellular tumor spheroids applicable to a wide variety of cell types. Biotechnology and Bioengineering. 2003;**83**(2):173-180. DOI: 10.1002/bit.10655

[43] Breslin S, O'Driscoll L. Three-dimensional cell culture: The missing link in drug discovery. Drug Discovery Today. 2013;**18**(5–6):240-249. DOI: 10.1016/j.drudis.2012.10.003

[44] Tan W, Krishnaraj R, Desai TA. Evaluation of nanostructured composite collagen—chitosan matrices for tissue engineering. Tissue Engineering. 2001;**7**(2):203-210. DOI: 10.1089/107632701300062831

[45] Kunz-Schughart LA, Heyder P, Schroeder J, Knuechel R. A heterologous 3-D coculture model of breast tumor cells and fibroblasts to study tumor-associated fibroblast differentiation. Experimental Cell Research. 2001;**266**(1):74-86. DOI: 10.1006/excr.2001.5210

[46] Rama-Esendagli D, Esendagli G, Yilmaz G, Guc D. Spheroid formation and invasion capacity are differentially influenced by co-cultures of fibroblast and macrophage cells in breast cancer. Molecular Biology Reports. 2014;**41**(5):2885-2892. DOI: 10.1007/s11033-014-3144-3

[47] Takagi A, Watanabe M, Ishii Y, Morita J, Hirokawa Y, Matsuzaki T, et al. Three-dimensional cellular spheroid formation provides human prostate tumor cells with tissue-like features. Anticancer Research. 2007;**27**(1A):45-53

[48] Alvarez-Perez J, Ballesteros P, Cerdan S. Microscopic images of intraspheroidal pH by 1H magnetic resonance chemical shift imaging of pH sensitive indicators. Magma (New York, NY). 2005;**18**(6):293-301. DOI: 10.1007/s10334-005-0013-z

[49] Mueller-Klieser W. Method for the determination of oxygen consumption rates and diffusion coefficients in multicellular spheroids. Biophysical Journal. 1984;**46**(3):343-348. DOI: 10.1016/s0006-3495(84)84030-8

[50] Douple EB, Cate CC, Curphey TJ, Pettengill OS, Sorenson GD, Maurer LH. Evaluation of drug efficacy in vitro using human small cell carcinoma of the lung spheroids. Cancer. 1985;**56**(8):1918-1925

[51] Huh D, Hamilton GA, Ingber DE. From 3D cell culture to organs-on-chips. Trends in Cell Biology. 2011;**21**(12):745-754. DOI: 10.1016/j.tcb.2011.09.005

[52] Kerr DJ, Wheldon TE, Hydns S, Kaye SB. Cytotoxic drug penetration studies in multicellular tumour spheroids. Xenobiotica. 1988;**18**(6):641-648. DOI: 10.3109/00498258809041702

[53] Gupta SK, Torrico Guzman EA, Meenach SA. Coadministration of a tumor-penetrating peptide improves the therapeutic efficacy of paclitaxel in a novel air-grown lung cancer 3D spheroid model. International Journal of Cancer. 2017;**141**(10):2143-2153. DOI: 10.1002/ijc.30913

[54] Mitchison TJ. The proliferation rate paradox in antimitotic chemotherapy. Molecular Biology of the Cell. 2012;**23**(1):1-6. DOI: 10.1091/mbc.E10-04-0335

[55] Kennedy KA. Hypoxic cells as specific drug targets for chemotherapy. Anti-Cancer Drug Design. 1987;**2**(2):181-194

[56] Meng F, Evans JW, Bhupathi D, Banica M, Lan L, Lorente G, et al. Molecular and cellular pharmacology of the hypoxia-activated prodrug TH-302. Molecular Cancer Therapeutics. 2012;**11**(3):740-751. DOI: 10.1158/1535-7163.mct-11-0634

[57] Gerweck LE, Vijayappa S, Kozin S. Tumor pH controls the in vivo efficacy of weak acid and base chemotherapeutics. Molecular Cancer Therapeutics. 2006;**5**(5):1275-1279. DOI: 10.1158/1535-7163.mct-06-0024

[58] Barrera-Rodriguez R, Fuentes JM. Multidrug resistance characterization in multicellular tumour spheroids from two human lung cancer cell lines. Cancer Cell International. 2015; **15**:47. DOI: 10.1186/s12935-015-0200-6

[59] Aaberg-Jessen C, Norregaard A, Christensen K, Pedersen CB, Andersen C, Kristensen BW. Invasion of primary glioma- and cell line-derived spheroids implanted into corticostriatal slice cultures. International Journal of Clinical and Experimental Pathology. 2013;**6**(4):546-560

[60] Liao J, Qian F, Tchabo N, Mhawech-Fauceglia P, Beck A, Qian Z, et al. Ovarian cancer spheroid cells with stem cell-like properties contribute to tumor generation, metastasis and chemotherapy resistance through hypoxia-resistant metabolism. PLoS One. 2014;**9**(1): e84941. DOI: 10.1371/journal.pone.0084941

[61] Steadman K, Stein WD, Litman T, Yang SX, Abu-Asab M, Dutcher SK, et al. PolyHEMA spheroids are an inadequate model for the drug resistance of the intractable solid tumors. Cell Cycle 2008;**7**(6):818-829

[62] Reynolds BA, Weiss S. Clonal and population analyses demonstrate that an EGF-responsive mammalian embryonic CNS precursor is a stem cell. Developmental Biology. 1996;**175**(1):1-13. DOI: 10.1006/dbio.1996.0090

[63] Singh SK, Clarke ID, Terasaki M, Bonn VE, Hawkins C, Squire J, et al. Identification of a cancer stem cell in human brain tumors. Cancer Research. 2003;**63**(18):5821-5828

[64] Burleson KM, Casey RC, Skubitz KM, Pambuccian SE, Oegema TR, Skubitz AP. Ovarian carcinoma ascites spheroids adhere to extracellular matrix components and mesothelial cell monolayers. Gynecologic Oncology. 2004;**93**(1):170-181. DOI: 10.1016/j.ygyno.2003.12.034

[65] Bussolati B, Bruno S, Grange C, Ferrando U, Camussi G. Identification of a tumor-initiating stem cell population in human renal carcinomas. The FASEB Journal. 2008;**22**(10):3696-3705. DOI: 10.1096/fj.08-102590

[66] Dontu G, Abdallah WM, Foley JM, Jackson KW, Clarke MF, Kawamura MJ, et al. In vitro propagation and transcriptional profiling of human mammary stem/progenitor cells. Genes & Development. 2003;**17**(10):1253-1270. DOI: 10.1101/gad.1061803

[67] Ricci-Vitiani L, Lombardi DG, Pilozzi E, Biffoni M, Todaro M, Peschle C, et al. Identification and expansion of human colon-cancer-initiating cells. Nature. 2007;**445**(7123):111-115. DOI: 10.1038/nature05384

[68] Simeone DM. Pancreatic cancer stem cells: Implications for the treatment of pancreatic cancer. Clinical Cancer Research. 2008;**14**(18):5646-5648. DOI: 10.1158/1078-0432.ccr-08-0584

[69] Chen L, Xiao Z, Meng Y, Zhao Y, Han J, Su G, et al. The enhancement of cancer stem cell properties of MCF-7 cells in 3D collagen scaffolds for modeling of cancer and anti-cancer drugs. Biomaterials. 2012;**33**(5):1437-1444. DOI: 10.1016/j.biomaterials.2011.10.056

[70] Palomeras S, Rabionet M, Ferrer I, Sarrats A, Garcia-Romeu ML, Puig T, et al. Breast cancer stem cell culture and enrichment using poly(epsilon-Caprolactone) scaffolds. Molecules (Basel, Switzerland). 2016;**21**(4):537. DOI: 10.3390/molecules21040537

[71] Rao W, Zhao S, Yu J, Lu X, Zynger DL, He X. Enhanced enrichment of prostate cancer stem-like cells with miniaturized 3D culture in liquid core-hydrogel shell microcapsules. Biomaterials. 2014;**35**(27):7762-7773. DOI: 10.1016/j.biomaterials.2014.06.011

[72] Su G, Zhao Y, Wei J, Han J, Chen L, Xiao Z, et al. The effect of forced growth of cells into 3D spheres using low attachment surfaces on the acquisition of stemness properties. Biomaterials. 2013;**34**(13):3215-3222. DOI: 10.1016/j.biomaterials.2013.01.044

[73] Cao D, Kishida S, Huang P, Mu P, Tsubota S, Mizuno M, et al. A new tumorsphere culture condition restores potentials of self-renewal and metastasis of primary neuroblastoma in a mouse neuroblastoma model. PLoS One. 2014;**9**(1):e86813. DOI: 10.1371/journal.pone.0086813

[74] Kaushik V, Azad N, Yakisich JS, Iyer AK. Antitumor effects of naturally occurring cardiac glycosides convallatoxin and peruvoside on human ER+ and triple-negative breast cancers. Cell Death Discovery. 2017;**3**:17009. DOI: 10.1038/cddiscovery.2017.9

[75] Gower A, Wang Y, Giaccone G. Oncogenic drivers, targeted therapies, and acquired resistance in non-small-cell lung cancer. Journal of Molecular Medicine. 2014;**92**(7):697-707. DOI: 10.1007/s00109-014-1165-y

[76] Hrustanovic G, Lee BJ, Bivona TG. Mechanisms of resistance to EGFR targeted therapies. Cancer Biology & Therapy. 2013;**14**(4):304-314. DOI: 10.4161/cbt.23627

[77] Kobayashi S, Boggon TJ, Dayaram T, Janne PA, Kocher O, Meyerson M, et al. EGFR mutation and resistance of non-small-cell lung cancer to gefitinib. The New England Journal of Medicine. 2005;**352**(8):786-792. DOI: 10.1056/NEJMoa044238

[78] Zhang Z, Lee JC, Lin L, Olivas V, Au V, LaFramboise T, et al. Activation of the AXL kinase causes resistance to EGFR-targeted therapy in lung cancer. Nature Genetics. 2012;**44**(8): 852-860. DOI: 10.1038/ng.2330

[79] Levina V, Marrangoni AM, DeMarco R, Gorelik E, Lokshin AE. Drug-selected human lung cancer stem cells: Cytokine network, tumorigenic and metastatic properties. PLoS One. 2008;**3**(8):e3077. DOI: 10.1371/journal.pone.0003077

[80] Hsieh JL, Lu CS, Huang CL, Shieh GS, Su BH, Su YC, et al. Acquisition of an enhanced aggressive phenotype in human lung cancer cells selected by suboptimal doses of cisplatin following cell deattachment and reattachment. Cancer Letters. 2012;**321**(1):36-44. DOI: 10.1016/j.canlet.2012.03.019

[81] Freitas DP, Teixeira CA, Santos-Silva F, Vasconcelos MH, Almeida GM. Therapy-induced enrichment of putative lung cancer stem-like cells. International Journal of Cancer. 2014; **134**(6):1270-1278. DOI: 10.1002/ijc.28478

[82] Chang KJ, Yang MH, Zheng JC, Li B, Nie W. Arsenic trioxide inhibits cancer stem-like cells via down-regulation of Gli1 in lung cancer. American Journal of Translational Research. 2016;**8**(2):1133-1143

[83] Zhu JY, Yang X, Chen Y, Jiang Y, Wang SJ, Li Y, et al. Curcumin suppresses lung cancer stem cells via inhibiting Wnt/beta-catenin and Sonic hedgehog pathways. Phytotherapy Research. 2017;**31**(4):680-688. DOI: 10.1002/ptr.5791

[84] Xiao Z, Sperl B, Ullrich A, Knyazev P. Metformin and salinomycin as the best combination for the eradication of NSCLC monolayer cells and their alveospheres (cancer stem cells) irrespective of EGFR, KRAS, EML4/ALK and LKB1 status. Oncotarget. 2014;**5**(24): 12877-12890. DOI: 10.18632/oncotarget.2657

[85] Cao X, Zou H, Cao J, Cui Y, Sun S, Ren K, et al. A candidate Chinese medicine preparation-Fructus Viticis Total flavonoids inhibits stem-like characteristics of lung cancer stem like cells. BMC Complementary and Alternative Medicine. 2016;**16**:364. DOI: 10.1186/s12906-016-1341-4

[86] Kaushik V, Yakisich JS, Azad N, Kulkarni Y, Venkatadri R, Wright C, et al. Anti-tumor effects of cardiac glycosides on human lung cancer cells and lung Tumorspheres. Journal of Cellular Physiology. 2017;**232**(9):2497-2507. DOI: 10.1002/jcp.25611

[87] Shen J, Ma B, Zhang X, Sun X, Han J, Wang Y, et al. Thioridazine has potent antitumor effects on lung cancer stem-like cells. Oncology Letters. 2017;**13**(3):1563-1568. DOI: 10.3892/ol.2017.5651

[88] Suwei D, Liang Z, Zhimin L, Ruilei L, Yingying Z, Zhen L, et al. NLK functions to maintain proliferation and stemness of NSCLC and is a target of metformin. Journal of Hematology & Oncology. 2015;**8**:120. DOI: 10.1186/s13045-015-0203-8

[89] Huang Y, Zeng F, Xu L, Zhou J, Liu X, Le H. Anticancer effects of cinnamic acid in lung adenocarcinoma cell line h1299-derived stem-like cells. Oncology Research. 2013;**20**(11): 499-507. DOI: 10.3727/096504013x13685487925095

[90] Moro M, Bertolini G, Pastorino U, Roz L, Sozzi G. Combination treatment with all-trans retinoic acid prevents Cisplatin-induced enrichment of CD133+ tumor-initiating cells and reveals heterogeneity of cancer stem cell compartment in lung cancer. Journal of Thoracic Oncology. 2015;**10**(7):1027-1036. DOI: 10.1097/jto.0000000000000563

[91] Yakisich JS, Azad N, Kaushik V, O'Doherty GA, Iyer AK. Nigericin decreases the viability of multidrug-resistant cancer cells and lung tumorspheres and potentiates the effects of cardiac glycosides. Tumour Biology. 2017;**39**(3):1010428317694310. DOI: 10.1177/1010428317694310

[92] Yeh CT, Wu AT, Chang PM, Chen KY, Yang CN, Yang SC, et al. Trifluoperazine, an antipsychotic agent, inhibits cancer stem cell growth and overcomes drug resistance of lung cancer. American Journal of Respiratory and Critical Care Medicine. 2012;**186**(11):1180-1188. DOI: 10.1164/rccm.201207-1180OC

[93] Mehta G, Hsiao AY, Ingram M, Luker GD, Takayama S. Opportunities and challenges for use of tumor spheroids as models to test drug delivery and efficacy. Journal of Controlled Release. 2012;**164**(2):192-204

3

Immunotherapy in Advanced Lung Cancer Treatment

Alexandru C. Grigorescu

Abstract

Despite the improvement in overall survival (OS) by platinum-based chemotherapy (NSCLC Meta-Analyses Collaborative Group, 2008), prognosis remains unsatisfactory for patients with advanced non-small cell lung cancer (NSCLC). We discuss in this chapter the new era of advanced lung cancer systemic therapy represented by immunotherapy. First of all I presented one of the modalities of immunological diagnostics based on new technology. The mechanism of action of the immunoagents is shortly described. In the in most part of the chapter, the main immunotherapeutic agents used in lung cancer immunotherapy are analyzed: vaccines, cytotoxic T lymphocyte-associated protein 4 (CTLA-4) inhibitors, and checkpoint inhibitors. In the end of the chapter, the combination between immunotherapeutic agents is discussed.

Keywords: lung cancer, systemic treatment, immunotherapy

1. Immunotherapeutic diagnosis

In order to have a therapy, it is known that we must first have a correct diagnosis. In this respect, we present an evolved oncology diagnostic system (http://www.carismolecularintelligence.com/i-o/). First of all, immunotherapy options should be sought through the development of complex immunoregulatory pathways. One of the systems that can be used in immunological diagnosis is Caris Molecular Intelligence. This system provides oncologists with reliable molecular information to make decisions about the use of immunotherapy. The tests are validated for testing PD-L1, MSI, and tumor mutation load (TML). Programmable cell death-ligand 1 (PD-L1) is one of the most important control immune proteins that mediates tumor-induced suppression by T-cell downregulation. Expression of PD-L1 may indicate a more likely response to immunotherapy. Of course, a perfect marker to predict the response to PD-L1 inhibitor therapy has not been validated for the moment, but with these tests, we have an important orientation (Cochrane Collaboration Guidelines).

Microsatellite instability (MSI) is caused by the failure of the mismatch repair (MMR) system. MSI-High correlates with the increase in neoantigenic burden, which is more likely to respond favorably to immunotherapy.

Tumor mutation load (TML) measures the total number of non-sinusoidal somatic mutations identified on the megabase of the genome coding region. High TML supports neoantigens and responds favorably to immunotherapy.

2. Immuno-oncological agents: action mechanism

The immune system is capable of recognizing and destroying tumor cells as well as pathogens. However, one of the hallmarks of cancer is its ability to avoid the immune system [1].

There are a lot of complex interactions between the cells presenting the antigen, the lymphocytes, and the tumor cells. The most studied is the cell membrane T-cell receptor binding, called programmed cell death 1 (PD-1), and its ligands 1 or 2 (PD-L1 or PD-L2) expressed by some tumor cells. This interaction results in inactivation of T lymphocytes in an effort to avoid the immune response against tumor cells [2, 3]. Inhibition of this pathway is the target of inhibitors of immune control points. There are two types of agents: anti-PD-1 and anti-PD-L1 monoclonal antibodies.

Among these, anti-PD-1 agents that bind the lymphocyte receptor and block both PD-L1 and PD-L2 bindings are considered to be more toxic than anti-PD-L1 due to their broad spectrum of clinical activity. However, this has not been confirmed by recent clinical trials [4, 5]. Pembrolizumab and nivolumab, two monoclonal antibodies against PD-1, as well as avelumab monoclonal IgG1 anti-PD-L1 antibodies, atezolizumab and MEDI4736, showed consistent antitumor activity against NSCLC [6].

3. Lung cancer immunotherapy

Despite an improvement in overall survival (OS) by platinum-based chemotherapy (NSCLC Meta-analyses Collaborative Group, 2008), prognosis remains unsatisfactory for patients with advanced NSCLC, with a median survival of 8–12 months [7, 8].

In 2006, there was a plateau for chemotherapy in a study that none of the four chemotherapy regimens compared offered a significant advantage over the others in the treatment of advanced non-small cell lung cancer [8].

The development in molecular characterization of NSCLC, especially in histological subtypes of adenocarcinoma, has allowed the identification of key genetic aberrations in NSCLC, which can be addressed with molecular targeted therapy. Genetic aberrations in EGFR, ALK, ROS1, RET, BRAF, and NTRK have a predictive value for susceptibility to receptor tyrosine kinase inhibitors [9–11]. Despite the success of molecular diagnostics, acquired resistance and disease progression are inevitable [9–11].

Treatment options for patients with small-cell lung cancer (SCLC) where the disease progressed after platinum-based chemotherapy are even more limited.

Immunotherapy in cancer has been described as any therapy that interacts with immunity. Immunotherapy in cancer can be classified into passive and active types. Passive immunotherapy has been described as administration of an active agent produced or generated outside the patient's body. Theoretically, such an approach does not depend on the host's own immune system to have an effect. Examples of passive immunotherapy include the use of monoclonal antibodies, such as trastuzumab [12, 13], and adoptive cell therapy, such as tumor-infiltrating lymphocytes (CAR-T cell) [14]. This new approach of therapy has and specific toxicity: cytokine release syndrome, neurologic toxicity, "on target/off tumor" recognition, and anaphylax [15].

Active immunotherapy involves stimulating or determining the host's immune system to recognize a tumor as a foreign. Examples of active immunotherapy include vaccination against cancer with tumor antigens and an adjuvant enhancement of immune cell function with cytokines, as well as targeting of immune control regulators with immune control inhibitor control.

Inhibitors targeting cytotoxic T-lymphocyte-associated protein 4 (CTLA-4) and programmed cell death 1 (PD-1)/programmed cell death-ligand 1 (PD-L1) are used in NSCLC and SCLC.

Studies that examine the efficacy of cytokines such as interferon alpha and interleukin-2 (IL-2) in lung cancer patients were negative and will not be discussed [16].

3.1. Vaccines against cancer

Therapeutically acting vaccines in cancer are designed to eliminate cancer cells by increasing their own immune responses. This type of vaccine contrasts with prophylactic vaccines, which are usually administered to healthy people. Cancer vaccines can be classified into several major types, such as cellular vaccines, peptide vaccines, and genetic vaccines [17].

Vaccines against cancer, despite despite setbacks attempt to harness the patient's immune system to fight tumor cells and show a promise in clinical trials.

Cellular vaccines may be either autologous or allogeneic. Autologous tumor cell vaccines are developed by isolating tumor cells from an individual (patient), creating a vaccine that is administered back to the same patient, usually in combination with an adjuvant that stimulates the immune system. These vaccines have been among the first types of cancer vaccines tested and have the advantage of provoking an immune response to a wide range of tumors. Antigens expressed by the patient's own tumor result in tumor destruction. Although similar to autologous vaccines, allogeneic vaccines are obtained by administering tumor cells to a patient, creating a vaccine that is then administered to another patient with the same type of cancer [18].

Unlike cellular vaccines that are made directly from patient tumors, peptide vaccines are often synthesized in vitro to mimic tumor-associated proteins in order to elicit an immune response against tumor cells expressing that protein [19].

Genetic vaccines are composed of DNA molecules or synthetic RNAs encoding tumor-associated proteins and are administered either alone or packaged in a nonpathogenic virus. The genetic material is taken up by the recipient cells, translated into proteins encoded, processed, and presented to the immune system to elicit the immune response against tumor-associated proteins [20].

DNA vaccination has suddenly become a favored strategy for inducing immunity. The molecular precision offered by gene-based vaccines, together with the facility to include additional genes to direct and amplify immunity, has always been attractive. However, the apparent failure to translate operational success in preclinical models to the clinic, for reasons that are now rather obvious, reduced initial enthusiasm. Recently, novel delivery systems, especially electroporation, have overcome this translational block. Here, we assess the development, current performance, and potential of DNA vaccines for the treatment of cancer.

Early studies on Calmette-Guerin adjuvant Calmette-Guerin adjuvant and neoadjuvant bacillus vaccine therapy were negative [21, 22].

In the modern age, multiple-stage, locally advanced, and advanced NSCLC vaccine studies have been conducted. The recombinant protein-associated anti-melanoma-antigen-associated antigen (MAGE)-A3 vaccine has been extensively studied in adjuvant therapy after complete resection. A randomized phase II trial showed that for patients with stage IB–II, MAGE-A3 in NSCLC, who did not receive any adjuvant chemotherapy, there was a tendency toward survival gain. And, survival without signs of disease was positively influenced by the MAGE-A3 vaccine compared to placebo after a median follow-up to 70 months (HR, 0.75; 95% CI, 0.46–1.23; p = 0.254) [23].

However, clinical benefit was not found in the randomized, double-blind, placebo-controlled phase III (MAGRIT) study in fully resected NSCLC IB–IIIA MAGE-A3, with or without adjuvant chemotherapy. Subsequently, for the total population in this study, median disease-free survival was 60.5 months for the MAGE-A3 vaccine group and 57.9 months for the placebo group (HR, 1.02; 95% CI, 0.89–1.18; p = 0.74). In the subgroup that performed adjuvant chemotherapy, median disease-free survival was 58.0 months in the vaccine group and 56.9 months in the placebo group (HR, 0.97; 95% CI, 0.80–1.18; p = 0.76) [24].

Tecemotide (L-BLP25) is a peptide vaccine based on a 25 amino acid sequence of mucin-1 (MUC1), which has shown promising activity in locally advanced NSCLC in a phase II study [25].

Subsequently, the result led to the initiation of two randomized trials. One was a complete phase III trial, START, in which the placebo tecemotide was compared for patients with stage III NSCLC without disease progression after chemoradiation therapy [26].

The second study, INSPIRE, was a randomized phase II study of Asian patients that did not have convincing results after the Asian phase [27].

Analysis of the START study showed that there was no significant difference in median overall survival between the tecemotide arm and placebo arms (25.6 months vs. 22.3 months; HR adjusted, 0.88; 95% CI, 0.75–1.03; p = 0.123). However, following a prespecified subgroup analysis, median overall survival was different between the vaccine arm and the placebo arm for patients receiving concomitant chemoradiation therapy (30.8 months vs. 20.6 months; HR, 0.78; 95% CI, 0.64–0.95; p = 0.016) compared with patients receiving sequential chemoradiation therapy (19.4 months vs. 24.6 months; HR, 1.12; 95% CI, 0.87–1.44; p = 0.38) [28].

In the advanced stage of the disease, the TG4010, another vaccine targeting MUC1, used a viral vector to express both MUC1 and IL-2 (a T-cell stimulus). The results were promising.

In a phase IIb study (TIME) results (part of the randomized, double-blind, placebo-controlled, phase IIb/III study), showed that in the overall population, disease-free survival was 5.9 months for the TG4010 group and 5.1 months for placebo (HR, 0.74; 95% CI, 0.55–0.98; p = 0.019) [29].

Belagenpumatucel-L is an allogeneic tumor cell tumor vaccine derived from four cell lines of NSCLC with different histologies, also express an antisense transgene for transforming beta2 growth factor that reduces the regulation of its immunosuppressive transformation. The results of a phase II study suggested clinical efficacy in patients with advanced NSCLC, and a randomized phase III (STOP) study was initiated. Patients with stage III/IV NSCLC in whom the disease did not progress after platinum-based chemotherapy received either belagenpumatucel-L or placebo [30]. There was no significant difference in overall survival between the two arms (20.3 months vs. 17.8 months; HR, 0.94; p = 0.594); there was also no difference in progression-free survival (PFS) (4.3 months vs. 4.0 months; HR, 0.99; p = 0.947) [30].

The epidermal growth factor receptor (EGFR) is an important signaling pathway in NSCLC, and a vaccine has been developed against its related EGF ligand, using recombinant human EGF coupled to a carrier protein. In a randomized phase II trial, patients with stage IIIB/IV NSCLC were randomly assigned to receive the best supportive treatment or EGF vaccines after first-line chemotherapy [31]. In the global population, there was a trend toward improved overall survival and a significant survival advantage for patients who had a good antibody response to the EGF [31].

A subsequent phase III study included patients with stage IIIB/IV NSCLC who were randomly assigned to the first line of chemotherapy to make the vaccine or the best supportive care. In the safety population, overall survival was 10.83 months for the vaccine arm and 8.86 months for the control arm [32]. For patients who received at least four doses of vaccine, overall survival differed significantly between the vaccine group and the supportive treatment group (12.43 months vs. 9.43 months; HR, 0.77; p = 0.036). In addition, overall survival was longer (14.66 months) for patients vaccinated with high concentrations of EGF at the baseline [32].

3.2. CTLA-4 inhibitors

Ipilimumab in combination with chemotherapy has been studied in patients with advanced NSCLC who have not received the previous treatment. In this phase II triple-arm study, patients were randomly assigned to chemotherapy (carboplatin plus paclitaxel), sequential chemotherapy with ipilimumab, or chemotherapy with concomitant ipilimumab. The primary endpoint of the study was overall survival and progression-free survival, which was 4.6 months for the chemotherapy arm, 5.7 months for the sequential ipilimumab chemo arm

(HR, 0.72; p = 0.05), and 5.5 months for the ipilimumab arm concomitantly with chemotherapy (HR, 0.81; p = 0.13) [33]. Progression-free survival was better in NSCLC patients with squamous histology than patients with nonsquamous NSCLC. To confirm these results, a larger phase III trial (NCT02279732) was initiated for patients with squamous cell NSCLC.

Conclusion of the study was that phased ipilimumab plus paclitaxel and carboplatin improved irPFS and PFS, which supports additional investigation of ipilimumab in NSCLC [33].

In the Govindan study ipilimumab added to chemotherapy (carboplatin plus paclitaxel) did not improve the survival of patients with advanced NSCLC [34].

3.3. PD-1 and PD-L1 inhibitors

PD-1 inhibitors include agents such as nivolumab and pembrolizumab. Nivolumab is a fully human immunoglobulin G4 (IgG4) monoclonal antibody that disrupts PD-1-mediated signaling, thus releasing T cells from their inhibitory interaction with PD-L1 and PD-L2. Pembrolizumab is a monoclonal antibody, the humanized IgG4/kappa isotype, which also blocks the binding of PD-L1 and PD-L2 to PD-1 on T cells, resulting in activation of tumor-specific cytotoxic T cells. Cytotoxicity is complement-dependent (CDC) (Alsaab) [35].

Action may be important because cytotoxicity can cause an exhaustion of activated T cells and infiltrating lymphocytes into tumors. PD-1 is expressed on effector T cells and other immune cells [36].

Checkmate 026 did not show a benefit in PFS for nivolumab versus chemotherapy. The authors reveal the fact that nivolumab monotherapy did not result in longer progression-free survival than platinum-based chemotherapy as first-line treatment for stage IV or recurrent NSCLC in a broad population of patients with a PD-L1 expression level of 5% or more. Overall survival with single-agent nivolumab was similar to overall survival with platinum-doublet chemotherapy. Nivolumab had a favorable safety profile as compared with chemotherapy, and no new safety signals were observed [37].

The new data from the phase 1b CA209-003 study were presented at the American Association for Cancer Research annual meeting: "The longest follow-up to date on patients treated with nivolumab for advanced non-small cell lung cancer (NSCLC) shows a 16% 5-year overall survival (OS) rate, according to new results presented here at the American Association for Cancer Research annual meeting." Suzanne Topalian, from Johns Hopkins University, and a coinvestigator (April 03, 2017): "the 5-year overall survival really quadrupled the survival that we would otherwise expect if these same patients had received chemotherapy" (April 03, 2017) (https://www.medscape.com/viewarticle/878148).

Nivolumab provides a long-term clinical benefit and a favorable tolerability profile compared to docetaxel in previously treated patients with advanced NSCLC [38]. FDA approved of nivolumab for second-line treatment of patients with advanced NSCLC.

In a single-arm phase II study (CheckMate 063) with nivolumab for patients with squamous cell NSCLC who were treated with third-line therapy and beyond, the partial response rate was 14.5, and 26% of patients had a stable disease [4]. Overall survival was 8.2 months, and 1-year survival was about 41%. Noteworthy, the study population was very refractory to treatment, with 65% of patients treated with at least three previous systemic therapy lines. In addition, 61% of patients had disease progression as the best response to the latest therapy [39].

In another phase II trial (CheckMate 153), 824 patients with advanced NSCLC were treated for 1 year with nivolumab. The partial response and stable disease rates were 12 and 44%, respectively. The answers were independent of the PD-L1 expression [40].

The second-line treatment with nivolumab was superior to docetaxel in two subsequent phase III randomized phases in advanced NSCLC patients receiving double-blind platinum chemotherapy.

In a study of 272 patients with squamous NSCLC (CheckMate 017), median overall survival and 1-year survival were better for nivolumab than for docetaxel. The risk for death was 0.59 with nivolumab ($p < 0.001$) [6].

In the study (CheckMate 057), which included patients with advanced nonsquamous NSCLC histology, nivolumab in line 2 was also associated with better overall survival and survival over 1 year, also better than docetaxel (HR, 0.73) [41]. In subset analysis of subset biomarker values, PD-L1 expression ≥1, ≥5, and ≥10% corresponded to an improvement in PFS with a HR of 0.70, 0.54, and 0.52, respectively, and in OS with a HR of 0.58, 0.43, and 0.40. In contrast, in tumors with a low PD <1, <5, and <10% PD-L1 expression, HR for PFS was 1.19, 1.31, and 1.24, respectively, and for OS was 0.87, 0.96, and 0.96 [41].

The safety and efficacy of single-agent nivolumab in first-line treatment of patients with advanced NSCLC have been reported in CheckMate 012 adverse events occurred in 71% of patients, the most common being fatigue (29%), rash (19%), nausea (14%), diarrhea (12%), pruritus (12%), and arthralgia (10%). The overall confirmed response was 23%, and progression-free survival and overall survival were 3.6 months and 19.4 months. The nonprogression-free survival rate of 24 weeks was 41%. The survival rate at 1 year was 73% [42].

Recently, in a phase III study, first-line nivolumab compared to a platinum-based chemotherapy for tumors with a PD-L1 expression of 5% or greater (CheckMate 026) showed progression-free survival greater for the chemotherapy arm, but overall survival was better for the nivolumab arm [43]. The objective response rate was lower for the nivolumab arm. In conclusion, nivolumab monotherapy did not result in longer progression-free survival than platinum-based chemotherapy as first-line treatment for stage IV or recurrent NSCLC. In this study the PD-L1 expression level was 5% or more [43].

3.4. Activity in SCLC

SCLC is most often an extended stage disease at the time of diagnosis. Although the first line of platinum-based chemotherapy has activity, the disease progresses inevitably, and response rates in the second-line treatment are low and are not sustainable. The activity and safety of nivolumab with or without ipilimumab in previously treated SCLCs were evaluated in CheckMate 032. The objective response rate was 10% with nivolumab 3 mg/kg alone, 23% with 1 mg/kg of nivolumab in combination with 3 mg/kg of ipilimumab, and 19% with 3 mg/kg of nivolumab in combination with 1 mg/kg of ipilimumab. PD-L1 expression was not associated with responses [44].

Patients with small-cell lung cancer (SCLC) and a high tumor mutation burden had an important increase in survival (near doubling in response rate and 1-year overall survival) with ipilimumab combined with nivolumab versus nivolumab alone.

The efficacy and safety of pembrolizumab at two different doses in previously untreated patients, advanced NSCLC, were reported in the Keynote-001 study. The objective response rate was 19.4%, and the median response time was 12.5 months. The progression-free survival was 3.7 months, and overall survival was 12.0 months [45]. The objective response rate was 18% in those treated previously and 24.8% of untreated patients. The objective response rate was 45.2%, and no time to progression was 6.3 months. The objective response rate was similar regardless of dose, schedule, and histology subtype. The response rate was higher among smokers than nonsmokers. Treatment-related adverse events of any grade occurred in 70.9% of patients, 9.5% having a grade 3 or higher adverse event [45].

Pembrolizumab was evaluated in a phase II/III study of patients previously treated with advanced NSCLC (Keynote-010). A total of 1034 patients were randomized to receive either 2 mg/kg dose or 10 mg/kg of pembrolizumab or 75 mg/m^2 of docetaxel every 3 weeks [46]. All patients had at least 1% tumor cells that were positive for PD-L1. Overall survival was improved with both doses of pembrolizumab compared to docetaxel. Among patients with at least 50% of the tumor cells expressing PD-L1, overall survival rates were 14.9 and 17.3 months with pembrolizumab at doses of 2 mg/kg and 10 mg/kg, respectively, compared to 8.2 months with docetaxel. Any degree of treatment-related adverse events occurred in 63% of pembrolizumab 2 mg/kg and 66% of patients receiving 10 mg/kg. The treatment-related toxicity was higher (81%) in the docetaxel arm.

Grade 3–5 treatment-related adverse events were less common in pembrolizumab-treated patients (2 mg/kg (13%), 10 mg/kg (16%)) versus docetaxel (35%) [46].

The Keynote-024 phase 3 clinical trial was the basis for pembrolizumab approval as a first-line treatment for patients with a diagnosis of metastatic NSCLC for whom PD-L1 expression is in 50% or more of tumor cells. Keynote-024 is a randomized, open-label phase 3 study evaluating pembrolizumab monotherapy at a fixed dose of 200 mg compared to the platinum-based chemotherapy standard for the treatment of patients with metastatic NSCLC with both squamous and unscrupulous histologies.

In phase III trial for first-line therapy of patients with advanced NSCLC (Keynote-024), with a PD-L1 tumor expression of 50% or greater, patients were randomly assigned to pembrolizumab- or platinum-based chemotherapy doublets, and progression-free survival was significantly better for pembrolizumab (HR, 0.50, 95% CI, 0.37–0.68; $p < 0.001$) median 10.4 months [47].

Overall survival was 0.60 (95% CI, 0.41–0.89; $p = 0.005$). The estimated percentage of patients in life at 12 months with pembrolizumab was 70%. In addition, the response rate was higher for pembrolizumab than for chemotherapy. Adverse events associated with pembrolizumab therapy were fewer than chemotherapy. The results are innovative because this is the first to demonstrate the superiority of anti-PD-1 therapy to platinum [47].

3.5. Activity in SCLC

Preliminary data from a multicohort phase Ib study on pembrolizumab with previously treated PD-L1-positive subjects include a 25% objective response rate and a 31% disease control rate [48].

3.6. PD-L1 inhibitors

3.6.1. *Avelumab and atezolizumab*

PD-L1 inhibitors also inhibit PD-1/PD-L1 interactions. PD-L1 inhibitors include atezolizumab, durvalumab, and avelumab. Atezolizumab and durvalumab are human IgG1 anti-PD-L1 antibodies with mutations in their Fc domains to eliminate both antibody-dependent cell-mediated cytotoxicity (ADCC) activity and complement-dependent cytotoxicity (CDC) activity. Avelumab is a fully human IgG1 anti-PD-L1 monoclonal antibody and, unlike another PD-1/PD-L1 inhibitor, has been shown to retain ADCC and CDC activity in preclinical studies [49].

In a single-arm phase II study (IMpower 110 study), the objective response rate for atezolizumab was 16%, regardless of PD-L1 expression in immune cells, and 28% in patients with 5% or more high expression PD-L1 [50]. Atezolizumab (MDPL3280A) clearly is an added value in the treatment of advanced-stage pretreated NSCLC. Its interest in contrast with other immune checkpoint inhibitors relies on its efficacy, even in low or no PD-L1 expression subgroups. Considering that the efficacy of anti-PD-1 such as pembrolizumab or nivolumab is overall higher in PD-L1-positive patients, atezolizumab might be preferable in PD-L1-negative patients. It will be necessary to consider other variant methods of PD-L1 testing used for each therapy to further explore this hypothesis [51].

In a randomized phase II (Poplar) study in patients receiving platinum-based chemotherapy, atezolizumab was associated with a higher overall survival (HR, 0.73; CI 95%, 0.53–0.99; $p = 0.04$) [52]. In another phase II trial (BIRCH), advanced NSCLC patients who were selected for PD-L1 expression received atezolizumab as first-line or as a subsequent therapy. Response rates ranged from 17 to 27% [53], and median overall survival was 14 months for patients receiving atezolizumab as the first line of therapy. Overall survival has not yet been achieved for patients receiving atezolizumab as a subsequent therapy [53]. In the OAK study, a phase III trial of previously treated NSCLC patients randomly assigned to atezolizumab or docetaxel, the overall survival was significantly better for atezolizumab (13.8 months vs. 9.6 months; HR, 0.73; 95% CI, 0.62–0.87; $p = 0.0003$) [54]. The OAK study led to the FDA approval of atezolizumab for second-line therapy of advanced NSCLC [54].

3.6.2. *Durvalumab*

In a phase I/II study with durvalumab in 2009 in the first-line treatment in NSCLC patients irrespective of PD-L1 status, the overall response rate was 27 and 29% for PD-L1-positive tumors (defined as ≥25% of tumor cells expressing PD-L1) and 11% in PD-L1-negative tumors [55]. In a phase II trial of patients with advanced NSCLC who received at least two previous systemic therapy lines, the activity was extremely encouraging. The objective response rate and survival rate at 1 year increased according to the PD-L1 expression: 7.5% (PD-L1 expression less than 25%), 16.4% (more than 25% expression), and 30.9% (greater than 90% expression). The corresponding 1-year survival rates were 34.5, 47.7, and 50.8% [56].

The study PACIFIC was presented to the ESMO Congress 2017 and was a randomized, double-blind, international, phase 3 study comparing durvalumab as consolidation therapy with placebo in patients with stage III, locally advanced, unresectable NSCLC that had not progressed after platinum-based chemoradiotherapy. Median progression-free survival as assessed by means of blinded independent central review was 16.8 months (95% confidence interval [CI], 13.0–18.1) with durvalumab versus 5.6 months (95% CI, 4.6–7.8) with placebo (stratified hazard ratio for disease progression or death, 0.52; 95% CI, 0.42–0.65; two-sided $p < 0.001$). Authors consider that this study will change the clinical practice [57].

3.7. Combinations of immunotherapy agents

CTLA-4 and PD-1/PD-L1 are combination. CTLA-4 inhibitors are also studied in conjunction with PD-1 and PD-L1 inhibitors. Results of preclinical studies indicate that this combination can work synergistically to produce improved antitumor activity [58].

Nivolumab was combined with ipilimumab for first-stage NSCLC in setting up in a phase I (CheckMate 12) study. The results included objective response rates ranging from 13 to 39%.

In NSCLC, the first-line nivolumab plus ipilimumab had a tolerable safety profile and showed an encouraging clinical activity characterized by a high response rate and durable response. In our study, the results of this study are the first suggestion of improved benefit compared with anti-PD-1 monotherapy in patients with NSCLC, supporting further evaluation of this combination in a phase 3 study [59].

Durvalumab was combined with the tremelimumab CTLA-4 inhibitor in a phase Ib study of patients with advanced NSCLC. Although many adverse events occurred during the study dose phase, the antitumor activity (23% objective response rate) was evident regardless of the PD-L1 status in the evaluable patients in the dose study—the expansion phase of the study [60].

In a phase III randomized study, the frontline durvalumab, either in combination with tremelimumab or as a single agent, did not improve progression-free survival (PFS) in patients with stage IV metastatic non-small cell lung cancer (NSCLC) compared with standard platinum-based chemotherapy [61].

4. Conclusions

Immunotherapy has become one of the most important therapeutic tools in advanced lung cancer. Existing studies have revealed a response rate of between 13 and 39%. It is also important that this therapy, unlike TKI-targeted therapy, also responds to smokers who make up most of the lung cancer patients.

Another important benefit from immunotherapy in advanced lung cancer is that squamous non-small cell lung cancer also responds to this therapy. Some promising results are and in treatment of small-cell lung cancer.

From existing studies, it is trembling that immunotherapy can improve survival compared to chemotherapy in a selected patient population, both in the first line and in the second line.

There is not yet a valid predictive marker that can be used to choose patients who will respond to immunotherapy. Currently, the only marker used is PD-1 expression that does not have a good validity. For the moment, there are not criteria to select patients for treatment with PD-1 or PD-L1 inhibitor because data to compare these two pathways is lacking. Better results were however obtained with a percent of PD-L1more then 50%. More study are needed to define the best combination of immunotherapy with chemotherapy or radiotherapy.

Vaccine therapy is promising but needs additional evaluation. Vaccine in combination with other therapeutic modalities especially checkpoint inhibitors is possible to have some benefits and must be studied.

Many guidelines are developed to treat side effects of immunotherapy. Despite a correct supportive therapy, some side effects are life-threatening. But generally, the quality of life of patients treated with immunotherapy is improved.

Author details

Alexandru C. Grigorescu

Address all correspondence to: alexgrigorescu2004@yahoo.com

Department of Medical Oncolog, Institute of Oncology Bucharest, Romania

References

[1] Hanahan D, Weinberg RA. Hallmarks of cancer: The next generation. Cell. 2011; **144**(5):646-674

[2] Pilotto S, Kinspergher S, Peretti U, et al. Immune checkpoint inhibitors for non-small-cell lung cancer: Does that represent a 'new frontier'? Anti-Cancer Agents in Medicinal Chemistry. 2015;**15**(3):307-313

[3] De Mello RA, Pousa I, Pereira D. Nivolumab for advanced squamous cell lung cancer: What are the next steps? The Lancet Oncology. 2015;**16**(3):234-235

[4] Rizvi NA, Mazières J, Planchard D, et al. Activity and safety of nivolumab, an anti-PD-1 immune checkpoint inhibitor, for patients with advanced, refractory squamous non-small-cell lung cancer (CheckMate 063): A phase 2, single-arm trial. The Lancet Oncology. 2015;**16**(3):257-265

[5] Brahmer JR, Drake CG, Wollner I, et al. Phase I study of single-agent anti-programmed death-1 (MDX-1106) in refractory solid tumors: Safety, clinical activity, pharmacodynamics, and immunologic correlates. Journal of Clinical Oncology. 2010;**28**(19):3167-3175

[6] Brahmer J, Reckamp KL, Baas P, et al. Nivolumab versus docetaxel in advanced squamous-cell non-small-cell lung cancer. The New England Journal of Medicine. 2015; **373**(2):123-135

[7] Schiller JH, Harrington D, Belani CP, Langer C, Sandler A, Krook J, et al. Comparison of four chemotherapy regimens for advanced non-small-cell lung cancer. The New England Journal of Medicine. 2002;**346**(2):92-98

[8] Sandler A, Gray R, Perry MC, Brahmer J, Schiller JH, Dowlati A, Lilenbaum R, Johnson DHN. Paclitaxel-carboplatin alone or with bevacizumab for non-small-cell lung cancer. New England Journal of Medicine. 2006;**355**(24):2542-2550

[9] Mok TS, Wu YL, Thongprasert S, Yang CH, Chu DT, Saijo N, Sunpaweravong P, Han B, Margono B, Ichinose Y, Nishiwaki Y, Ohe Y, Yang JJ, Chewaskulyong B, Jiang H, Duffield EL, Watkins CL, Armour AA, Fukuoka M. Gefitinib or carboplatin-paclitaxel in pulmonary adenocarcinoma. The New England Journal of Medicine. 2009;**361**(10): 947-957. DOI: 10.1056/NEJMoa0810699. Epub 2009 Aug 19

[10] Shaw AT, Ou SH, Bang YJ, Camidge DR, Solomon BJ, Salgia R, Riely GJ, Varella-Garcia M, Shapiro GI, Costa DB, Doebele RC, Le LP, Zheng Z, Tan W, Stephenson P, Shreeve SM, Tye LM, Christensen JG, Wilner KD, Clark JW, Iafrate AJ. Crizotinib in ROS1-rearranged non-small-cell lung cancer. New England Journal of Medicine. 2014;**371**(21):1963-1971. DOI: 11.1056/NEJMoa1406766. Epub 2014 Sep 27

[11] Planchard D, Besse B, Groen HJM, Souquet PJ, Quoix E, Baik CS, Barlesi F, Kim TM, Mazieres J, Novello S, Rigas JR, Upalawanna A, D'Amelio AM Jr, Zhang P, Mookerjee B, Johnson BE. Dabrafenib plus trametinib in patients with previously treated BRAF(V600E)-mutant metastatic non-small cell lung cancer: An open-label, multicentre phase 2 trial. Lancet Oncology. 2016;**17**(7):984-993. DOI: 10.1016/S1470-2045(16)30146-2. Epub 2016 Jun 6

[12] Chan BA, Hughes BGM. Targeted therapy for non-small cell lung cancer: Current standards and the promise of the future. Translational Lung Cancer Research. 2015;**4**(1):36-54

[13] Mazières J, Barlesi F, Filleron T, Besse B, Monnet I, Beau-Faller M, Peters S, Dansin E, Früh M, Pless M, et al. Lung cancer patients with *HER2* mutations treated with chemotherapy and *HER2*-targeted drugs: Results from the European EUHER2 cohort. Annals of Oncology. 2016;**27**(2):281-286. DOI: 10.1093/annonc/mdv573

[14] Johnson LA, Heemskerk B, Powell DJ Jr, Cohen CJ, Morgan RA, Dudley ME, Robbins PF, Rosenberg SA. Gene transfer of tumor-reactive TCR confers both high avidity and tumor reactivity to nonreactive peripheral blood mononuclear cells and tumor-infiltrating lymphocytes. Journal of Immunology. 2006;**177**(9):6548-6559. DOI: 10.4049/jimmunol.177.9.6548

[15] Bonifant CL, Jackson HJ, Brentjens RJ, Curran KJ. Toxicity and management in CAR T-cell therapy. Molecular Therapy—Oncolytics. 2016;**3**:16011

[16] Testera WJ, Kim KM, Krigel RL, Bonomi PD, Glick JH, Asbury RF, Kirkwood JM, Blumg RH, Schillerb JH. A randomized Phase II study of interleukin-2 with and without beta-interferon for patients with advanced non-small cell lung cancer. Lung Cancer. 1999; **25**(3):199-206

[17] Cuppens K, Vansteenkiste J. Vaccination therapy for non-small-cell lung cancer. Current Opinion in Oncology. 2014;**26**(2):165-170

[18] de Gruijl TD, Van den Eertwegh AJM, Pinedo HM, Scheper RJ. Whole-cell cancer vaccination: From autologous to allogeneic tumor- and dendritic cell-based vaccines. Cancer Immunology, Immunotherapy. 2008;**57**:1569

[19] Rosenberg SA, Yang JC, Schwartzentruber DJ, Hwu P, Marincola FM, Topalian SL, Restifo NP, Dudley ME, Schwarz SL, Spiess PJ, Parkhurst MR, Kawakami Y, Seipp CA, Einhorn JH. Immunologic and therapeutic evaluation of a synthetic peptide vaccine for the treatment of patients with metastatic melanoma. Nature Medicine. 1998;**4**:321-327. DOI: 10.1038/nm0398-321

[20] Rice J, Ottensmeier CH, Stevenson FK. DNA vaccines: Precision tools for activating effective immunity against cancer. Nature Reviews Cancer. 2008;**8**:108-120. DOI: 10.1038/nrc2326

[21] Giaccone G, Debruyne C, Felip E, Chapman PB, Grant SC, Millward M. Phase III study of adjuvant vaccination with Bec2/Bacille Calmette-Guerin in responding patients with limited-disease small-cell lung cancer (European Organisation for Research and Treatment of Cancer 08971-08971B; Silva Study). Journal of Clinical Oncology. 2005;**23**(28):6854-6864. DOI: 10.1200/JCO.2005.17.186

[22] Al-Moundhri M, O'Brien M, Souberbielle BE. Immunotherapy in lung cancer. British Journal of Cancer. 1998;**78**:282-288. DOI: 10.1038/bjc.1998.486

[23] Vansteenkiste JF, Cho BC, Vanakesa T, De Pas T, Zielinski M, Kim MS, Jassem J, Yoshimura M, Dahabreh J, Nakayama H, Havel L, Kondo H, Mitsudomi T, Zarogoulidis K, Gladkov OA, Udud K, Tada H, Hoffman H, Bugge A, Taylor P, Gonzalez EE, Liao ML, He J, Pujol JL, Louahed J, Debois M, Brichard V, Debruyne C, Therasse P, Altorki N. Efficacy of the MAGE-A3 cancer immunotherapeutic as adjuvant therapy in patients with resected MAGE-A3-positive non-small-cell lung cancer (MAGRIT): A randomised, double-blind, placebo-controlled, phase 3 trial. The Lancet Oncology. 2016;**17**(6):822-835. DOI: 10.1016/S1470-2045(16)00099-1

[24] Tyagi P, Mirakhur B. MAGRIT: The largest-ever phase III lung Cancer trial aims to establish a novel tumor-specific approach to therapy. Clinical Lung Cancer. 2009;**10**(5):371-374

[25] Nokihara H, Katakami N, Hida T, Imamura F, Sakai H, Atagi S. Phase I/II study of tecemotide cancer immunotherapy for Japanese patients with unresectable stage III non-small cell lung cancer (NSCLC). Journal of Clinical Oncology. 2015;**33**(15_suppl):3036-3036

[26] Butts C, Socinski MA, Mitchell PL, Thatcher N, Havel L, Krzakowski M, Nawrocki S, Ciuleanu TE, Bosquée L, Trigo JM, Spira A, Tremblay L, Nyman J, Ramlau R, Wickart-Johansson G, Ellis P, Gladkov O, Pereira JR, Eberhardt WE, Helwig C, Schröder A, Shepherd FA, START trial team. Tecemotide (L-BLP25) versus placebo after chemoradiotherapy for stage III non-small-cell lung cancer (START): A randomised, double-blind, phase 3 trial. The Lancet. 2014;**15**(1):59-68

[27] Wu Y-L, Park K, Soo RA, Sun Y, Tyroller K, Wages D, Ely G, Yang JC-H, Mok T. INSPIRE: A phase III study of the BLP25 liposome vaccine (L-BLP25) in Asian patients with unresectable stage III non-small cell lung cancer. BMC Cancer. 2011;**11**:430. DOI: 10.1186/1471-2407-11-430

[28] Mitchell P, Thatcher N, Socinski MA, Wasilewska-Tesluk E, Horwood K, Szczesna A, Martín C, Ragulin Y, Zukin M, Helwig C, Falk M, Butts C, Shepherd FA. Tecemotide in unresectable stage III non-small-cell lung cancer in the phase III START study: Updated overall survival and biomarker analyses. Annals of Oncology. 2015;**26**(6):1134-1142. DOI: 10.1093/annonc/mdv104. Epub 2015 Feb 26

[29] Quoix E, Lena H, Losonczy G, Forget F, Chouaid C, Papai Z, Gervais R, Ottensmeier C, Szczesna A, Kazarnowicz A, Beck JT, Westeel V, Felip E, Debieuvre D, Madroszyk A, Adam J, Lacoste G, Tavernaro A, Bastien B, Halluard C, Palanché T, Limacher JM. TG4010 immunotherapy and first-line chemotherapy for advanced non-small-cell lung cancer (TIME): Results from the phase 2b part of a randomised, double-blind, placebo-controlled, phase 2b/3 trial. The Lancet Oncology. 2016;**17**(2):212-223. DOI: 10.1016/S1470-2045(15)00483-0. Epub 2015 Dec 23

[30] Giaccone G, Bazhenova LA, Nemunaitis J, Tan M, Juhász E, Ramlau R, van den Heuvel MM, Lal R, Kloecker GH, Eaton KD, Chu Q, Dunlop DJ, Jain M, Garon EB, Davis CS, Carrier E, Moses SC, Shawler DL, Fakhrai H. A phase III study of belagenpumatucel-L, an allogeneic tumour cell vaccine, as maintenance therapy for non-small cell lung cancer. European Journal of Cancer. 2015;**51**(16):2321-2329. DOI: 10.1016/j.ejca.2015.07.035. Epub 2015 Aug 14

[31] García B, Neninger E, de la Torre A, Leonard I, Martínez R, Viada C, González G, Mazorra Z, Lage A, Crombet T. Effective inhibition of the epidermal growth factor/epidermal growth factor receptor binding by anti-epidermal growth factor antibodies is related to better survival in advanced non-small-cell lung cancer patients treated with the epidermal growth factor cancer vaccine. Clinical Cancer Research. 2008;**14**(3):840-846. DOI: 10.1158/1078-0432.CCR-07-1050

[32] Rodriguez PC, Popa X, Martínez O, Mendoza S, Santiesteban E, Crespo T, Amador RM, Fleytas R, Acosta SC, Otero Y, Romero GN, de la Torre A, Cala M, Arzuaga L, Vello L, Reyes D, Futiel N, Sabates T, Catala M, Flores YI, Garcia B, Viada C, Lorenzo-Luaces P, Marrero MA, Alonso L, Parra J, Aguilera N, Pomares Y, Sierra P, Rodríguez G, Mazorra Z, Lage A, Crombet T, Neninger E, A phase III clinical trial of the epidermal growth factor vaccine CIMAvax-EGF as switch maintenance therapy in advanced non-small cell lung

cancer patients. Clinical Cancer Research. 2016;**22**(15):3782-3790. DOI: 10.1158/1078-0432.CCR-15-0855. Epub 2016 Feb 29

[33] Lynch TJ, Bondarenko I, Luft A, Serwatowski P, Barlesi F, Chacko R, Sebastian M, Neal J, Lu H, Cuillerot JM, Reck M. Ipilimumab in combination with paclitaxel and carboplatin as first-line treatment in stage IIIB/IV non-small-cell lung cancer: Results from a randomized, double-blind, multicenter phase II study. Journal of Clinical Oncology. 2012;**30**(17):2046-2054. DOI: 10.1200/JCO.2011.38.4032. Epub 2012 Apr 30

[34] Govindan R, Szczesna A, Ahn MJ, Schneider CP, Gonzalez Mella PF, Barlesi F, Han B, Ganea DE, Von Pawel J, Vladimirov V, Fadeeva N, Lee KH, Kurata T, Zhang L, Tamura T, Postmus PE, Jassem J, O'Byrne K, Kopit J, Li M, Tschaika M, Reck M. Phase III trial of Ipilimumab combined with paclitaxel and carboplatin in advanced squamous non-small-cell lung cancer. Journal of Clinical Oncology. 2017;**35**(30):3449-3457. DOI: 10.1200/JCO.2016.71.7629. Epub 2017 Aug 30

[35] Alsaab HO, Sau S, Alzhrani R, Tatiparti K, Bhise K, Kashaw SK, Iyer AK. PD-1 and PD-L1 checkpoint signaling inhibition for cancer immunotherapy: Mechanism, combinations, and clinical outcome. Frontiers in Pharmacology. 2017;**8**:561. DOI: 10.3389/fphar.2017.00561

[36] Chen J, Feng Y, Lu L, Wang H, Dai L, Li Y, Zhang P. Interferon-γ-induced PD-L1 surface expression on human oral squamous carcinoma via PKD2 signal pathway. Immunobiology. 2012;**217**(4):385-393. DOI: 10.1016/j.imbio.2011.10.016. Epub 2011 Nov 3

[37] Carbone DP, Reck M, Paz-Ares L, Creelan B, Horn L, Steins M, Felip E, van den Heuvel MM, Ciuleanu T-E, Badin F, Ready N, Jeroen T, Hiltermann N, Nair S, Juergens R, Peters S, Minenza E, Wrangle JM, Rodriguez-Abreu D, Borghaei H, Blumenschein GR Jr, Villaruz LC, Havel L, Krejci J, Jaime JC, Chang H, Geese WJ, Bhagavatheeswaran P, Chen AC, Socinski MA, for the CheckMate 026 Investigators. First-line Nivolumab in stage IV or recurrent non–small-cell lung Cancer. The New England Journal of Medicine. 2017;**376**:2415-2426. DOI: 10.1056/NEJMoa1613493

[38] Horn L, Spigel DR, Vokes EE, Holgado E, Ready N, Steins M, More S. Nivolumab versus docetaxel in previously treated patients with advanced non-small-cell lung cancer: Two-year outcomes from two randomized, open-label, phase III trials (CheckMate 017 and CheckMate 057). Journal of Clinical Oncology. 2017;**35**(35):3924-3933. DOI: 10.1200/JCO.2017.74.3062

[39] http://www.esmo.org/Conferences/Past-Conferences/ELCC-2016-Lung-Cancer/News-Press-Releases/Updates-from-CheckMate-063-and-017-Trials-Confirm-Nivolumab-Efficacy-in-Patients-with-Advanced-Platinum-Refractory-Squamous-NSCLC

[40] Spigel D, Schwartzberg L, Waterhouse D, Chandler J, Hussein M, Jotte R, Stepanski E, Mccleod M, Page R, Sen R, Mcdonald J, Bennett K, Korytowsky B, Aanur N, Reynolds C. P3.02c-026 is nivolumab safe and effective in elderly and PS2 patients with non-small cell lung cancer (NSCLC)? Results of checkmate 153. Journal of Thoracic Oncology. 2017;**12**(1, Supplement):S1287-S1288

[41] Borghaei H, Paz-Ares L, Horn L, Spigel DR, Steins M, Ready NE, Chow LQ, Vokes EE, Felip E, Holgado E, Barlesi F, Kohlhäufl M, Arrieta O, Burgio MA, Fayette J, Lena H, Poddubskaya E, Gerber DE, Gettinger SN, Rudin CM, Rizvi N, Crinò L, Blumenschein GR Jr, Antonia SJ, Dorange C, Harbison CT, Finckenstein FG, Brahmer JR. Nivolumab versus docetaxel in advanced nonsquamous non-small-cell lung cancer. The New England Journal of Medicine. 2015, 2015;**373**:1627-1639. DOI: 10.1056/NEJMoa1507643

[42] Antonia SJ, Gettinger SN, Goldman J, Brahmer J, Borghaei H, Chow LQ, Ready NE, Gerber DE, Juergens R, Shepherd F, Laurie SA, Young T, Geese WJ, Agrawal S, Li X, Hellmann MD. ORAL01.03: CheckMate 012: Safety and efficacy of first-line Nivolumab and Ipilimumab in advanced NSCLC. Journal of Thoracic Oncology;**11**(11, Supplement):S250-S251

[43] Carbone DP, Reck M, Paz-Ares L, Creelan B, Horn L, Steins M, Felip E, van den Heuvel MM, Ciuleanu T-E, Badin F, Ready N, Hiltermann TJN, Nair S, Juergens R, Peters S, Minenza E, Wrangle JM, Rodriguez-Abreu D, Borghaei H, Blumenschein GR Jr, Villaruz LC, Havel L, Krejci J, Jaime JC, Chang H, Geese WJ, Bhagavatheeswaran P, Chen AC, Socinski MA, for the CheckMate 026 Investigators. First-line Nivolumab in stage IV or recurrent non-small-cell lung Cancer. The New England Journal of Medicine. 2017;**376**:2415-2426. DOI: 10.1056/NEJMoa1613493

[44] Antonia SJ, Lopez-Martin JA, Bendell JC, Ott PA, Taylor MH, Eder JP. Checkmate 032: Nivolumab (N) alone or in combination with ipilimumab (I) for the treatment of recurrent small cell lung cancer (SCLC). Journal of Clinical Oncology. 2016;**34**(15_suppl):100-100

[45] Garon EB, Rizvi NA, Hui R, Leighl N, Balmanoukian AS, Eder JP, Patnaik A, Aggarwal C, Gubens M, Horn L, Carcereny E, Ahn M-J, Felip E, Lee J-S, Hellmann MD, Hamid O, Goldman JW, Soria J-C, Dolled-Filhart M, Rutledge RZ, Zhang J, Lunceford JK, Rangwala R, Lubiniecki GM, Charlotte Roach BS, Emancipator K, Gandhi L, for the KEYNOTE-001 Investigators. Pembrolizumab for the treatment of non–small-cell lung cancer. The New England Journal of Medicine. 2015, 10.1056/NEJMoa1501824;**372**:2018-2028

[46] Herbst RS, Herbst RS, Baas P, Kim D-W, Felip E, Pérez-Gracia JL, Han J-Y, Molina J, Kim J-H, Arvis CD, Ahn M-J, Majem M, Fidler MJ, Gilberto de Castro MG Jr, Lubiniecki GM, Shentu Y, Im E, Dolled-Filhart M, Garon EB. Pembrolizumab versus docetaxel for previously treated, PD-L1-positive, advanced non-small-cell lung cancer (KEYNOTE-010): A randomised controlled trial. The Lancet. 2016;**387**(10027):1540-1550

[47] Reck M, Rodríguez-Abreu D, Robinson AG, Hui R, Csőszi T, Fülöp A, Gottfried M, Peled N, Tafreshi A, Cuffe S, O'Brien M, Rao S, Hotta K, Leiby MA, Lubiniecki GM, Shentu Y, Rangwala R, Brahmer JR, for the KEYNOTE-024 Investigators. Pembrolizumab versus chemotherapy for PD-L1–positive non-small-cell lung cancer. The New England Journal of Medicine. 2016;**375**:1823-1833. DOI: 10.1056/NEJMoa1606774

[48] Ott PA, Elez E, Hiret S, Kim DW, Morosky A, Saraf S, Piperdi B, Mehnert JM. Pembrolizumab in patients with extensive-stage small-cell lung cancer: Results from the phase Ib KEYNOTE-028 study. Journal of Clinical Oncology. 2017;**35**(34):3823-3829. DOI: 10.1200/JCO.2017.72.5069. Epub 2017 Aug 16

[49] Boyerinas B, Jochems C, Fantini M, Heery CR, Gulley JL, Tsang KY, Schlom J. Antibody-dependent cellular cytotoxicity activity of a novel anti-PD-L1 antibody Avelumab (MSB0010718C) on human tumor cells. Cancer Immunology Research. 2015;**3**(10):1148-1157. DOI: 10.1158/2326-6066.CIR-15-0059. Epub 2015 May 26

[50] Herbst RS, de Marinis F, Jassem J, Spigel DR, Shankar G, Mocci S, Sandler A, Lopez-Chavez A, Li S, Giaccone G. Phase III clinical trials of atezolizumab compared with standard chemotherapy in PD-L1–selected chemotherapy-naïve patients with advanced NSCLC. Annals of Oncology. 2015;**26**(suppl_9):ix105-ix106

[51] Jean F, Tomasini P, Barlesi F. Atezolizumab: Feasible second-line therapy for patients with non-small cell lung cancer? A review of efficacy, safety and place in therapy. Therapeutic Advances in Medical Oncology. 2017;**9**(12):769-779

[52] Fehrenbacher L, Spira A, Ballinger M, Kowanetz M, Vansteenkiste J, Mazieres J, Park K, Smith D, Artal-Cortes A, Lewanski C, Braiteh F, Waterkamp D, He P, Zou W, Chen DS, Yi J, Sandler A, Rittmeyer A. Atezolizumab versus docetaxel for patients with previously treated non-small-cell lung cancer (POPLAR): A multicentre, open-label, phase 2 randomised controlled trial. The Lancet. 2016;**387**(10030):1837-1846

[53] Besse B, Johnson M, Janne PA, Garassino M, Eberhardt WEE, Besse B, Johnson M, Janne PA, Garassino M, Eberhardt WEE, Peters S, Toh CK, Kurata T, Kowanetz ZLM, Mocci S, Sandler A, Rizvi NA. Phase II, single-arm trial (BIRCH) of atezolizumab as first-line or subsequent therapy for locally advanced or metastatic PD-L1-selected non-small cell lung cancer (NSCLC). European Journal of Cancer. **51, 3**(Supplement 3):S717-S718

[54] Rittmeyer A, Barlesi F, Waterkamp D, Park K, Ciardiello F, von Pawel J, Gadgeel SM, Hida T, Kowalski DM, Dols MC, Cortinovis DL, Leach J, Polikoff J, Barrios C, Kabbinavar F, Frontera OA, De Marinis F, Turna H, Lee JS, Ballinger M, Kowanetz M, He P, Chen DS, Sandler A, Gandara DR, OAK Study Group. Atezolizumab versus docetaxel in patients with previously treated non-small-cell lung cancer (OAK): A phase 3, open-label, multicentre randomised controlled trial. Lancet. 2017;**389**(10066):255-265. DOI: 10.1016/S0140-6736(16)32517-X. Epub 2016 Dec 13

[55] Antonia S, Goldberg SB, Balmanoukian A, Chaft JE, Sanborn RE, Gupta A, Narwal R, Steele K, Gu Y, Karakunnel JJ, Rizvi NA. Safety and antitumour activity of durvalumab plus tremelimumab in non-small cell lung cancer: A multicentre, phase 1b study. The Lancet Oncology. 2016;**17**(3):299-308. DOI: 10.1016/S1470-2045(15)00544-6. Epub 2016 Feb 6

[56] Garassino M, Vansteenkiste J, Kim J-H, Léna H, Mazières J, Powderly J, Dennis P, Huang Y, Wadsworth C, Rizvi N. PL04a.03: Durvalumab in ≥3rd-line locally advanced or metastatic, EGFR/ALK wild-type NSCLC: Results from the phase 2 ATLANTIC study. Journal of Thoracic Oncology. 2017;**12**(1, Supplement):S10-S11

[57] Antonia SJ, Villegas A, Daniel D, Vicente D, Murakami S, Hui R, Yokoi T, Chiappori A, Lee KH, de Wit M, Cho BC, Bourhaba M, Quantin X, Tokito T, Mekhail T, Planchard D, Kim Y-C, Karapetis CS, Hiret S, Ostoros G, Kubota K, Gray JE, Paz-Ares L, de Castro Carpeño J, Wadsworth C, Melillo G, Jiang H, Huang Y, Dennis PA, Özgüroğlu M, for the

PACIFIC Investigators. Durvalumab after chemoradiotherapy in stage III non–small-cell lung cancer. The New England Journal of Medicine. 2017;**377**:1919-1929. DOI: 10.1056/NEJMoa1709937

[58] Curran MA, Montalvo W, Yagita H, Allison JP. PD-1 and CTLA-4 combination blockade expands infiltrating T cells and reduces regulatory T and myeloid cells within B16 melanoma tumors. Proceedings of the National Academy of Sciences of the United States of America. 2010;**107**(9):4275-4280

[59] Hellmann MD, Rizvi NA, Goldman JW, Gettinger SN, Borghaei H, Brahmer JR, Ready NE, Gerber DE, Chow LQ, Juergens RA, Shepherd FA, Laurie SA, Geese WJ, Agrawal S, Young TC, Li X, Antonia SJ. Nivolumab plus ipilimumab as first-line treatment for advanced non-small-cell lung cancer (CheckMate 012): Results of an open-label, phase 1, multicohort study. Lancet Oncology. 2017;**18**(1):31-41. DOI: 10.1016/S1470-2045(16)30624-6. Epub 2016 Dec 5

[60] Antonia S, Goldberg SB, Balmanoukian A, Chaft JE, Sanborn RE, Gupta A, Narwal R, Steele K, Gu Y, Karakunnel JJ, Rizvi NA. Safety and antitumour activity of durvalumab plus tremelimumab in non-small cell lung cancer: A multicentre, phase 1b study. The Lancet Oncology. 2016;**17**(3):299-308. DOI: 10.1016/S1470-2045(15)00544-6. Epub 2016 Feb 6

[61] http://www.onclive.com/web-exclusives/frontline-durvalumabtremelimumab-falls-short-in-phase-iii-nsclc-trial. 2017

4

Precise Diagnosis of Histological Type of Lung Carcinoma: The First Step in Personalized Therapy

Jelena Stojšić

Abstract

This chapter is a combination of personal experience of a pulmonary pathologist and available references in the diagnosis of non-small cell lung cancer (NSCLC) types. The morphological appearance of poorly differentiated lung carcinoma is not characteristic, so immunohistochemical staining is used for further differentiation. In order to save tumor tissue from paraffin blocks, the most rational way is to use only two antibodies, p40 for squamous cell carcinoma and TTF-1 for adenocarcinoma of the lung, and if necessary or if cancer growth is organoid, also one of two neuroendocrine markers (CD56 or Synaptophysin) can be used. If there is enough tumor tissue in the paraffin block to confirm the diagnosis, NapsinA, p63, Cytokeratin5/6 or Cytokeratin5 can be used. It should be kept in mind that no antibody is highly specific for one histological type of carcinoma or its origin and if the immunohistochemical finding is unspecific, it should be concluded that this is "not otherwise specified" (NOS) carcinoma. The rest of tissue must be preserved for current and future molecular testing and predictive immunohistochemical staining for the purpose of personalized NSCLC therapy.

Keywords: non-small cell lung cancer, diagnosis, immunohistochemical staining, paraffin block, TTF-1, p40, p63, CD56, Synaptophysin, NapsinA, Cytokeratin5/6, Cytokeratin5

1. Introduction

1.1. Epidemiology as basis for developing a strategy in the treatment of advanced non-small cell lung cancer

Lung carcinoma is the most commonly diagnosed malignancy worldwide. There is a different lung cancer incidence and mortality statistics throughout the world. In male population, lung cancer has the highest incidence rate, especially in developing countries, while in developed countries, it is immediately behind the prostate cancer. In female population, the incidence rate of lung cancer is rising, and it is higher than cervical carcinoma, but still lower than breast cancer. Lung carcinoma mortality rate is still alarmingly high, both in developing and developed countries [1–3].

This high mortality rate has led to research of drugs, which will, in the era of personalized therapy, prolong the survival of diseased patients for more than 5 years and also improve the quality of their lives during and after the treatment. Individual approach to the treatment of lung cancer is based on a precisely diagnosed pathohistological type of non-small cell lung cancer (NSCLC) [4, 5].

1.2. Types of biopsy specimens and pathohistological classification of lung cancer

Two most common histological types of NSCLC are adenocarcinoma and squamocellular carcinoma [6–8]. At the time of diagnosis, about 75% of lung cancer is in an inoperable, advanced stage and less than 15% of patients survive more than 5 years. As these patients cannot be surgically treated, diagnosis of NSCLC is based on bronchoscopic and fine-needle aspiration biopsy (*fnab*) or video-assisted thoracic surgery (*VATS*). That is why there is a huge responsibility on the shoulders of the pathologist to diagnose a histological type of NSCLC on a small biopsy specimen and preserve paraffin-embedded carcinoma tissue for further genetic and immunohistochemical testing in order to determine the effective personalized therapy. It aims at prolonging survival of patients and improving the quality of their lives during and after the therapy [9, 10].

In the final interpretation of the pathohistological findings, pathologists use the classification of the World Health Organization (WHO) from 2004 [6], that is, an improved version from 2015 [7].

According to WHO classification from 2004, histological subtypes of NSCLC are as follows:

- squamous cell carcinoma (**Figure 1**)
- adenocarcinoma (**Figure 2**)
- large-cell carcinoma
- adenosquamous carcinoma
- sarcomatoid carcinoma
- carcinoid tumors
- salivary gland tumors.

Each of these histological NSCLC subtypes has its own variants that are diagnosed based on their morphological picture and specific immunophenotype [6].

In the WHO classification of lung carcinoma from 2015, there have been some changes because adenocarcinoma took over the first place from squamous cell carcinoma, which previously had primacy. The greatest change in this classification compared to the previous one

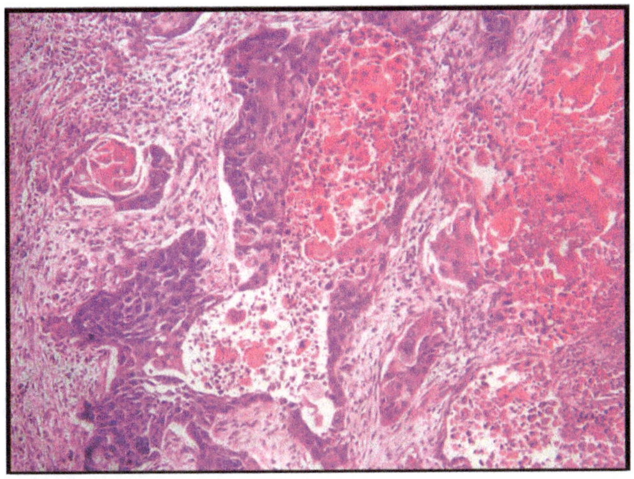

Figure 1. Keratinizing squamous cell carcinoma of the lung, H&E 100×.

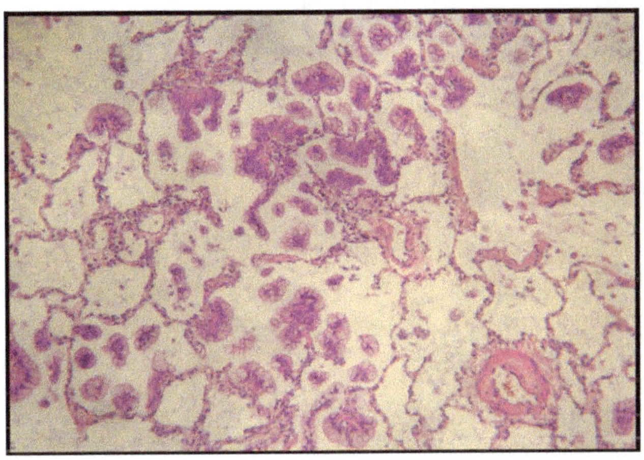

Figure 2. Adenocarcinoma of the lung with lepidic growth pattern, H&E 100×.

is a grouping of all carcinoma with neuroendocrine differentiation: carcinoid tumors, typical carcinomas (TC) and atypical carcinomas (AC), large-cell neuroendocrine carcinomas (LCC-NEC) and small-cell neuroendocrine carcinomas (SCLC) into one group of carcinomas due to specific biological behavior and special therapy, regardless of the different morphological picture. Remaining classification is identical to that of 2004 [7].

1.3. Processing of lung carcinoma tissue samples taken during bronchoscopy, FNA biopsy or VATS method

Bioptized lung samples obtained during bronchoscopy are fixed in 10% buffered formalin and brought to the laboratory. It is considered that sampling of tissue is representative if at least five biopsy samples have been delivered in diameter larger than 2 mm. Tissue samples taken during FNA biopsy should be delivered in 10% buffered formalin in the form of punctuate cylinder in order to use the whole tissue material for which is believed to contain lung cancer for morphological analysis and for immunohistochemical staining, while the rest of the tissue would be preserved for molecular testing (EGFR, optional KRAS), predictive immunohistochemical staining (ALK, ROS1 and PDL-1), as well as for fluorescent *in situ* hybridization (FISH) if this method is accepted by consensus [11].

Basic information about the patient which is to be submitted in the biopsy referral for the pathohistological laboratory is: name and surname, gender, age, place of residence, occupation and smoking status. It is necessary to deliver clear and concise clinical picture, for example, whether there is a suspect tumor shadow in the lung, mediastinal lymphadenopathy, superior vena cava syndrome (SVCS), and so on. Also, it is necessary to note that there is a previously diagnosed pulmonary or some other kind of malignancy in patient, which histological type of tumor is diagnosed on that occasion and how long before the current examination. This data help to set a new pathohistological diagnosis by applying a smaller number of immunohistochemical staining to prove metastatic malignancy or a new primary carcinoma of the lung. An endoscopic finding of the mode of tumor growth and its localization must also be given. In this way, we save tumor tissue for methods which would be used in personalized therapy for advanced lung cancer. If these data are not available, the pathologist should consider that this is a biopsy of primary lung cancer. Incomplete data because of sloppiness and lack of interest of the doctor who performed the biopsy can lead to vagueness and difficulty in diagnosing and thus, to disrespect of the patient and pathologist. Correct communication at the patient-clinician level and clinician-pathologist level is the basis for setting a precise diagnosis.

According to NSCLC morphology, many pathologists would not agree on a definitive diagnosis, but after immunohistochemical stainings, the same diagnosis should be made in a high percentage of them. Also, crush phenomenon that can appear on obtained tissue samples during bronchoscopy and inadequate fixation of them can put pathologist on misdiagnosis.

1.4. Routine treatment of biopsy samples when there is a suspicion of NSCLC

Biopsy samples are routinely fixed in a 10% buffered formalin and then dehydrated in xylol and rising alcohol concentrations, embedded into paraffin block, cut at thickness of 2 μm, using hematoxylin-eosin stained, covered with medium (Canada balsam) and analyzed under the microscope. There should be only one, two at most cross sections, on one object plate in order to determine whether there is cancer in the first two cross sections by routine hematoxylin-eosin (H&E) staining and also to assume a histological type of cancer, based on the morphological characteristics of malignant cells. The following sections are cut separately on two respective plates for immunohistochemical staining in order to determine the precise histological type of NSCLC. The pathologist concludes that there are no malignant cells on both cross sections and to report this in his definitive pathohistological finding. If NSCLC is found, two immunohistochemical stainings are applied, TTF-1 and p40, which determine the histological subtype of two most histological subtypes of NSCLC, adenocarcinoma and squamous cell carcinoma. In the end, it is desirable for the pathologist to indicate in his report whether there is enough and how much tissue material is left for the next molecular testings. The number of plates is 4: for EGFR molecular testing and ALK, ROS1 and PDL-1 immunohistochemical evaluation (**Figure 2**). In the era of personalized therapy, it is desirable to cut eight tissue sections at the same time from paraffin block: two for morphological analysis based on H&E stained preparations, two for basic immunohistochemical staining (TTF-1 and p40) and the last four for molecular and immunohistochemical predictive staining only in the case that NSCLC is found on H&E stained cross sections [12, 13].

2. Immunohistochemistry

2.1. Immunohistochemical staining method

The labeled streptavidin-biotin staining method uses a highly "refined" avidin-biotin complex (ABC) three-stage technique in which a biotinylated secondary antibody reacts with several streptavidin molecules conjugated by peroxidase or alkaline phosphatase [12].

2.2. Immunohistochemical staining procedure

Tissue samples for immunohistochemical staining are deparaffined according to the prescribed procedure of the manufacturer and then incubated with a specific serum at room temperature in a damp chamber for a prescribed duration. It is used the labeled streptavidin-biotin (LSAB) technique. The antigen-antibody complex is visualized by 3-amino-9-ethylcarbazole or diaminobenzidine hydrochloride solution. Mayer's hematoxylin is used as a counterstain. A "positive control" is used to evaluate the effectiveness of a method or reaction.

As already stated, "internal positive control" is used, since there are normal tissue structures on the preparation itself, in this case, lung, which express the administered antibodies. In the part of the chapter in which we analyze individual monoclonal antibodies, we will also indicate which lung structures are expressing them regularly [12, 14, 15].

3. Monoclonal antibodies in the diagnosis of non-small cell lung cancer

There is a question, which two monoclonal antibodies should be rationally applied in order to establish the exact diagnosis of the histological subtype of NSCLC. Currently, these are thyreoid-transcription-factor-1 (TTF-1) and p40. These two antibodies have a role in distinguishing two most common histological subtypes, adenocarcinoma and squamous cell carcinoma. TTF-1 (clone 8G7G3/1, DAKO Cytomation, Denmark) is a diagnostic marker for adenocarcinoma of the lung and p40 (BC28, Ventana, USA) for squamous cell carcinoma [16, 17].

However, in the past, other less specific antibodies were used in the differentiation of histological subtypes of NSCLC. They can also be used now as an additional confirmation about histological subtype of NSCLC and differentiation of primary from secondary lung cancer. The following antibodies are also useful for differentiation: NapsinA (clone IP64, Novocastra™ HD, Leica Biosystems, UK), p63 (clone 7JUL, Novocastra™ HD, Leica Biosystems, UK), Cytokeratin5/6 (cloneD5/16B4 DAKO Cytomation, Denmark) or Cytokeratin5 (clone EP1601Y, Cell Marque RUO, USA) and Cytokeratin7 (clone OV-TL 12/30 DAKO Cytomation, Denmark) [18, 19]. If the morphological picture of NSCLC has organoid appearance, there is a suspicion that this is large cell lung carcinoma with neuroendocrine differentiation (LCC-NEC). To confirm this suspicion, it is necessary to use at least one of two neuroendocrine markers, CD56 (clone NCAM-1 Ab-2, Thermo Scientific LabVision, USA) or Synaptophysin (clone 27G1 Novocastra ™ HD, Leica Biosystems, UK) [18, 20]. If TTF-1, p40 and optionally CD56 were not expressed, for the purpose of storing malignant tissue for molecular testing, it should be concluded that this is non-small-cell lung carcinoma, or "not otherwise specified" (NOS) carcinoma [7, 16]. It should be noted that no antibody is not highly specific for one organ or one histological type of cancer, that is, each antibody is specific for more than one histological types of cancer or more organs [21].

For precise pathohistological diagnosis of histological subtype of NSCLC, it is necessary to use two antibodies, TTF-1 and p40. If it is estimated that there is enough tumor tissue in a paraffin mold, it is possible to use additional antibodies to confirm the diagnosis and to preserve it for molecular testing [22, 23].

The advantages and disadvantages of each of these antibodies are discussed in the next section.

3.1. Thyroid transcription factor-1 (TTF-1)

Thyroid Transcription factor-1 (TTF-1) is a nucleic specific protein transcriptional factor expressed by thyroid gland and thyroid tumors as well as adenocarcinoma of the lung (**Figures 3** and **4**). This marker is expressed in the majority of lung adenocarcinoma (75%), but also in about 10% of squamous cell carcinoma. TTF-1 is significant in the differential diagnosis between primary and metastatic adenocarcinoma. At a time, when less antibodies were known, if TTF-1 with Cytokeratin7 was positive and Cytokeratin20 negative, diagnosis of adenocarcinoma of the lung was established [5, 24–28]. Diagnostic algorithms in the diagnosis of adenocarcinoma and differentiation of adenocarcinoma from squamous cell carcinoma are shown in papers of IASLC/ATS/ERS and Terry et al. [29, 30]. In various studies, TTF-1 was specific from 88 to 97% [6, 30, 31]. This marker is also expressed in lung cancer with neuroendocrine differentiation, in typical and atypical carcinoids, as well as in more than 90% of small cell lung carcinomas with neuroendocrine differentiation and in 50% of large cell lung carcinomas with neuroendocrine differentiation [30]. Literature reveals that TTF-1 can be expressed in breast and ovarian carcinoma [31, 32].

In one of our studies, we found that TTF-1 was expressed in 85.2% and in the other study, in 86% of lung adenocarcinomas [12, 33]. We also found that TTF-1 was also expressed in benign lung tumors [34, 35].

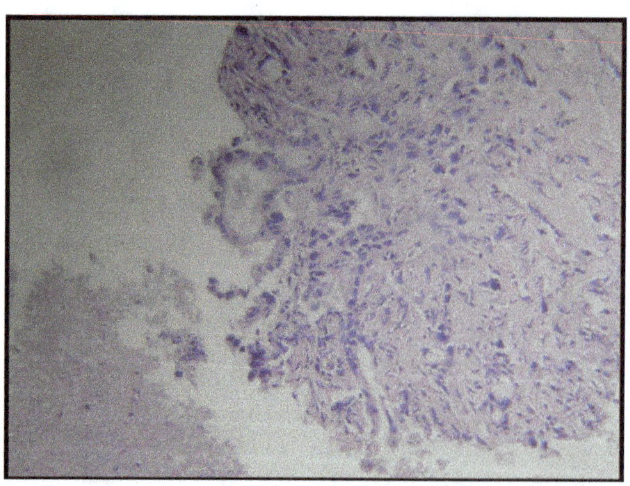

Figure 3. Adenocarcinoma of the lung with acinar growth, fnab, H&E 100×.

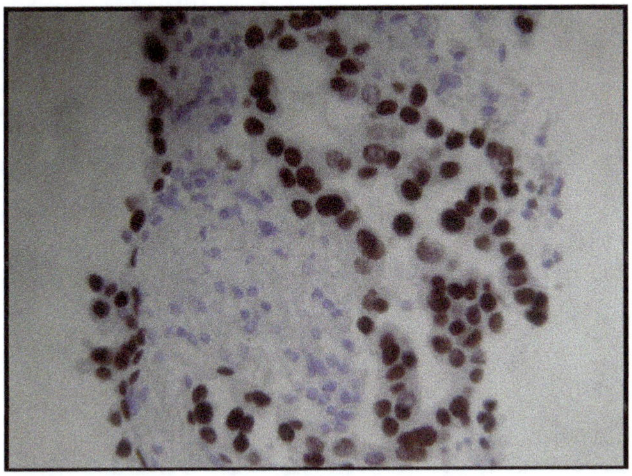

Figure 4. Adenocarcinoma of the lung, nucleic expression, TTF-1 200×.

3.2. p40

Role of p40 is to distinguish adenocarcinomas from squamous cell carcinomas in small samples (**Figure 5**) as well as on cytological smears. Squamous cell carcinoma is confirming with p40 antibody which is also known as DNp63. p40 is expressed in the nucleus of malignant cells of squamous cell carcinoma (**Figure 6**). This antibody is more specific for squamous cell lung carcinoma from p63. p40 is expressed in a smaller number of lung adenocarcinoma cells than p63. That is why it is recommended to use p40 instead of p63 for diagnostics of squamous cell carcinoma [36, 37]. If in malignant cells of carcinoma are not expressed TTF-1 and p40, diagnosis of non-small cell lung carcinoma -not otherwise specified (NSCLC-NOS) on a small biopsy sample will be established [16].

However, p40 is not a highly specific marker for only squamous cell lung carcinoma. It is also highly specific marker for urothelial carcinoma. This means that metastatic urothelial carcinoma in the lung is difficult to distinguish from primary squamous cell lung carcinoma both for morphological similarity these two carcinomas and similar immunophenotype [38]

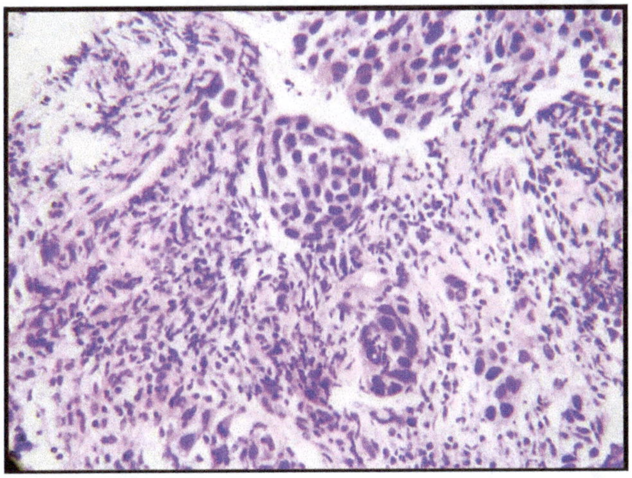

Figure 5. Moderately differentiated squamous cell carcinoma of the lung on bronchoscopic biopsy, H&E 20×.

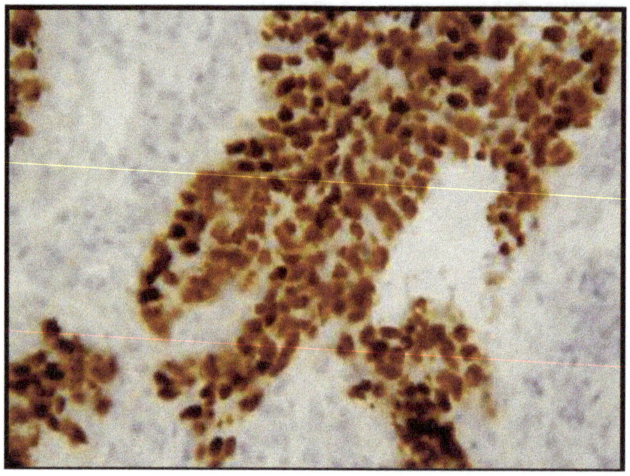

Figure 6. p40 expression in the squamous cell lung nuclei, 400×.

(**Figures** 7 and **8**). Therefore, for definitive differentiation lung squamous cell carcinomafrom urotothelial carcinoma is also required clinical data on current local status in previously operated patients with urothelial carcinomas (degree of cancer invasion at the time of surgery, presence of angioinvasion, state of resection margins, the presence of metastases in local and remote lymph nodes).

p40 is also expressed in squamous cell carcinoma of other localizations (head and neck, larings, trachea, cervix, skin). That is why it is not possible to differentiate primary squamous cell lung carcinoma from metastatic lung carcinoma of the same histological type by using p40. Differentiation of primary from secondary squamous cell carcinoma in the lung is possible only in clinicopathological correlation [39].

3.3. NapsinA

NapsinA is expressed in the cytoplasm of preserved lung parenchyma in the form of functional aspartic proteinase, homologous to the polypeptide Tao2 and included in maturation of the

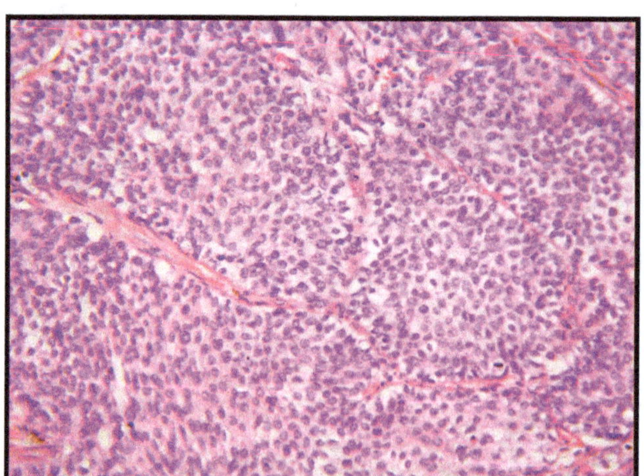

Figure 7. Urothelial carcinoma metastases in the lung, 400×.

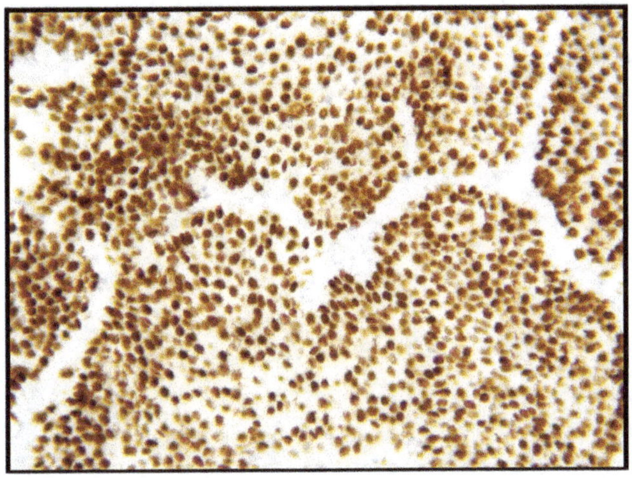

Figure 8. p40 expression in urothelial carcinoma metastases in the lung, 400×.

biologically active surfactant protein B. It also consists of 38-kDa protein, protein chain which is expressed in type II pneumocytes, alveolar macrophages and renal tubules, secretion channels of exocrine glands and pancreas. NapsinA is staining as coarse-grained intracytoplasmic marker [40].

There are papers that favor the use of NapsinA in regard to TTF-1 in differentiation of lung adenocarcinoma from other histological subtypes of NSCLC. Papers were done on a large number of lung adenocarcinomas wherein NapsinA showed higher specificity compared to the TTF-1. It is even recommended double immunohistochemical staining, so-called cocktail, which would beside NapsinA for cytoplasmic staining, contain and p40 for nuclear staining for squamous cell lung carcinoma [17, 36, 40, 41]. A simple diagnostic algorithm from 2010 recommends that NapsinA should be applied in order to diagnose adenocarcinoma, if TTF-1 is not exposed in NSCLC and if squamous cell carcinoma is not proved [30]. Our study on 50 adenocarcinomas showed a greater specificity of TTF-1 as compared to NapsinA [34]. If NapsinA is not expressed and the presence of mucin has not been proven, it should be concluded that it is about NSCLC-NOS. The definitive conclusion is that NapsinA is supplemental to TTF-1 which serves as the main marker for proving of lung adenocarcinoma (**Figure 9**).

3.4. p63

This antibody is known in the two isoforms, DNp63 and TAp63. It is expressed in the nucleus of the malignant cells. According to previous diagnostic algorithms, before occurrence of p40, p63 was the main marker in the differentiation of NSCLC on small biopsy samples beside TTF-1 [29]. Beside TTF-1, NapsinA and Cytokeratin5/6 are considered to be useful markers for the diagnosis of NSCLC on small biopsy samples [28]. The degree of p63 expression increases with the decrease in the degree of keratinization, that is, differentiation of squamous cell carcinoma [25] (**Figure 10** 200×; **Figure 11** 400×).

However, p63 as well as p40 is not a highly specific marker only for squamous cell carcinoma. It is also a marker for urothelial carcinoma. That is why it is hard to differentiate metastatic carcinoma of urothelial type from primary squamous cell lung carcinoma [39] (**Figure 12** 200×; **Figure 13** 400×).

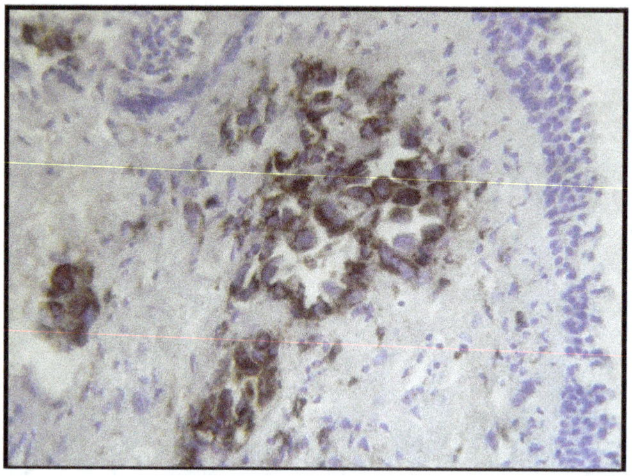

Figure 9. Bronchoscopic biopsy, infiltrate of the acinar adenocarcinoma of the lung in the mucosallayer of the bronchi, proven by using NapsinA 200×.

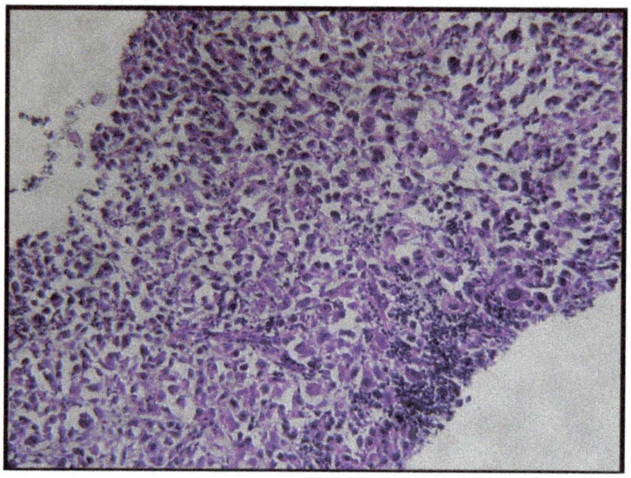

Figure 10. NSCLC deposit in the lymphatic tissue, where squamous cell carcinoma was immunohistochemically proven, H&E 200×.

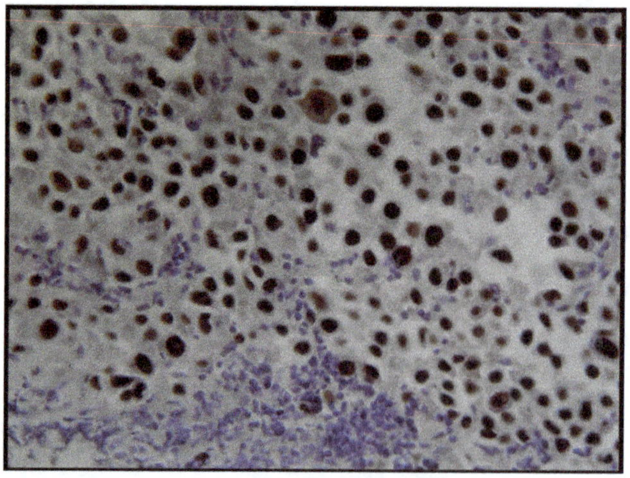

Figure 11. Strong nuclear expression of p63 in the cells of poorly differentiated squamous cell lung carcinoma, 400×.

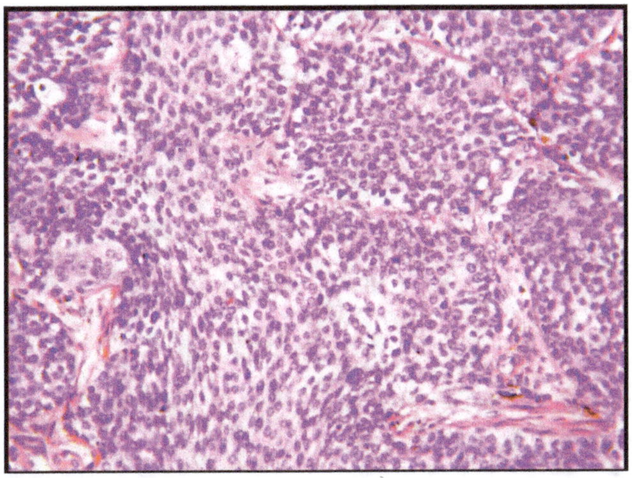

Figure 12. Urothelial carcinoma with lung metastases, H&E 400×.

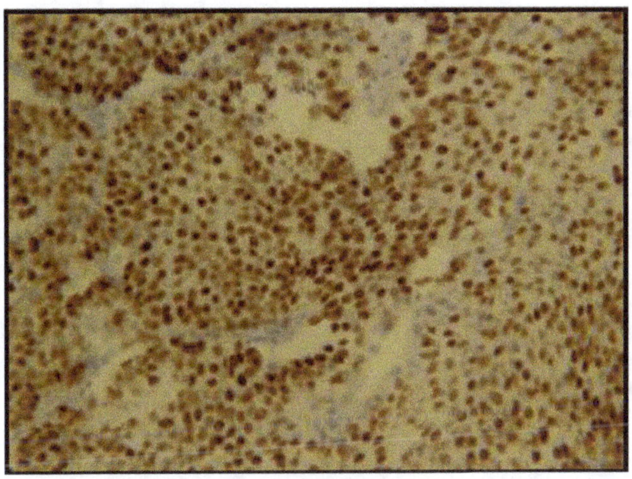

Figure 13. p63 expression in urothelial carcinoma with lung metastases, 400×.

3.5. Cytokeratin5/6 or Cytokeratin5

Cytokeratin 5/6 or Cytokeratin5 is a cytoplasmic marker. Its expression is present at squamous cell carcinoma (**Figure 14**). Because of that, this marker can be used as a confirmation for this histological type, together with p40 and p63, especially if there are no technical conditions for using one of these antibodies. Except in the regular epithelium of bronchial airways, Cytokeratin 5/6 or Cytokeratin5 is also expressed in regular and reactive mesothelioma cells, but also in the epithelium cells of the malignant pleural mesothelioma. Ovarian carcinomas, especially those of serous type, are cytoplasmically expressed antibody [21, 28, 42].

3.6. Neuroendocrine markers

According to WHO recommendations about the classification of lung carcinoma from 2004, in order to establish the diagnosis of large cell lung carcinoma with neuroendocrine differentiation, it is necessary for the cells to be large and round in an organoidal arrangement, with a

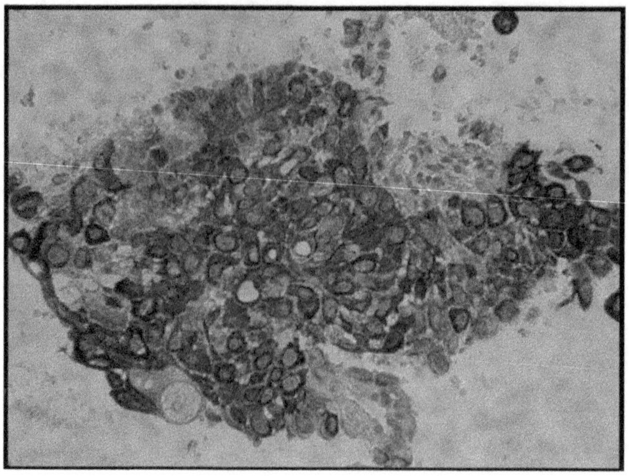

Figure 14. Expression of Cytokeratina5/6 in squamous cell carcinoma, fnab, 200×.

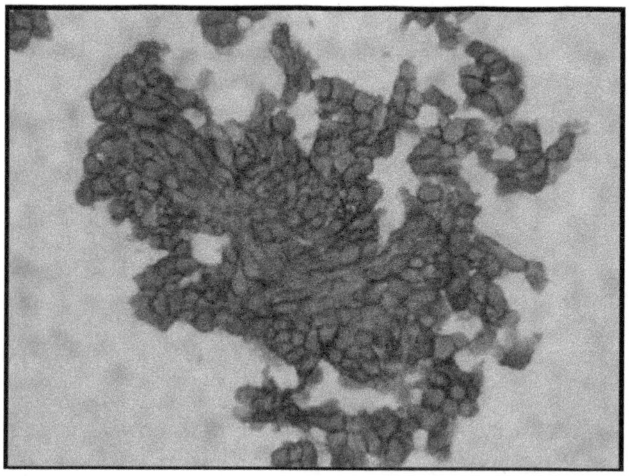

Figure 15. Membrane expression of CD56 into LCLC-NEC cells, 200×.

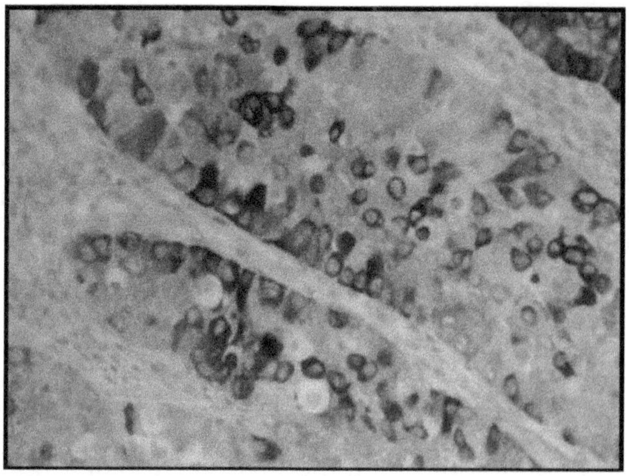

Figure 16. Cytoplasmic expression of Synaptophysin into NSCLC with partly adenoid growth pattern 200×.

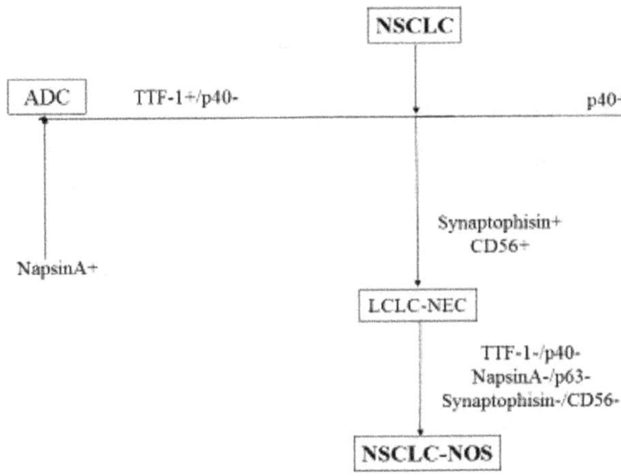

Figure 17. The proposed algorithm for the differential diagnosis of non-small cell lung carcinoma by using immunohistochemical stainings.

luminous and large nucleus and noticeable nucleolus and to express at least one neuroendocrine marker: CD56 (**Figure 15**), Synaptophysin (**Figure 16**) or ChromograninA [5, 6]. It means that if on a small biopsy sample, non-small cell lung cancer is showing organoid, trabecular or acinar growth pattern, and two neuroendocrine markers, preferably CD56 and Synaptohysin [43], should be used to confirm this type of cancer (LCLC-NEC) (**Figure 17**).

4. Discussion

Finally, someone may ask why it is necessary to know of which histological type of non-small cell lung cancer is about and to save enough malignant tissue in paraffin block for molecular testings at the same time.

The answer is that it is necessary to know how to apply certain tests for the application of personalized oncology therapy. If the evaluation of the tests showed that a positive response on therapy is expected, the same will be applied.

Globally, adenocarcinoma of the lungs is the most common histologic type of lung cancer. EGFR molecular testing is used to assess the response to tyrosine kinase inhibitors (TKI) therapy in patients with adenocarcinoma. Positive response to the TKI therapy is more commonly expected in young nonsmoking woman. It is also recommended that this testing is done in young nonsmoking woman with squamous cell lung cancer because it showed positive results. The result of this molecular testing depends on the sensitivity of the method and number of cells remaining after morphological and immunohistochemical diagnostics, more than 5% of malignant cells in relation to the total number of cells on the cross section. EGFR mutations are diagnosed in 10–15% of Caucasians patients with NSCLC [22, 44].

ALK testing (clone D5F3, Ventana, USA) is done in patients with adenocarcinoma of the lungs in which EGFR mutations have not been detected. There is no consensus on whether this test should be performed only in lung adenocarcinoma or it can be performed in all pathohistological subtypes of NSCLC. Namely, there are several diagnostic algorithms which include all histological types of NSCLC or only adenocarcinoma of the lungs. There are data indicating that this genetic rearrangement was detected only in about 4% of patients with adenocarcinoma of the lungs or in about 2% of patients with NSCLC. In order for this test to be valid, it is necessary that on the tissue cross section at least 50 malignant cells have to be present after primary diagnostics and EGFR testing. Then immunochemical testing would be valid and where there is this type of consensus, to confirm the presence of rearrangements, FISH test should also be done [13, 45, 46].

It is necessary to know the fact that about 70% of LCC-NEC is ALK positive, but that its expression is not in correlation with personalized ALK inhibitors. If NSCLC have an organoid morphological picture, it is necessary to apply CD56 and Synaptophysin on small biopsy samples in order to exclude LCC-NEC [13, 45, 46].

ROS1 testing (clone D4D6, Ventana, USA) is also done in adenocarcinoma of the lungs where EGFR and ALK tests did not show positive results. This fusion is present only in 1–2%, predominantly younger patients, nonsmokers, with adenocarcinoma of the lungs. The presence of fusion is immunohistochemically determined, and it is necessarily confirmed by the FISH method, so it is necessary to preserve tissue for these methods after diagnosis of adenocarcinoma [13, 46].

If any of these tests fail to give results, for the application of immunotherapy, it is applied PDL-1 testing (clone 22C3, DAKO Cytomation, Denmark), mainly in squamous cell lung cancer, but also in adenocarcinomas in which previous test did not show positive results. For this immunohistochemical testing, it is recommended that tissue cross section contains at least 100 malignant cells [47, 48].

The future of personalized lung cancer treatment is next-generation sequencing (NGS), polymerase chain reaction (PCR) method, in which, from the remaining of paraffin block in which NSCLS was diagnosed, at the same time is detecting all druggable mutations [23].

Liquid biopsy is a method that detects DNA tumor cells in whole or in its parts. This method is useful in early detection of lung cancer, but it is false negative if circulating malignant cells do not possess a mutation [49].

5. Conclusions

Precise diagnosis of NSCLC histological type is based only on morphological characteristics of the tumor, cell appearance and their growth pattern on H&E stained preparation is rarely possible. Based on morphological findings, keratinizing squamous cell carcinoma can be diagnosed with great certainty, without immunohistochemistry. The main disadvantage of all used antibodies is not highly specificity only for one histological type of cancer or originates from more than one organ. In order to preserve tumor tissue for molecular testing, one must use only one, the most specific antibody for one histological type of carcinoma. For adenocarcinoma of the lung, highly specific is TTF-1, and for squamous cell carcinoma, it is p40. Other additional antibodies can be applied only if there is a greater amount of bioptic tumor material (*fnab* biopsy or *VATS* biopsy). NapsinA is an additional antibody, which can be applied in proving adenocarcinoma of the lung and p63 for squamous cell carcinoma. When LCLC-NEC is suspected, it is recommended to use only one neuroendocrine marker, and the most reliable is CD56. For saving, in order to apply all the appropriate antibodies and to preserve tissue for molecular testing, it is necessary to cut only one cross section on one plate.

Author details

Jelena Stojšić

Address all correspondence to: dr.jelenastoj@sezampro.rs

Department of Thoracopulmonary Pathology, Service of Pathology, Clinical Centre of Serbia, Belgrade, Serbia

References

[1] Ferlay J, Shin HR, Bray F, Forman D, Mathers C, Parkin DM. Estimates of worldwide burden of cancer in 2008: GLOBOCAN 2008. International Journal of Cancer. 2010; **127**(12):2893-2917. DOI: 10.1002/ijc.25516

[2] Jemal A, Bray F, Center MM, Ferlay J, Ward E, Forman D. Global cancer statistics. CA: A Cancer Journal for Clinicians. 2011;**61**(2):69-90. DOI: 10.3322/caac.20107

[3] Ferlay J, Soerjomataram I, Dikshit R, Eser S, Mathers C, Rebelo M, Parkin DM, Forman D, Bray F. Cancer incidence and mortality worldwide: Sources, methods and major patterns in GLOBOCAN 2012. International Journal of Cancer. 2015;**136**(5):E359-E386. DOI: 10.1002/ijc.29210

[4] Mollberg N, Surati M, Demchuk C, Fathi R, Salama AK, Husain AN, Hensing T, Salgia R. Mind-mapping for lung cancer: towards a personalized therapeutics approach. Advances in Therapy. 2011;**28**(3):173-194. DOI: 10.1007/s12325-010-0103-9

[5] Kerr KM. Personalized medicine for lung cancer: New challenges for pathology. Histopathology. 2012;**60**(4):531-546. DOI: 10.1111/j.1365-2559.2011.03854.x

[6] Travis WD, Brambilla E, Müller-Hermelink HK, Harris CC, editors. World Health Organisation Classification of Tumours. Pathology and Genetics of Tumours of the Lung, Pleura, Thymus and Heart. Lyon: IARC; 2004. ISBN: 9283224183

[7] Travis WD, Brambilla E, Burke AP, Marx A, Nicholson AG, editors. World Health Organisation Classification of Tumours of the Lung, Pleura, Thymus and Heart. Lyon: IARC; 2015. ISBN: 9789283224365

[8] Janssen-Heijnen M, Coebergh JW. The chainging epidemiology in Europe. Lung Cancer. 2003;**41**(3):245-258. DOI: 10.1016/S0169-5002(03)00230-7

[9] Cagle PT, Allen TC, Dacic S, Beasley MB, Borczuk AC, Chirieac LR, Laucirica R, Ro JY, Kerr KM. Revolution in lung cancer: New challenges for the surgical pathologist. Archives of Pathology & Laboratory Medicine. 2011;**135**(1):110-116. DOI: 10.1043/2010-0567-RA.1

[10] Hirsch FR, Franklin WA, Gazdar AF, Bunn PA Jr. Early detection of lung cancer: Clinical perspectives of recent advances in biology and radiology. Clinical Cancer Research. 2001; **7**(1):5-22. PMID: 11205917

[11] Cheng L, Alexander RE, Maclennan GT, Cummings OW, Montironi R, Lopez-Beltran A, Cramer HM, Davidson DD, Zhang S. Molecular pathology of lung cancer: Key to personalized medicine. Modern Pathology. 2012;**25**(3):347-369. DOI: 10.1038/modpathol. 2011.215

[12] Dabbs DJ. Diagnostic Immunohistochemistry Theranostic and Genomic Applications. 3rd ed. Philadelphia: Saunders Elsevier; 2010. ISBN: 9781416057666

[13] Sound TM, Hirsch ER, Yatabe Y, editors IASLC Atlas of ALK and ROS1 testing in lung cancer. North Fort Myers, FL; Editorial Rx Press; 2016

[14] Shi SR, Key ME, Kalra KL. Antigen retrieval in formalin-fixed, paraffin-embedded tissues: An enhancement method for immunohistochemical staining based on microwave oven heating of tissue sections. The Journal of Histochemistry and Cytochemistry. 1991;**3449**(6):741-748. DOI: 10.1177/39.6.1709656

[15] Stojsic J, Jovanic I, Markovic J, Gajic M. Contribution of immunohistochemistry in the differential diagnosis of non-small cell lung carcinomas on small biopsy samples. Journal of BUON. 2013;**18**(1):176-187. PMID: 23613404

[16] Walia R, Jain D, Madan K, Sharma MC, Mathur SR, Mohan A, Iyer VK, Kumar L. p40 & thyroid transcription factor-1 immunohistochemistry: A useful panel to characterize non-small cell lung carcinoma-not otherwise specified (NSCLC-NOS) category. The Indian Journal of Medical Research. 2017;**146**(1):42-48. DOI: 10.4103/ijmr.IJMR_1221_15

[17] Ikeda S, Naruse K, Nagata C, Kuramochi M, Onuki T, Inagaki M, Suzuki K. Immunostaining for thyroid transcription factor 1, Napsin A, p40, and cytokeratin 5 aids in differential diagnosis of non-small cell lung carcinoma. Oncology Letters. 2015;**9**(5):2099-2104. DOI: 10.3892/ol.2015.3045

[18] Micke P, Mattsson JS, Djureinovic D, Nodin B, Jirström K, Tran L, Jönsson P, Planck M, Botling J, Brunnström H. The impact of the fourth edition of the WHO classification of lung tumours on histological classification of resected pulmonary NSCCs. Journal of Thoracic Oncology. 2016;**11**(6):862-872. DOI: 10.1016/j.jtho.2016.01.020

[19] Travis WD, Brambilla E, Noguchi M, Nicholson AG, Geisinger KR, Yatabe Y, Beer DG, Powell CA, Riely GJ, Van Schil PE, Garg K, Austin JH, Asamura H, Rusch VW, Hirsch FR, Scagliotti G, Mitsudomi T, Huber RM, Ishikawa Y, Jett J, Sanchez-Cespedes M, Sculier JP, Takahashi T, Tsuboi M, Vansteenkiste J, Wistuba I, Yang PC, Aberle D, Brambilla C, Flieder D, Franklin W, Gazdar A, Gould M, Hasleton P, Henderson D, Johnson B, Johnson D, Kerr K, Kuriyama K, Lee JS, Miller VA, Petersen I, Roggli V, Rosell R,

Saijo N, Thunnissen E, Tsao M, Yankelewitz D. International association for the study of lung cancer/American Thoracic Society/European Respiratory Society: International multidisciplinary classification of lung adenocarcinoma. Journal of Thoracic Oncology. 2011;**6**(2):244-285. DOI: 10.1513/pats.201107-042ST

[20] Fasano M, Della Corte CM, Papaccio F, Ciardiello F, Morgillo F. Pulmonary large-cell neuroendocrine carcinoma: From epidemiology to therapy. Journal of Thoracic Oncology. 2015;**10**(8):1133-1141. DOI: 10.1097/JTO.0000000000000589

[21] Stojsic J, Spasic Z, Velinovic M, Adzic T, Maric D, Todorovic V, Drndarevic N. Diagnostic procedures in pleural malignant mesothelioma: Our experience. Journal of BUON. 2004;**9**:423-426 17415849

[22] Penzel R, Sers C, Chen Y, Lehmann-Mühlenhoff U, Merkelbach-Bruse S, Jung A, Kirchner T, Büttner R, Kreipe HH, Petersen I, Dietel M, Schirmacher P. EGFR mutation detection in NSCLC — Assessment of diagnostic application and recommendations of the German Panel for Mutation Testing in NSCLC. Virchows Archiv. 2011;**458**:95-98. DOI: 10.1007/s00428-010-1000-y

[23] Padmanabhan V, Steinmetz HB, Rizzo EJ, Erskine AJ, Fairbank TL, de Abreu FB, Tsongalis GJ, Tafe LJ. Improving adequacy of small biopsy and fine-needle aspiration specimens for molecular testing by next-generation sequencing in patients with lung cancer: A quality improvement study at Dartmouth-Hitchcock Medical Center. Archives of Pathology & Laboratory Medicine. 2017;**141**(3):402-409. DOI: 10.5858/arpa.2016-0096-OA

[24] Stojsić J, Adzić T, Marić D, Subotić D, Milovanović I, Milenković B, Radojicić J, Marković J, Dimitrijević D. Histological types and age distribution of lung cancer operated patients over a 20-year period: A pathohistological based study. Srpski Arhiv za Celokupno Lekarstvo. 2011;**139**(9-10):619-624. DOI: 10.1097/JTO.0b013e3181d40fac

[25] Loo PS, Thomas SC, Nicolson MC, Fyfe MN, Kerr KM. Subtyping of undifferentiated non-small cell carcinomas in bronchial biopsy specimens. Journal of Thoracic Oncology. 2010;**5**(4):442-447

[26] Conde E, Angulo B, Redondo P, Toldos O, Garsia-Garsia E, Suarez A, Rubio-Viqueira B, Marron C, et al. The use of p63 immunohistochemistry for the identification of squamous cell carcinoma of the lung. PLoS One. 2010;**5**(8):e12209. DOI: 10.1371/journal.pone.0012209

[27] Tan D, Zander DS. Immunohistochemistry for assessment of pulmonary and pleural neoplasms: A review and update. International Journal of Clinical and Experimental Pathology. 2008;**1**:19-31. PMCID: PMC2480532

[28] Mukhopadhyay S, Katzenstein A-LA. Subclassification of non-small cell lung carcinomas lacking morphologic differentiation on biopsy specimens: Utility of an immunohistochemical panel containing TTF-1, Napsin A, p63, and CK5/6. The American Journal of Surgical Pathology. 2011;**35**:15-25. DOI: 10.1097/PAS.0b013e3182036d05

[29] Terry J, Leung S, Laskin J, Leslie KO, Gown AM, Ionescu DN. Optimal immunohistochemical markers for distinguishing lung adenocarcinomas from squamous cell carcinomas in small tumor samples. The American Journal of Surgical Pathology. 2010; **34**:1805-1811. DOI: 10.1097/PAS.0b013e3181f7dae3

[30] Sterlacci W, Fiegl M, Hilbe W, Auberger J, Mikuz G, Tzankov A. Clinical relevance of neuroendocrine differentiation in non-small cell lung cancer assessed by immunohistochemistry: A retrospective study on 405 surgically resected cases. Virchows Archiv. 2009;**455**(2):125-132. DOI: 10.1007/s00428-009-0812-0

[31] Klingen TA, Chen Y, Gundersen MD, Aas H, Westre B, Sauer T. Thyroid transcription factor-1 positive primary breast cancer: A case report with review of the literature. Diagnostic Pathology. 2010;**5**:37-41. DOI: 10.1186/1746-1596-5-37

[32] Graham AD, Williams AR, Salter DM. TTF-1 expression in primary ovarian epithelial neoplasia. Histopathology. 2006;**48**(6):764-765. DOI: 10.1111/j.1365-2559.2006.02365.x

[33] Stojsic J. Immunohistochemical approach to the diagnosis of adenocarcinoma of the lung. Journal of Cytology and Histology. 2014;**5**(3):229. DOI: 10.4172/2157-7099.1000229

[34] Stojsić J, Milenković B, Radojicić J, Percinkovski M. Alveolar adenoma—A rare lung tumour. Srpski Arhiv Za Celokupno Lekarstvo. 2007;**135**(7-8):461-464. Serbian. PMID: 17929540

[35] Stojsić J, Milenković V, Radojicić J, Percinkovski M. Pulmonary sclerosing haemangioma—Case report. Srpski Arhiv Za Celokupno Lekarstvo. 2007;**135**(9-10):569-571. Serbian. PMID: 18088044

[36] Nishino M, Mai P, Hoang MP, Della Pelle P, Morales-Oyarvide V, Huynh TG, Mark EJ, Mino-Kenudson M. Napsin A/p40 antibody cocktail for subtyping non-small cell lung carcinoma on cytology and small biopsy specimens. Cancer Cytopathology. 2016; **124**:472-478. DOI: 10.1002/cncy.21707

[37] Bishop JA, Teruya-Feldstein J, Westra WH, Pelosi G, Travis WD, Rekhtman N. p40 (ΔNp63) is superior to p63 for the diagnosis of pulmonary squamous cell carcinoma. Modern Pathology. 2012;**25**(3):405-415. DOI: 10.1038/modpathol.2011.173

[38] Leivo MZ, Elson PJ, Tacha DE, Delahunt B, Hansel DE. A combination of p40, GATA-3 and uroplakin II shows utility in the diagnosis and prognosis of muscle-invasive urothelial carcinoma. Pathology. 2016;**48**(6):543-549. DOI: 10.1016/j.pathol.2016.05.008

[39] Tacha D, Bremer R, Haas T, Qi W. An immunohistochemical analysis of a newly developed, mouse monoclonal p40 (BC28) antibody in lung, bladder, skin, breast, prostate, and head and neck cancers. Archives of Pathology & Laboratory Medicine. 2014;**138**(10):1358-1364. DOI: 10.5858/arpa.2013-0342-OA

[40] Turner BM, Cagle PT, Sainz IM, Fukuoka J, Shen SS, Jagirdar J. Napsin A, A new marker for lung adenocarcinoma, is complementary and more sensitive and specific than thyroid transcription factor 1 in the differential diagnosis of primary pulmonary carcinoma. Evaluation of 1674 cases by tissue microarray. Archives of Pathology & Laboratory Medicine. 2012;**136**:163-171. DOI: 10.5858/arpa.2011-0320-OA

[41] Jagirdar J. Application of immunohistochemistry to the diagnosis of primary and metastatic carcinoma to the lung. Archives of Pathology & Laboratory Medicine. 2008;**132**:384-396. DOI: 10.1043/1543-2165(2008)132[384:AOITTD]2.0.CO;2

[42] Ricciardelli C, Lokman NA, Pyragius CE, Ween MP, Macpherson AM, Ruszkiewicz A, Hoffmann P, Oehler MK. Keratin 5 overexpression is associated with serous ovarian cancer recurrence and chemotherapy resistance. Oncotarget. 2017;**8**(11):17819-17832. DOI: 10.18632/oncotarget.14867

[43] Wallace WA. The challenge of classifying poorly differentiated tumours in the lung. Histopathology. 2009;**54**(1):28-42. DOI: 10.1111/j.1365-2559.2008.03181.x. Review

[44] Chan BA, Brett GM, Hughes BGM. Targeted therapy for non-small cell lung cancer: Current standards and the promise of the future. Translational Lung Cancer Research. 2015;**4**(1):36-54. DOI: 10.3978/j.issn.2218-6751.2014.05.01

[45] Thunnissen E, Bubendorf L, Dietel M, Elmberger G, Kerr K, Lopez-Rios F, Moch H, Olszewski W, Pauwels P, Penault-Llorca F, Rossi G. EML4-ALK testing in non-small cell carcinomas of the lung: A review with recommendations. Virchows Archiv. 2012;**461**:245-257. DOI: 10.1007/s00428-012-1281-4

[46] Scarpinoa S, Vinciguerraa GLR, Di Napolia A, Fochettia F, Uccinia S, Iaconob D, Marchettib P, Rucoa L. High prevalence of ALK+/ROS1+ cases in pulmonary adenocarcinomaof adoloscents and young adults. Lung Cancer. 2016;**97**:95-98. DOI: 10.1016/j.lungcan.2016.04.022

[47] Ilie M, Hofman V, Dietel M, Soria J-C, Hofman P. Assessment of the PD-L1 status by immunohistochemistry: Challenges and perspectives for therapeutic strategies in lung cancer patients. Virchows Archiv. 2016;**468**:511-525. DOI: 10.1007/s00428-016-1910-4

[48] Tsao MS, Kerr KM, Dacic S, Yatabe Y, Hirsch FR. IASLC Atlas of PD-L1 Immunohistochmeistry Testing in Lung Cancer. North Fort Myers, FL, Editorial Rx Press; 2017. ISBN: 978-0-9832958-7-7

[49] Duréndez-Sáez E, Azkárate A, Meri M, Calabuig-Fariñas S, Aguilar-Gallardo C, Blasco A, Jantus-Lewintre E, Camps C. New insights in non-small-cell lung cancer: Circulating tumor cells and cell-free DNA. Journal of Thoracic Disease. 2017;**9**(Suppl 13):S1332-S1345. DOI: 10.21037/jtd.2017.06.112

5

The Immune Regulatory Role of Cytokine-Induced Killer Cells Treatment on Non-Small Cell Lung Cancer Patients

Li Zhang and Yanyan Pan

Abstract

Although a great progress has been made in surgery, radiotherapy and chemotherapy for non-small cell lung cancer (NSCLC), the 5-year overall survival rate (OS) remains unsatisfactory (approximately 15%). Recently, cytokine-induced killer (CIK) cells treatment as an adoptive immunotherapy has great promises in the scenario of potential new approaches for the treatment of lung tumors. Adaptive and innate cellular immunity are all important for inhibiting tumor growth and the clearance of cancer. The abilities to efficiently kill tumor cells and promote immune responses are the ultimate basic ability requested to CIK cells treatment. Therefore, we conducted a systematic review to evaluate the immunoregulation of CIK cells treatment in NSCLC patients to provide an objective reference for clinical decision-making.

Keywords: CIK, immune regulatory, NSCLC

1. Introduction

Lung cancer is a major cause of diagnosed cancer worldwide with a 5-year survival rate of less than 15% [1, 2]. Non-small cell lung cancer (NSCLC) accounts for about 80–85% of lung malignancies and shows high morbidity, high mortality and low survival rates. Most of these NSCLC patients are diagnosed at the late stage leading to a poor prognosis.

So far, the predominant applied cancer treatment methods are still surgery, radiation and chemotherapy; however, the effectiveness of these treatments is not completely satisfactory. These methods often have limited effects and often fail to completely remove minimal residual cancer cells. Surgery is the predominant treatment method against for NSCLC; however, 60–70% of patients who receive surgery may eventually develop loco-regional recurrence or distant metastasis [3]. Chemotherapy may be useful, but drug resistance and adverse effects still remain; therefore, chemotherapy cannot be used for most of the patients due to the poor tolerance of the majority of later stage patients. Thus, the more effective and safer treatments are urgently needed [4], and tremendous efforts had been done to find new method that can offer better prospects to eradicate tumors.

Recently, adoptive immunotherapy is an evolving treatment approach based on the use of the immune system to treat cancer. Immunotherapy has become a hot area in cancer research and treatment in China. The rapid ex vivo generation of adoptive immune cells is a simpler, cheaper, and more efficient way to generate a potent immunotherapeutic product [5, 6]. Since the 1980s, there are different forms of adoptive immunotherapy used in clinical trials: lymphokine-activated killer cells (LAK), tumor-infiltrating lymphocytes cells (TIL), natural killer (NK), $\gamma\ \delta$ T-cells and cytokine-induced killer (CIK) cells, tumor-associated antigen (TAA)-specific cytotoxic T-cell (CTL), and other forms of cells have been extensively employed in adoptive immunotherapy [7].

Among them, CIK cells are a heterogeneous population of ex-vivo expanded T lymphocytes with diverse T-cell receptor (TCR) specificities and are endowed with nonmajor histocompatibility complex (MHC)-restricted activities against tumor cells. The antitumor activity is mainly, even if not exclusively, associated with the $CD3^{+}CD56^{+}$ cells [8]. The antitumor effects of CIK cells have been described against a number of hematologic and solid malignancies both in vitro and vivo. In vitro, CIK cells can kill tumor cells directly [9–11] and improve apoptosis of tumor cells [12], CIK cells also can reverse the drug resistance of A549/DDP [13], and other study found that CIK can alter the cytokine secretion profiles of some immune cells [14]. In vivo, CIK cells also showed significant antitumor activity in animal studies and clinical trials. In the severe combined immunodeficiency (SCID) mouse model, human CIK cells infusion significantly prolongs the survival of SCID mice when compared with control animals or animals infused with LAK cells [15]. In other studies, using the SCID model, CIK cells have in vivo antitumor activity against a number of hematopoietic and solid tumors [16]. Since 1991, CIK cells were reported by Schmidt-Wolf [15], and several clinical trials have been studied. The application of CIK cells as an adoptive immunotherapy is important for the treatment of cancer, since several clinical studies have confirmed the safety of CIK therapy for patients [17, 18]. Numerous clinical studies have been recently performed, whereby adjuvant infusions of CIK cells following surgical resection or chemotherapy demonstrated a significant increase in survival time [19, 20]. The first clinical study included 10 patients with metastatic renal carcinoma, colorectal cancer and lymphoma. One patient with lymphoma obtained a complete response while six patients had progressive diseases and three patients did not experience any change [21, 22]. Other clinical trials subsequently confirmed the safety and benefit of CIK cell-based therapy along with demonstration of initial clinical activity [23, 24]. But, in a recent review, it is reported that patients with localized NSCLC (stages I–III) using immunotherapy (excluding checkpoint inhibitors) did not get a survival benefit [25].

The host immune system plays a critical role in tumor surveillance and rejection. Innate and adaptive cellular immunity are all important for against tumor growth and the clearance of cancer. Lung cancer is not typically regarded as an "immunogenic" malignancy, a growing body of evidence suggests that immune responses to lung tumors might be present, and their magnitude might correlate with patient outcome. According to previous studies, cancer patients have some dysfunctions in cellular immunity, including innate and adaptive immune responses [26]. Because of the low immune functions of lung cancer patients, effective immune response cannot be achieved. That is one of the reasons that malignant tumors are incurable [27, 28]. Autoimmune disorders in peripheral blood of lung cancer patients are demonstrated by lower levels of CD4$^+$T, NK cells, DCs and higher levels of CD8$^+$T cells [29–31]. Several studies showed that in peripheral blood, increased number of inhibitory cells such as regulatory T-cells (Tregs) and myeloid-derived suppressor cells (MDSCs) and inhibitory molecular such as PD-1 TIM-3 expressed on lymphocytes has been observed in patients with NSCLC, and other cancers [32–34]. Otherwise, in tumors tissue there are local immunological changes. Tumor-infiltrating lymphocytes (TILs) may play an important role in cell-mediated immunological destruction of tumors. Many studies demonstrated that there are more T-cells in tumors tissue in NSCLC compared with that in normal tissue [35, 36]. Accumulating evidence shows that levels of TILs are associated with improved recurrence-free survival in NSCLC patients as well as a reduced likelihood of systemic recurrence [37, 38]. A high density of tumor-infiltrating Tregs was reported to be associated with the recurrence of resected NSCLC [39].

The abilities to efficiently kill tumor cells and promote immune responses are the ultimate basic ability requested to adoptive immunotherapy. The number of immune cells particularly Th1 cells, CD8$^+$ T-cells, and NK, NK T-cells is associated with the survival of cancer patients. Such antitumor cellular immune responses can be greatly enhanced by adoptive transfer of CIK cells [40, 41]. However, the immune regulation role of CIK cells treatment remains controversial. Therefore, in the present study, we conducted a review to evaluate the immunoregulation of CIK cells treatment in NSCLC patients, in order to provide an objective reference for clinical decision-making.

2. Immunoregulation of CIK cells treatment in NSCLC patients

2.1. The changes of lymphocytes of NSCLC patients in peripheral blood

According to previous studies, cancer patients exhibit certain dysfunctions in cellular immunity, including innate and adaptive immune responses [26]. Due to the low immune function displayed by patients with lung cancer, effective immune response cannot be achieved, and this is one of the reasons why malignant tumors are incurable [27, 28]. Autoimmune disorders in patients with lung cancer are demonstrated by reduced levels of CD4$^+$ and CD3$^+$CD56$^+$ cells, and increased levels of CD8$^+$ cells [29, 30]. The response of the human immune system against tumors mainly depends on cellular immunity [42]. CD3$^+$ T-cells are mature T-cells, while CD4$^+$ T-cells are considered to have a predefined role as Th cells [43]. It has been demonstrated that cytotoxicity against tumors is dependent on an appropriate interaction between CD4$^+$ and CD8$^+$ T-cells [44]. However, the ratios of T lymphocyte subsets in peripheral blood are usually disordered in cancer patients [45, 46]. The proportion of these cells in the human body must remain constant in order to maintain its optimal state of balance and participate in cellular immune surveillance [47]. NK and NK T-cells are effector cells, which are involved in the immune response against tumors during the early stages of tumor development [48]. These cells do not require any specific antibodies or presensitized lymphocytes to exert their function and may be rapidly activated to suppress and destroy a variety of tumor cells [49]. In addition, NK and NK T-cells are more lethal upon being activated by lymphokines [49].

Many studies including our study found that the average percentage of $CD3^+CD4^+$, $CD3^+$ and NK T-cells, as well as the levels of IFN-γ following several treatment courses, were significantly higher than the values observed prior to CIK cells treatment [50–52]. Of course, there are studies found that there are no changes after CIK cells treatment [25]. Here, we have to discuss about the course of CIK cells treatment. Fan et al. found that the median OS of the CIK cells treatment more than four cycles subgroup was significantly longer than that of less than four cycles subgroup [53]. Shi et al. [54] observed that the percentage of $CD3^+$ and $CD4^+$ cells, and the ratio of $CD4^+/CD8^+$ cells were significantly higher following the first course of CIK cells therapy, compared with the values prior to treatment. However, in our study, the percentages of $CD3^+$ and $CD3^+CD4^+$ cells were observed to be no change following only one course of CIK cells therapy, which may be due to the difference in the detection time point (1 month in our study vs. 2 weeks in the study by Shi et al. subsequent to each course), and this result was consistent with others. Jin et al. [55] reported that only one treatment course of CIK cells treatment was unable to improve the immune function in patients with lung cancer. Several researches have reported that $CD3^+$, $CD3^+CD4^+$ and other immune cells peaked at 4 weeks following CIK cells treatment, while circulating CIK cells persisted for ≤2 weeks following infusion [22]. Those studies suggested that several courses of CIK cells treatment would be required to achieve a stable effect [22, 55]. Therefore, to gain therapeutic efficacy, multiple courses of therapy should be administered to the patients.

Otherwise, the treatment done before CIK cells treatment may affect the immune status of NSCLS patients [50]. Thus, the treatments administered to the patients prior to CIK cells therapy seemed to affect the outcome, since more courses were required to achieve effective antitumor immune responses. At present, there is controversy regarding the number of cells required to be infused in CIK cells therapy, since the antitumor activity of CIK cells is mainly associated with the $CD3^+CD56^+$ fraction, rather than the $CD8^+$ fraction, which constitutes the highest percentage of CIK cells [56]. A previous study suggested that the improvements in immune function exerted by CIK cells were affected by the number of CIK cells [22]. In our study, we found that the number of $CD3^+CD4^+$ and $CD3^+$ T lymphocytes did not change following each course of CIK cells treatment. These demonstrated that the number of CIK cells did not affect lymphocyte-associated functions. By contrast, the number of NK and NK T-cells increased with the increase in the percentage of $CD3^+CD56^+$ cells, which enabled the patients to effectively kill tumor cells.

In most studies, patients received autologous CIK cells, allogeneic CIK cells may be applicable in the combination treatment in NSCLC [57, 58], median progression-free survival (mPFS) of allogeneic CIK cells treatment group was significantly longer that of control group [57]. The study found that the levels of IL-2 and IFN-γ in serum did not differ significantly between the two groups both before and after the treatment. Moreover, there were no obvious changes in the percentage of $CD3^+$, $CD3^+CD4^+$, $CD3^+CD8^+$, $CD4^+/CD8^+$ T-cell ratio and NK cells before and after treatment. Wang et al. found that after allogeneic CIK cells treatment, the outcomes of immune function remained unchanged, but the median OS was higher in NSCLC patients receiving allogeneic CIK cells than control group [58]. The CIK cells used in clinical treatment are mostly induced by PBMC in the peripheral blood of patients with tumors. Autologous CIK cells may have the ability to recognize the surface markers of tumor cells and have strong anti-tumor activity. However, in recent years, it has been suggested that low immunity and poor activity of immune cell in patients with tumors may affect the efficacy of CIK cell therapy. Comparative studies of autologous and allogeneic CIK cells treatment have not been reported in lung cancer clinical study. One study had found that semi-allogeneic DC-CIK cells had a stronger anti-tumor effect than did autologous CIK cells in vitro [59]. The reason for this is that the immune function of cancer patients is broken. The CIK cells induced by PBMC in tumor patients are significantly reduced in both quantity and biological activity.

2.2. The changes of Tregs and MDSCs of NSCLC patients in peripheral blood

The response of the human immune system against tumors mainly depends on cellular immunity [42]. However, our immune system does not work effectively in the setting of malignancy. The reason for this may be the existence of immune suppression [60–62].

Tregs have an important role in suppressing adaptive immune responses and maintaining immune tolerance [63]. At the same time, the existence of Tregs may downregulate tumor-specific immunity. Tregs interact with various immune cell types, $CD8^+$ T-cells [64], natural killer (NK) cells [65], and natural killer T (NKT) cells [66], thus, Tregs may have an important impact on cancer immune escape. Several studies have reported that the number of Tregs has increased in patients with NSCLC and other cancers [33, 67, 68]. It was reported that the percentage of Tregs was significantly reduced at week 2 after CIK cells treatment compared with the baseline and remained low at week 4 [51]. The decreasing of Treg was related with treatment cycle. Baodan Yu et al. found that significant reduction of Tregs frequency were presented in patients received with more than three cycles of CIK cells treatment compared with patients with less than three cycles of treatment [69]. In addition, inhibitory cytokines TGF-β as well as IL-10 were also decreased [51, 69].

MDSCs are heterogeneous population of myeloid cells known to exhibit potent suppression of T-cell proliferation and cytokine production [70–72]. Several evidence showed that MDSCs have a role in lung tumor growth and progression [73, 74]. In NSCLC patients MDSCs were reported in the peripheral blood [75, 76] and MDSCs were significantly higher compared with the healthy volunteers and were associated with poorer PFS [77]. In case of SCLC, preliminary results from a randomized phase II trial have shown that all-trans-retinoic acid (ATRA)-induced depletion of MDSCs may increase the immune response to DC-based vaccination to 42% [78]. Two Chinese articles found that CIK cells treatment can decrease the level of MDSCs in peripheral blood in malignant melanoma and gastrointestinal carcinomas patients. But, we did not find any literature to study the role of CIK cells on MDSCs in NSCLC patients.

2.3. The changes of immune cells of NSCLC patients in tumor tissue

A malignant tumor is not merely an accumulation of neoplastic cells, but also constitutes a microenvironment including endothelial cells, fibroblasts, structural components, and infiltrating immune cells that impact tumor development, invasion, metastasis, and outcome [79]. More recently, Fridman et al. reviewed that TILs was associated with clinical outcome in several cancers, including lung cancer [80]. All immune cell types might be found in a tumor such as $CD4^+$ T-cells, $CD8^+$ T-cells, macrophages, dendritic cells (DCs), mast cells, NK cells, memory cells, Tregs cells.

$CD4^+$ T and $CD8^+$ cells are the two major subsets of T lymphocytes and have different roles on tumor immunity within the tumor tissue [81]. Wakabayashi et al. [82] found that $CD4^+$ T-cells but not $CD8^+$ T-cells in cancer cell nests are associated with a better prognosis in NSCLC patients. Another study found that infiltrating $CD8^+$ T-cells and $CD4^+$ T-cells in NSCLC may work together to suppress cancer progression [83]. MDSCs were found in lymph nodes and tumor tissue of patients with NSCLC [84]. In mouse model, researchers found that CIK cells can inhibit the accumulation of MDSCs in the tumor [85]. But, we did not find any literature to study the role of CIK cells on infiltrating T-cells and MDSCs in patients with NSCLC. This may have been the result of the difficult access to tumor tissue, and relatively little research was done in vivo about the CIK cells, especially the studies published in high-level journals. Our research team may add these studies to their work in the future.

2.4. Immune checkpoint in NSCLC patients

In the setting of malignancy, immune suppression exists. Except the abovementioned aspects, immune checkpoint is another essential mechanism of immune suppression. These immune checkpoint included cytotoxic T lymphocyte antigen 4 (CTLA4), programmed death protein 1 (PD-1), lymphocyte activation gene 3 protein (LAG3), T-cell immunoglobulin domain and mucin domain 3 (TIM3), T-cell immunoreceptor with Ig and ITIM domains (TIGIT), and B and T lymphocyte attenuator (BTLA) [86]. They can inhibit the development and proliferation of lymphocytes [87]. These checkpoint expressed on T-cells was found in peripheral blood and tumor tissue have limited ability to effectively eliminate tumors, have gained considerable attention and PD-1 expression on peripheral blood T-cell subsets correlates with prognosis in non-small cell lung cancer [88, 89]. These molecules were found expressed on CIK cells [60]. The majority of these molecules, except BTLA were increased during CIK cells culture. But articles about the effect of CIK cells treatment on these molecules was very little in NSCLC patients, we only found one Chinese article found that after CIK cells treatment, the expression of PD-1 in peripheral blood decreased, and the decreasing was associated with the clinical stage of NSCLC.

2.5. Cytokines in NSCLC patients

In the process of ex-vivo expansion, cytokines play a decisive role in the differentiation and function of CIK. Only the addition of cytokines in vitro can induce peripheral blood monocytes (PBMCs) to differentiate into CIK cells. Importantly, different cultures affected the toxicity of CIK cells [15]. In the process of killing tumors in vivo, CIK can secrete a large number of

IL-2, IFN-γ, TNF-α, and GM-CSF and other cytokines. It can not only play an anti-tumor role directly, but also regulate the immune system of the body, and to stimulate cell proliferation and differentiation, and further enhance the cytotoxic activity of immune cells. Immune balance is controlled by the balance of cytokines produced by two distinct helper T-cell subsets, Th1 and Th2 cells [90, 91]. Our study found that the levels of IFN-γ following several treatment courses were significantly higher than the values observed prior to CIK cells treatment. The levels of IL-2, in vitro and in vivo, were elevated in CIK cells treatment group [12]. The serum levels of IL-4 and IL-6 in tumor-bearing patients were elevated after immunotherapy, and IFN-γ and IL-6 levels in patients with resected NSCLC were significantly increased. Otherwise, Li et al. have also shown that CIK cells treatment increased Th1 cytokines in patients who have no progression, but in patients who had developed metastasis had no change [92]. Successful immunotherapeutic interventions should overcome Th2 immunity by promoting and restoring antitumor Th1 immune response to achieve better clinical benefits [93].

3. Conclusion

In recent years, with the gradual clearer of tumor immunity regulation mechanism and the continuous improvement of gene transformation technology, tumor immunotherapy has been developed unprecedentedly. From the nonspecific immune stimulating agent to tumor vaccine, then monoclonal antibody and adoptive cellular immunotherapy for immune checkpoint blockade, therapeutic immune technology innovation provides more weapons for the human resistance tumor. Especially in the recent 5 years, with the rise of immunotherapy for immunological checkpoints and CAR-T-cell, immunotherapy has become more and more popular. Nonspecific immunotherapy, such as CIK, DC-CIK or NK cells, is widely used in China at present. These kinds of innate immune cells as the first immune defense cells, although the specific killing effect may be less than CAR-T, TCR-T, but these nonspecific cells play a positive role in lowering recurrence rate, improving tolerance of chemotherapy, improving life quality and prolonging the period of survival. However, the curative effect of recurrent and refractory tumors is limited to a small number of typical cases, and there is no evidence-based supports for prospective, randomized controlled trials. Besides, the combination of PD-1 antibody and CTLA-4 antibody is also easy to cause autoimmunity. The instability of tumor cells is also easy to form tumor heterogeneity. There is some progress in the research of CAR-T in the hematologic malignancies, but there are many problems in the treatment of solid tumors for CAR-T. Generally speaking, tumor immunotherapy is progressing faster and has many advantages. But if we want to apply for large-scale clinical application, we need to do a lot of research work.

Several articles had reported the safety and efficacy of CIK-cell therapy. Current studies on the immunomodulatory effects of CIK-cell therapy have focused on T lymphocytes and Treg in peripheral blood. It is much more challenging to study the relationship between CIK cells and immune system. Immune system is dynastic and complex, and a lot of other aspects are in the volume of the complex. The role of CIK cells on immune responses was associated with host factors. Not only cellular immunity we mentioned above but also humoral immunity get involved in tumor immunity. Tumor is characterized by distinct individual differences, the same disease, different stages, and different pathological types, resulting in different outcomes. Immune system had important roles in these processes. Thus, we evaluate the immune function of the patient and analyze the status of each patient itself, which are significantly related to the final outcome. The ultimate goal of precision immunology for cancer is to select the patients who are most likely to benefit from a particular immunotherapy.

With the development of new technologies to dynamically detect the cancer-immune system interaction and at the same time taking into account the particularity of different groups of people, precision cancer immunology and the evaluation of immune function will be applied more widely, improving diagnosis and treatment of NSCLC patients.

Author details

Li Zhang* and Yanyan Pan

*Address all correspondence to: tyouri19652004@hotmail.com

Department of Central Laboratory, Dalian Municipal Central Hospital, Dalian, Liaoning, China

References

[1] Ahn SH, Han MS, Yoon JH, Jeon SY, Kim CH, Yoo HJ, Lee JC. Treatment of stage I non-small cell lung cancer with CyberKnife, image-guided robotic stereotactic radiosurgery. Oncology Reports. 2009 Mar;**21**(3):693-696

[2] Zheng YW, Li RM, Zhang XW, Ren XB. Current adoptive immunotherapy in non-small cell lung cancer and potential influence of therapy outcome. Cancer Investigation. 2013 Mar;**31**(3):197-205. DOI: 10.3109/07357907.2013.775294

[3] Hirsh V. Review of the treatment of metastatic non small cell lung carcinoma: A practical approach. World J Clin Oncol. 2011 Jun;**2**(6):262-271. DOI: 10.5306/wjco.v2.i6.262

[4] Kobayashi K, Hagiwara K. Epidermal growth factor receptor (EGFR) mutation and personalized therapy in advanced nonsmall cell lung cancer (NSCLC). Targeted Oncology. 2013 Mar;**8**(1):27-33. DOI: 10.1007/s11523-013-0258-9. Epub 2013 Jan 30

[5] Barrett J, Bollard CM. T-cell therapy for cancer. Immunotherapy. 2012 Apr;**4**(4):347-350. DOI: 10.2217/imt.12.12

[6] Vera JF, Brenner LJ, Gerdemann U, Ngo MC, Sili U, Liu H, Wilson J, Dotti G, Heslop HE, Leen AM, Rooney CM. Accelerated production of antigen-specific T-cells for preclinical and clinical applications using gas-permeable rapid expansion cultureware (G-Rex). Journal of Immunotherapy. 2010 Apr;**33**(3):305-315. DOI: 10.1097/CJI.0b013e3181c0c3cb

[7] Ruella M, Kalos M. Adoptive immunotherapy for cancer. Immunological Reviews. 2014 Jan;**257**(1):14-38. DOI: 10.1111/imr.12136

[8] Sangiolo D, Martinuzzi E, Todorovic M, Vitaggio K, Vallario A, Jordaney N, Carnevale-Schianca F, Capaldi A, Geuna M, Casorzo L, Nash RA, Aglietta M, Cignetti A. Alloreactivity and anti-tumor activity segregate within two distinct subsets of cytokine-induced killer (CIK) cells: Implications for their infusion across major HLA barriers. International Immunology. 2008 Jul;**20**(7):841-848. DOI: 10.1093/intimm/dxn042. Epub 2008 May 9

[9] Zhang YS, Yuan FJ, Jia GF, Zhang JF, Hu LY, Huang L, Wang J, Dai ZQ. CIK cells from patients with HCC possess strong cytotoxicity to multidrug-resistant cell line Bel-7402/R. World Journal of Gastroenterology. 2005 Jun;**11**(22):3339-3345

[10] Rombo R, Weiher H, Schmidt-Wolf IG. Effect of chaetocin on renal cell carcinoma cells and cytokine-induced killer cells. German Medical Science. 2016 Apr;**14**:Doc04. DOI: 10.3205/000231. eCollection 2016

[11] Tita-Nwa F, Moldenhauer G, Herbst M, Kleist C, Ho AD, Kornacker M. Cytokine-induced killer cells targeted by the novel bispecific antibody CD19xCD5 (HD37xT5.16) efficiently lyse B-lymphoma cells. Cancer Immunology, Immunotherapy. 2007 Dec;**56**(12):1911-1920. Epub 2007 May 9

[12] Fan XY, Wang PY, Zhang C, Zhang YL, Fu Y, Zhang C, Li QX, Zhou JN, Shan BE, He DW. All-trans retinoic acid enhances cytotoxicity of CIK cells against human lung adenocarcinoma by upregulating MICA and IL-2 secretion. Scientific Reports. 2017 Nov;**7**(1):16481. DOI: 10.1038/s41598-017-16745-z

[13] Yang L, Du C, Wu L, Yu J, An X, Yu W, Cao S, Li H, Ren X. Cytokine-induced killer cells modulates resistance to cisplatin in the A549/DDP cell line. Journal of Cancer. 2017 Sep;**8**(16):3287-3295. DOI: 10.7150/jca.19426. eCollection 2017

[14] Li D, Guo S, Li H, Zhu G, Gao L, Xin X, Yan D, Li X, Geng S, Hou H, Yang Y. Effect of inhibition proliferation in human lung adenocarcinoma A549 cells by cytokine-induced killer cells. Thoracic Cancer. 2015 Jul;**6**(4):458-463. DOI: 10.1111/1759-7714.12205. Epub 2014 Dec 29

[15] Schmidt-Wolf IG, Negrin RS, Kiem HP, Blume KG, Weissman IL. Use of a SCID mouse/human lymphoma model to evaluate cytokine-induced killer cells with potent antitumor cell activity. The Journal of Experimental Medicine. 1991 Jul;**174**(1):139-149

[16] Thanendrarajan S, Nowak M, Abken H, Schmidt-Wolf IG. Combining cytokine-induced killer cells with vaccination in cancer immunotherapy: More than one plus one? Leukemia Research. 2011 Sep;**35**(9):1136-1142. DOI: 10.1016/j.leukres.2011.05.005. Epub 2011 Jun 8

[17] Wang Y, Lv B, Li K, Zhang A, Liu H. Adjuvant immunotherapy of dendritic cells and cytokine-induced killer cells is safe and enhances chemotherapy efficacy for multiple myeloma in China: A meta-analysis of clinical trials. Drug Design, Development and Therapy. 2017 Nov;**11**:3245-3256. DOI: 10.2147/DDDT.S146959. eCollection 2017

[18] Hu J, Hu J, Liu X, Hu C, Li M, Han W. Effect and safety of cytokine-induced killer (CIK) cell immunotherapy in patients with breast cancer: A meta-analysis. Medicine (Baltimore). 2017 Oct;**96**(42):e8310. DOI: 10.1097/MD.0000000000008310

[19] Zhang J, Li H, Gao D, Zhang B, Zheng M, Lun M, Wei M, Duan R, Guo M, Hua J, Liu Q, Bai J, Liu H, Zheng J, Yao H. A prognosis and impact factor analysis of DC-CIK cell therapy for patients with hepatocellular carcinoma undergoing postoperative TACE. Cancer Biology & Therapy. 2018 Jun 3;**19**(6):475-483. DOI: 10.1080/15384047.2018.1433501

[20] Zhang Y, Zhu Y, Zhao E, He X, Zhao L, Wang Z, Fu X, Qi Y, Ma B, Song Y, Gao Q. Autologous cytokine-induced killer cell immunotherapy may improve overall survival in advanced malignant melanoma patients. Immunotherapy. 2017 Nov;**9**(14):1165-1174. DOI: 10.2217/imt-2017-0061

[21] Schmidt-Wolf IG, Finke S, Trojaneck B, Denkena A, Lefterova P, Schwella N, Heuft HG, Prange G, Korte M, Takeya M, Dorbic T, Neubauer A, Wittig B, Huhn D. Phase I clinical study applying autologous immunological effector cells transfected with the interleukin-2 gene in patients with metastatic renal cancer, colorectal cancer and lymphoma. British Journal of Cancer. 1999 Nov;**81**(6):1009-1016

[22] Sangiolo D. Cytokine induced killer cells as promising immunotherapy for solid tumors. Journal of Cancer. 2011;**2**:363-368. Epub 2011 Jun 15

[23] Zhu Y, Zhang H, Li Y, Bai J, Liu L, Liu Y, Qu Y, Qu X. Efficacy of postoperative adjuvant transfusion of cytokine-induced killer cells combined with chemotherapy in patients with colorectal cancer. Cancer Immunology, Immunotherapy. 2013 Oct;**62**(10):1629-1635. DOI: 10.1007/s00262-013-1465-z. Epub 2013 Aug 23

[24] Huang ZM, Li W, Li S, Gao F, Zhou QM, Wu FM, He N, Pan CC, Xia JC, Wu PH, Zhao M. Cytokine-induced killer cells in combination with transcatheter arterial chemoembolization and radiofrequency ablation for hepatocellular carcinoma patients. Journal of Immunotherapy. 2013 Jun;**36**(5):287-293. DOI: 10.1097/CJI.0b013e3182948452

[25] Zhu J, Li R, Tiselius E, Roudi R, Teghararian O, Suo C, Song H. Immunotherapy (excluding checkpoint inhibitors) for stage I to III non-small cell lung cancer treated with surgery or radiotherapy with curative intent. Cochrane Database of Systematic Reviews. 2017 Dec;**12**:CD011300. DOI: 10.1002/14651858.CD011300.pub2

[26] Sun K, Wang L, Zhang Y. Dendritic cell as therapeutic vaccines against tumors and its role in therapy for hepatocellular carcinoma. Cellular & Molecular Immunology. 2006 Jun;**3**(3):197-203

[27] Méndez R, Ruiz-Cabello F, Rodríguez T, Del Campo A, Paschen A, Schadendorf D, Garrido F. Identification of different tumor escape mechanisms in several metastases from a

melanoma patient undergoing immunotherapy. Cancer Immunology, Immunotherapy. 2007 Jan;**56**(1):88-94. Epub 2006 Apr 19

[28] Wongkajornsilp A, Somchitprasert T, Butraporn R, Wamanuttajinda V, Kasetsinsombat K, Huabprasert S, Maneechotesuwan K, Hongeng S. Human cytokine-induced killer cells specifically infiltrated and retarded the growth of the inoculated human cholangiocarcinoma cells in SCID mice. Cancer Investigation. 2009 Feb;**27**(2):140-148. DOI: 10.1080/07357900802189832

[29] Chen KJ, Zhou L, Xie HY, Ahmed TE, Feng XW, Zheng SS. Intratumoral regulatory T cells alone or in combination with cytotoxic T cells predict prognosis of hepatocellular carcinoma after resection. Medical Oncology. 2012 Sep;**29**(3):1817-1826. DOI: 10.1007/s12032-011-0006-x. Epub 2011 Jun 16

[30] Lee WC, Wu TJ, Chou HS, Yu MC, Hsu PY, Hsu HY, Wang CC. The impact of CD4+ CD25+ T cells in the tumor microenvironment of hepatocellular carcinoma. Surgery. 2012 Feb;**151**(2):213-222. DOI: 10.1016/j.surg.2011.07.029. Epub 2011 Oct 5

[31] Hubo M, Trinschek B, Kryczanowsky F, Tuettenberg A, Steinbrink K, Jonuleit H. Costimulatory molecules on immunogenic versus tolerogenic human dendritic cells. Frontiers in Immunology. 2013 Apr;**4**(82). DOI: 10.3389/fimmu.2013.00082. eCollection 2013

[32] Woo EY, Chu CS, Goletz TJ, Schlienger K, Yeh H, Coukos G, Rubin SC, Kaiser LR, June CH. Regulatory CD4(+)CD25(+) T cells in tumors from patients with early-stage non-small cell lung cancer and late-stage ovarian cancer. Cancer Research. 2001 Jun; **61**(12):4766-4772

[33] Li JY, Duan XF, Wang LP, Xu YJ, Huang L, Zhang TF, Liu JY, Li F, Zhang Z, Yue DL, Wang F, Zhang B, Zhang Y. Selective depletion of regulatory T cell subsets by docetaxel treatment in patients with nonsmall cell lung cancer. Journal of Immunology Research. 2014;**2014**:286170. DOI: 10.1155/2014/286170. Epub 2014 Apr 28

[34] Li S, Li Y, Qu X, Liu X, Liang J. Detection and significance of TregFoxP3(+) and Th17 cells in peripheral blood of non-small cell lung cancer patients. Archives of Medical Science. 2014 May;**10**(2):232-239. DOI: 10.5114/aoms.2014.42573. Epub 2014 May 13

[35] Kataki A, Scheid P, Piet M, Marie B, Martinet N, Martinet Y, Vignaud JM. Tumor infiltrating lymphocytes and macrophages have a potential dual role in lung cancer by supporting both host-defense and tumor progression. The Journal of Laboratory and Clinical Medicine. 2002 Nov;**140**(5):320-328

[36] Tian C, Lu S, Fan Q, Zhang W, Jiao S, Zhao X, Wu Z, Sun L, Wang L. Prognostic significance of tumor-infiltrating $CD8^+$ or $CD3^+$ T lymphocytes and interleukin-2 expression in radically resected non-small cell lung cancer. Chinese Medical Journal. 2015 Jan;**128**(1):105-110. DOI: 10.4103/0366-6999.147828

[37] Al-Shibli KI, Donnem T, Al-Saad S, Persson M, Bremnes RM, Busund LT. Prognostic effect of epithelial and stromal lymphocyte infiltration in non-small cell lung cancer. Clinical Cancer Research. 2008 Aug;**14**(16):5220-5227. DOI: 10.1158/1078-0432.CCR-08-0133

[38] Onion D, Isherwood M, Shridhar N, Xenophontos M, Craze ML, Day LJ, García-Márquez MA, Pineda RG, Reece-Smith AM, Saunders JH, Duffy JP, Argent RH, Grabowska AM. Multicomponent analysis of the tumour microenvironment reveals low CD8 T cell number, low stromal caveolin-1 and high tenascin-C and their combination as significant prognostic markers in non-small cell lung cancer. Oncotarget. 2017 Jun;**9**(2):1760-1771. DOI: 10.18632/oncotarget.18880. eCollection 2018 Jan 5

[39] Petersen RP, Campa MJ, Sperlazza J, Conlon D, Joshi MB, Harpole DH Jr, Patz EF Jr. Tumor infiltrating Foxp3+ regulatory T-cells are associated with recurrence in pathologic stage I NSCLC patients. Cancer. 2006 Dec;**107**(12):2866-2872

[40] Wang XP, Xu M, Gao HF, Zhao JF, Xu KC. Intraperitoneal perfusion of cytokine-induced killer cells with local hyperthermia for advanced hepatocellular carcinoma. World Journal of Gastroenterology. 2013 May;**19**(19):2956-2962. DOI: 10.3748/wjg.v19.i19.2956

[41] Jiang J, Wu C, Lu B. Cytokine-induced killer cells promote antitumor immunity. Journal of Translational Medicine. 2013 Mar;**11**:83. DOI: 10.1186/1479-5876-11-83

[42] Perdicchio M, Cornelissen LA, Streng-Ouwehand I, Engels S, Verstege MI, Boon L, Geerts D, van Kooyk Y, Unger WW. Tumor sialylation impedes T cell mediated anti-tumor responses while promoting tumor associated-regulatory T cells. Oncotarget. 2016 Feb;**7**(8):8771-8782. DOI: 10.18632/oncotarget.6822

[43] Attallah AM, Tabll AA, El-Sadany M, Ibrahim TA, El-Dosoky I. Dysregulation of blood lymphocyte subsets and natural killer cells in schistosomal liver cirrhosis and hepatocellular carcinoma. Clinical and Experimental Medicine. 2003 Nov;**3**(3):181-185

[44] Motz GT, Coukos G. Deciphering and reversing tumor immune suppression. Immunity. 2013 Jul;**39**(1):61-73. DOI: 10.1016/j.immuni.2013.07.005

[45] Kiessling R, Wasserman K, Horiguchi S, Kono K, Sjöberg J, Pisa P, Petersson M. Tumor-induced immune dysfunction. Cancer Immunology, Immunotherapy. 1999 Oct;**48**(7): 353-362

[46] Rayman P, Uzzo RG, Kolenko V, Bloom T, Cathcart MK, Molto L, Novick AC, Bukowski RM, Hamilton T, Finke JH. Tumor-induced dysfunction in interleukin-2 production and interleukin-2 receptor signaling: A mechanism of immune escape. The Cancer Journal from Scientific American. 2000 Feb;**6**(Suppl 1):S81-S87

[47] Shepherd FA, Douillard JY, Blumenschein GR Jr. Immunotherapy for non-small cell lung cancer: Novel approaches to improve patient outcome. Journal of Thoracic Oncology. 2011;**6**:1763-1773. DOI: 10.1097/JTO.0b013e31822e28fc

[48] Subleski JJ, Wiltrout RH, Weiss JM. Application of tissue-specific NK and NKT cell activity for tumor immunotherapy. Journal of Autoimmunity. 2009 Nov-Dec;**33**(3-4):275-281. DOI: 10.1016/j.jaut.2009.07.010. Epub 2009 Aug 13

[49] Kuss I, Hathaway B, Ferris RL, Gooding W, Whiteside TL. Decreased absolute counts of T lymphocyte subsets and their relation to disease in squamous cell carcinoma of the head and neck. Clinical Cancer Research. 2004;**10**:3755-3762

[50] Pan Y, Wu Y, Ji J, Cai H, Wang H, Jiang Y, Sang L, Yang J, Gao Y, Liu Y, Yin L, Zhang LI. Effect of cytokine-induced killer cells on immune function in patients with lung cancer. Oncology Letters. 2016 Apr;**11**(4):2827-2834. Epub 2016 Feb 29

[51] Yu B, Wang J, He C, Wang W, Tang J, Zheng R, Zhou C, Zhang H, Fu Z, Li Q, Xu J. Cytokine-induced killer cell therapy for modulating regulatory T cells in patients with non-small cell lung cancer. Experimental and Therapeutic Medicine. 2017 Jul;**14**(1):831-840. DOI: 10.3892/etm.2017.4562. Epub 2017 Jun 8

[52] Zhou C, Liu D, Li J, Sun H, Zheng X, Wang S, Hong G, Mallampati S, Sun H, Zhou X, Cheng Z, Zhang H, Ma H. Chemotherapy plus dendritic cells co-cultured with cytokine-induced killer cells versus chemotherapy alone to treat advanced non-small-cell lung cancer: A meta-analysis. Oncotarget. 2016 Dec;**7**(52):86500-86510. DOI: 10.18632/oncotarget.13394

[53] Gu Y, Lv H, Zhao J, Li Q, Mu G, Li J, Wuyang J, Lou G, Wang R, Zhang Y, Huang X. Influence of the number and interval of treatment cycles on cytokine-induced killer cells and their adjuvant therapeutic effects in advanced non-small-cell lung ancer (NSCLC). International Immunopharmacology. 2017 Sep;**50**:263-269. DOI: 10.1016/j.intimp.2017.07.006. Epub 2017 Jul 12

[54] Shi L, Zhou Q, Wu J, Ji M, Li G, Jiang J, Wu C. Efficacy of adjuvant immunotherapy with cytokine-induced killer cells in patients with locally advanced gastric cancer. Cancer Immunology, Immunotherapy. 2012;**61**:2251-2259

[55] Jin CG, Chen XQ, Li J, Wu ZP, Liu X, Wang XC. Moderating effects and maintenance of lung cancer cellular immune functions by CIK cell therapy. Asian Pacific Journal of Cancer Prevention. 2013;**14**:3587-3592

[56] Kuçi S, Rettinger E, Voss B, Weber G, Stais M, Kreyenberg H, Willasch A, Kuçi Z, Koscielniak E, Klöss S, von Laer D, Klingebiel T, Bader P. Efficient lysis of rhabdomyosarcoma cells by cytokine-induced killer cells: Implications for adoptive immunotherapy after allogeneic stem cell transplantation. Haematologica. 2010 Sep;**95**(9):1579-1586. DOI: 10.3324/haematol.2009.019885. Epub 2010 Apr 7

[57] Zhang L, Xu Y, Shen J, He F, Zhang D, Chen Z, Duan Y, Sun J. Feasibility study of DCs/CIKs combined with thoracic radiotherapy for patients with locally advanced or metastatic non-small-cell lung cancer. Radiation Oncology. 2016 Apr;**11**:60. DOI: 10.1186/s13014-016-0635-5

[58] Wang S, Zhang H, Liu C, Jiao X, Liu D, DU W, He Y, Zhang Z, Wu X, Wang J, Liang C, Zhang L, Liu S. Human leukocyte antigen-haploidentical donor-derived cytokine-induced killer cells are safe and prolong the survival of patients with advanced non-small cell lung cancer. Oncology Letters. 2014 Dec;**8**(6):2727-2733. Epub 2014 Sep 24

[59] Wang QJ, Wang H, Pan K, Li YQ, Huang LX, Chen SP, He J, Ke ML, Zhao JJ, Li JJ, Sun JC, Liang XT, Ma HQ, Chen YB, Xia JC. Comparative study on anti-tumor immune response of autologous cytokine-induced killer (CIK) cells, dendritic cells-CIK (DC-CIK), and semi-allogeneic DC-CIK. Chinese Journal of Cancer. 2010 Jul;**29**(7):641-648

[60] Zhang L, Wang J, Wei F, Wang K, Sun Q, Yang F, Jin H, Zheng Y, Zhao H, Wang L, Yu W, Zhang X, An Y, Yang L, Zhang X, Ren X. Profiling the dynamic expression of checkpoint molecules on cytokine-induced killer cells from non-small-cell lung cancer patients. Oncotarget. 2016 Jul;**7**(28):43604-43615. DOI: 10.18632/oncotarget.9871

[61] Yu J, Du W, Yan F, Wang Y, Li H, Cao S, Yu W, Shen C, Liu J, Ren X. Myeloid-derived suppressor cells suppress antitumor immune responses through IDO expression and correlate with lymph node metastasis in patients with breast cancer. Journal of Immunology. 2013 Apr;**190**(7):3783-3797. DOI: 10.4049/jimmunol.1201449. Epub 2013 Feb 25

[62] Yu J, Wang Y, Yan F, Zhang P, Li H, Zhao H, Yan C, Yan F, Ren X. Noncanonical NF-κB activation mediates STAT3-stimulated IDO upregulation in myeloid-derived suppressor cells in breast cancer. Journal of Immunology. 2014 Sep;**193**(5):2574-2586. DOI: 10.4049/jimmunol.1400833. Epub 2014 Jul 25

[63] Nadkarni S, Mauri C, Ehrenstein MR. Anti-TNF-alpha therapy induces a distinct regulatory T cell population in patients with rheumatoid arthritis via TGF-beta. The Journal of Experimental Medicine. 2007 Jan;**204**(1):33-39. Epub 2007 Jan 2

[64] Antony PA, Piccirillo CA, Akpinarli A, Finkelstein SE, Speiss PJ, Surman DR, Palmer DC, Chan CC, Klebanoff CA, Overwijk WW, Rosenberg SA, Restifo NP. CD8+ T cell immunity against a tumor/self-antigen is augmented by CD4+ T helper cells and hindered by naturally occurring T regulatory cells. Journal of Immunology. 2005 Mar;**174**(5):2591-2601

[65] Jemal A, Siegel R, Xu J, Ward E. Cancer statistics, 2010. CA: A Cancer Journal for Clinicians. 2010 Sep-Oct;**60**(5):277-300. DOI: 10.3322/caac.20073. Epub 2010 Jul 7

[66] Ohki S, Shibata M, Gonda K, Machida T, Shimura T, Nakamura I, Ohtake T, Koyama Y, Suzuki S, Ohto H, Takenoshita S. Circulating myeloid-derived suppressor cells are increased and correlate to immune suppression, inflammation and hypoproteinemia in patients with cancer. Oncology Reports. 2012 Aug;**28**(2):453-458. doi: 10.3892/or.2012.1812. Epub 2012 May 14

[67] Duan MC, Han W, Jin PW, Wei YP, Wei Q, Zhang LM, Li JC. Disturbed Th17/Treg balance in patients with non-small cell lung cancer. Inflammation. 2015 Dec;**38**(6):2156-2165. DOI: 10.1007/s10753-015-0198-x

[68] Barua S, Fang P, Sharma A, Fujimoto J, Wistuba I, Rao AUK, Lin SH. Spatial interaction of tumor cells and regulatory T cells correlates with survival in non-small cell lung cancer. Lung Cancer. 2018 Mar;**117**:73-79. DOI: 10.1016/j.lungcan.2018.01.022

[69] Song H, Liu S, Zhao Z, Sun W, Wei X, Ma X, Zhao P, Gao D. Increased cycles of DC/CIK immunotherapy decreases frequency of Tregs in patients with resected NSCLC. International Immunopharmacology. 2017 Nov;**52**:197-202. DOI: 10.1016/j.intimp.2017.09.014. Epub 2017 Sep 21

[70] Gabrilovich DI, Nagaraj S. Myeloid-derived suppressor cells as regulators of the immune system. Nature Reviews. Immunology. 2009 Mar;**9**(3):162-174. DOI: 10.1038/nri2506

[71] Hanazawa A, Ito R, Katano I, Kawai K, Goto M, Suemizu H, Kawakami Y, Ito M, Takahashi T. Generation of human immunosuppressive myeloid cell populations in human Interleukin-6 transgenic NOG mice. Frontiers in Immunology. 2018 Feb;**9**:152. DOI: 10.3389/fimmu.2018.00152. eCollection 2018

[72] Draghiciu O, Lubbers J, Nijman HW, Daemen T. Myeloid derived suppressor cells-An overview of combat strategies to increase immunotherapy efficacy. Oncoimmunology. 2015 Feb;**4**(1):e954829. eCollection 2015 Jan

[73] Wang S, Fu Y, Ma K, Liu C, Jiao X, Du W, Zhang H, Wu X. The significant increase and dynamic changes of the myeloid-derived suppressor cells percentage with chemotherapy in advanced NSCLC patients. Clinical and Translational Oncology. 2014 Jul;**16**(7):616-622. DOI: 10.1007/s12094-013-1125-y. Epub 2013 Nov 6

[74] Zhang G, Huang H, Zhu Y, Yu G, Gao X, Xu Y, Liu C, Hou J, Zhang X. A novel subset of B7-H3+CD14+HLA-DR−/low myeloid-derived suppressor cells are associated with progression of human NSCLC. Oncoimmunology. 2015 Mar;**4**(2):e977164. eCollection 2015 Feb

[75] Jiang J, Guo W, Liang X. Phenotypes, accumulation, and functions of myeloid-derived suppressor cells and associated treatment strategies in cancer patients. Human Immunology. 2014 Nov;**75**(11):1128-1137. DOI: 10.1016/j.humimm.2014.09.025. Epub 2014 Oct 7

[76] Tian T, Gu X, Zhang B, Liu Y, Yuan C, Shao L, Guo Y, Fan K. Increased circulating CD14(+)HLA-DR−/low myeloid-derived suppressor cells are associated with poor prognosis in patients with small-cell lung cancer. Cancer Biomarkers. 2015;**15**(4):425-432. DOI: 10.3233/CBM-150473

[77] Hansen GL, Gaudernack G, Brunsvig PF, Cvancarova M, Kyte JA. Immunological factors influencing clinical outcome in lung cancer patients after telomerase peptide vaccination. Cancer Immunology, Immunotherapy. 2015 Dec;**64**(12):1609-1621. DOI: 10.1007/s00262-015-1766-5. Epub 2015 Oct 26

[78] Iclozan C, Antonia S, Chiappori A, Chen DT, Gabrilovich D. Therapeutic regulation of myeloid-derived suppressor cells and immune response to cancer vaccine in patients with extensive stage small cell lung cancer. Cancer Immunology, Immunotherapy. 2013 May;**62**(5):909-918. DOI: 10.1007/s00262-013-1396-8. Epub 2013 Apr 16

[79] Bremnes RM, Busund LT, Kilvær TL, Andersen S, Richardsen E, Paulsen EE, Hald S, Khanehkenari MR, Cooper WA, Kao SC, Dønnem T. The role of tumor-infiltrating lymphocytes in development, progression, and prognosis of non-small cell lung cancer. Journal of Thoracic Oncology. 2016 Jun;**11**(6):789-800. DOI: 10.1016/j.jtho.2016.01.015 Epub 2016 Feb 1

[80] Fridman WH, Pagès F, Sautès-Fridman C, Galon J. The immune contexture in human tumours: Impact on clinical outcome. Nature Reviews. Cancer. 2012 Mar;**12**(4):298-306. DOI: 10.1038/nrc3245

[81] Geng Y, Shao Y, He W, Hu W, Xu Y, Chen J, Wu C, Jiang J. Prognostic role of tumor-infiltrating lymphocytes in lung cancer: A meta-analysis. Cellular Physiology and Biochemistry. 2015;**37**(4):1560-1571. DOI: 10.1159/000438523. Epub 2015 Oct 30

[82] Sznurkowski JJ, Zawrocki A, Emerich J, Biernat W. Prognostic significance of CD4+ and CD8+ T cell infiltration within cancer cell nests in vulvar squamous cell carcinoma. International Journal of Gynecological Cancer. 2011 May;**21**(4):717-721. DOI: 10.1097/IGC.0b013e3182131f36

[83] Hiraoka K, Miyamoto M, Cho Y, Suzuoki M, Oshikiri T, Nakakubo Y, Itoh T, Ohbuchi T, Kondo S, Katoh H. Concurrent infiltration by CD8+ T cells and CD4+ T cells is a favourable prognostic factor in non-small-cell lung carcinoma. British Journal of Cancer. 2006 Jan;**94**(2):275-280

[84] Pogoda K, Pyszniak M, Rybojad P, Tabarkiewicz J. Monocytic myeloid-derived suppressor cells as a potent suppressor of tumor immunity in non-small cell lung cancer. Oncology Letters. 2016 Dec;**12**(6):4785-4794. DOI: 10.3892/ol.2016.5273. Epub 2016 Oct 18

[85] Shi S, Wang R, Chen Y, Song H, Chen L, Huang G. Combining antiangiogenic therapy with adoptive cell immunotherapy exerts better antitumor effects in non-small cell lung cancer models. PLoS One. 2013 Jun;**8**(6):e65757. DOI: 10.1371/journal.pone.0065757. Print 2013

[86] Nguyen LT, Ohashi PS. Clinical blockade of PD1 and LAG3--potential mechanisms of action. Nature Reviews. Immunology. 2015 Jan;**15**(1):45-56. DOI: 10.1038/nri3790

[87] Pardoll DM. The blockade of immune checkpoints in cancer immunotherapy. Nature Reviews. Cancer. 2012 Mar;**12**(4):252-264. DOI: 10.1038/nrc3239

[88] Waki K, Yamada T, Yoshiyama K, Terazaki Y, Sakamoto S, Matsueda S, Komatsu N, Sugawara S, Takamori S, Itoh K, Yamada A. PD-1 expression on peripheral blood T-cell subsets correlates with prognosis in non-small cell lung cancer. Cancer Science. 2014 Oct;**105**(10):1229-1235. DOI: 10.1111/cas.12502. Epub 2014 Sep 23

[89] Topalian SL, Drake CG, Pardoll DM. Targeting the PD-1/B7-H1(PD-L1) pathway to activate anti-tumor immunity. Current Opinion in Immunology. 2012 Apr;**24**(2):207-212. DOI: 10.1016/j.coi.2011.12.009. Epub 2012 Jan 9

[90] Hirahara K, Poholek A, Vahedi G, Laurence A, Kanno Y, Milner JD, O'Shea JJ. Mechanisms underlying helper T-cell plasticity: Implication for immune-mediated disease. The Journal of Allergy and Clinical Immunology. 2013 May;**131**(5):1276-1287

[91] Cui G, Florholmen J. Polarization of cytokine profile from Th1 into Th2 along colorectal adenoma-carcinoma sequence: Implications for the biotherapeutic target? Inflammation & Allergy—Drug Targets. 2008 Jun;**7**(2):94-97

[92] Li H, Wang C, Yu J, Cao S, Wei F, Zhang W, Han Y, Ren XB. Dendritic cell-activated cytokine-induced killer cells enhance the anti-tumor effect of chemotherapy on non-small cell lung cancer in patients after surgery. Cytotherapy. 2009;**11**(8):1076-1083

[93] Uno T, Takeda K, Kojima Y, Yoshizawa H, Akiba H, Mittler RS, Gejyo F, Okumura K, Yagita H, Smyth MJ. Eradication of established tumors in mice by a combination antibody-based therapy.Nature Medicine. 2006 Jun;**12**(6):693-698. Epub 2006 May 7

6

Targeted Photodynamic Therapy for Improved Lung Cancer Treatment

Anine Crous and Heidi Abrahamse

Abstract

Cancer develops from the outgrowth of a clonal population of cells with a genetic pathology to evade cell death and exponential proliferation. It has become a global burden with increasing mortality rates. Lung cancer is a major contributor to cancer fatalities. Conventional therapies have shown advances in treating lung cancer, but the successful eradication of cancer lies in targeting both cancer and cancer stem cells. Cancer stem cells (CSCs) are a ration of cells found within the tumour bulk, capable of cancer initiation, therapy resistance, metastasis and cancer relapse. Photodynamic therapy (PDT) has proven effective in treating lung cancer. PDT exerts selective cell death mechanisms toward cancerous cells. With the use of a photosensitizer (PS) which becomes excited upon irradiation with laser light at a specific wavelength, the PS forms reactive oxygen species (ROS) in turn killing neoplastic cells. Leading therapeutic sequel can be obtained by transcending PDT though combination therapies such as immunotherapy and nanotechnology which will enable PDT to target lung CSCs preventing lung cancer recurrence.

Keywords: lung cancer, lung cancer stem cells, PDT, targeted PDT

1. Introduction

Cancer is a global burden affecting millions of people. The yearly death toll for cancer surpasses AIDS, tuberculosis and malaria combined [1]. Cancer is characterised by mutational development of cells that lead to uncontrolled cell proliferation and tumour formation [2]. Tumours are classified according to tissue type and origin [3]. Lung cancer is one of the most frequently diagnosed diseases, having the highest fatality rate amongst all cancers [1]. Carcinoma of the lung arises due to risk factors; such as smoking, corrosive chemical inhalation and air pollution; leading to accumulated mutations of normal lung tissue. These mutations cause genetic modifications that can alter cell cycle regulation, leading to increased cell proliferation, tissue invasion, tumour formation and metastasis [4]. Lung cancer treatment options are: chemotherapy, radiation, surgery, targeted and immunotherapy [5].

It has been hypothesised that a small group of cells residing within a tumour are responsible for tumour initiation and development. These cells; called cancer stem cells (CSCs); arise from normal stem cells (SCs) that have acquired several mutations, due to their extended life span as compared to differentiated cells [6]. Dysregulation of pathways controlling SCs are seen in CSCs, which lead to exponential cell proliferation, evasion of apoptosis, infinite replication capacity, angiogenesis, metastasis and immune response evasion [7]. CSCs have been identified and characterised using various biochemical assays and techniques. Lung CSCs with tumorigenic potential have been identified [8]. They can be characterised and isolated using CSC identification methods [9, 10]. Due to the identification of CSCs in lung cancer it has become apparent to re-evaluate and develop target specific therapies for lung cancer. Evidence suggests that conventional therapies fail in complete cancer eradication due to lung CSCs and their abilities of drug efflux, treatment resistance and metastasis.

Photodynamic therapy (PDT) is a low cost, minimally invasive therapeutic model that has previously been used for lung cancer treatment. PDT uses a non-toxic photochemical dye/ photosensitizer (PS) that is administered orally or intravenously and absorbed by the cancer. The dye localises in the cellular organelles, whereby upon activation by light at a specific wavelength causes cell death [11, 12]. Even though PDT has shown many successes treating lung cancer [12], there are still some complications that need to be addressed such as photosensitivity and low tumour selectivity [13]. New advancements addressing the complications seen in PDT have been made by developing a PS that is cell specific which can target CSCs in particular by using immunoconjugates and carrier molecules in the form of antibodies (Abs) and nanoparticles (NPs), respectively.

2. Cancer

2.1. Cancer

Malignancy or cancer is a term used for diseased cells. These cells characteristically evade cell death through rapid proliferation and can metastasize by travelling through the blood and lymphatic systems invading distant tissues [14]. Collectively, cancer has more yearly fatalities than diseases such as AIDS, tuberculosis and malaria. According to the International Agency for Research on Cancer the most frequently diagnosed cancers were lung (1.8 million, 13.0% of the total), breast (1.7 million, 11.9%), and colorectal (1.4 million, 9.7%). The most prevalent cancer-related fatalities included lung (1.6 million, 19.4% of the total), liver (0.8 million, 9.1%), and stomach (0.7 million, 8.8%) malignancies. Population growth and ageing affects the cancer related outcome. By 2030, it could be expected that there would be 27 million cases of cancer, 17 million cancer deaths annually and 75 million persons living with cancer within 5 years of diagnosis [1]. Cancer arises from progressive transformation of normal cells that encounter genomic damages leading to mutations in their DNA sequence. Corruption of the DNA can be endogenous caused by errors in replication of DNA, the intrinsic chemical instability of certain DNA bases or from attack by free radicals generated during metabolism. Exogenous DNA damage can be caused by ionising radiation, UV radiation and chemical carcinogens. Although cells have the ability to repair unwanted changes in the genome, errors may occur leading to permanent mutations. Errors such as inactivation of regulatory genes maintaining genomic integrity facilitate additional mutations [15].

Tumorous cells can overpower their normal functioning neighbouring cells eventually forming a tumour as it overcomes normal regulation of cell growth leading to clonal evolution [2]. Neoplastic cells are self-sustainable, making them able to relocate to any space of the body and multiply. This is due to activation of certain enzymes, specifically telomerase, which is normally active only in SCs. Telomeres control cell death by shrinking during every mitoses until the cells eventually die. Therefore cancer cells are able to evade cell death through up regulation of telomerase as it avoids telomere shrinkage, preventing it from shortening leading to elongated telomeres. In addition, telomerase can prevent cell senescence and apoptosis [16].

Cancer classification is based on their tissue type and origin. Carcinomas encompass more than 80% of all cancer cases. These are cells that are epithelial in origin, and usually include breast, colon, prostate and lung. Carcinomas are subdivided into adenocarcinoma and squamous carcinoma [3].

2.2. Lung cancer

Lung carcinomas are neoplastic cells showing unrestrained development of mutated lung cells that are formed in the lung tissue lining the air passages. The mutated cells divide rapidly leading to tumour formation. As tumour formation progress, the numerous abnormal cells start undermining the lungs primary function preventing the lungs from providing the bloodstream with oxygen. Lung cancer can be categorised into two broad groups namely: Small cell lung cancer (SCLC), which is characterised by its neuroendocrine appearance. It encompasses 15% of lung cancer cases. Non-small cell lung cancer (NSCLC), accounts for the remaining 85% of cases. It is classified into subtypes including: adenocarcinoma (38.5%), squamous cell carcinoma (20%), and large cell carcinoma (2.9%). 52% of Patients have a 5 year expectancy when diagnosed with localised disease. Over 52% of patients with distant metastasis at diagnosis have a 5-year survival rate of 3.6% [17].

Regulatory circuits maintaining normal cell proliferation and homeostasis have defects in lung carcinoma. A multistep transformation is followed from a normal lung cell to malignant lung cancer phenotype, altered by a series of genetic and epigenetic modifications, leading to aggressive cancerous expansion. Subsequent to the primary cancer development, constant addition of genetic and epigenetic abnormalities follow during cancer proliferation, leading to tissue invasion, metastasis, and resistance to conventional therapies. Cancer prevention, early detection and treatment rely on the identification and characterisation of these molecular changes. Information on tumour characteristics and genetics will significantly advance prognosis and ideal treatment selection [18].

Contributing carcinogenic risk factors for lung cancer include: smoking, passive smoking and radon; occupational exposures such as asbestos; inhalation of corrosive chemicals like cadmium, silica and vinyl chloride; and long-term and accumulated exposure to air pollution. Lung cancer can also be congenital, where family history of lung cancer increases the risk of development [4].

Therapeutic modalities for NSCLC include: surgery, radiofrequency ablation (RFA), radiation therapy, chemotherapy, targeted therapies and immunotherapy. Therapeutic options depend on the cancer stage, patient's health and lung function and cancer characteristics. Treatments used for SCLC include: chemotherapy, radiation, surgery and palliative care. Surgery is less likely to be a primary treatment for SCLC as by the time diagnoses are made it would have metastasised [5].

3. Cancer stem cells

3.1. The CSC hypothesis

It is hypothesised that tumour development and progression is maintained by a small subset of cancer cells having SC characteristics. These CSCs are capable of self-renewal and differentiation, playing a significant role in malignant proliferation, invasion, metastasis, and tumour recurrence. Cancer cells have accumulated several mutations during their cell cycle, acquiring significant characteristics called the hallmarks of cancer. These specific traits include evasion of growth signalling pathways impeding proliferation, anti-apoptotic functions, infinite replication capacity, angiogenesis and metastasis with distant organ invasion, as well as immune response evasion. In order for a cell to acquire these mutations, its cell cycle needs to be longer than that of somatic cells. Cells that are maintained throughout an organism's lifespan are adult SCs, making them susceptible to neoplastic conversion [19]. SCs divide either symmetrically producing two daughter SCs, or asymmetrically producing one progenitor and one SC, having the ability to differentiate into multiple cell types while self-renewing and overcome senescence [6].

Dysregulation of the pathways maintaining SC function can lead to uncontrolled cell division and differentiation leading to CSC formation and tumour progenitors [7]. A major pathway involved in cell cycle proliferation and arrest is Wnt-β-catenin, which promotes SC renewal by signalling transcription genes. [20]. SC self-renewal is regulated by Notch signalling [21]. The Sonic Hedgehog (Shh) pathway promotes SC proliferation, activating various SCs [7]. Studies have found that these signalling pathways are not always activated in normal SCs but rather in CSCs where the genetic programs governing self-renewal are stimulated in SCs when the need for rejuvenation and repair arises where as in CSCs it is differentially active [22].

3.2. CSC identification and characterisation

Improved identification and isolation of CSCs will lead to enhanced studies on CSCs and targeted therapies. To date, various methods have been implicated in this regard, having different levels of success in common malignancies [23].

First identification of CSCs where made by Bonnet and Dick in 1997, who identified an arrangement of stem like cells that simulated the normal hierarchy of haematopoietic SCs. They identified rare carcinogenic cells in human acute myeloid leukaemia (AML) that was able to repopulate the entire original disease over serial transplantations. The subpopulation characterised by CD34 +ve and CD38 −ve had the capacity to self-renew and differentiate [24]. This study formed the basis for CSC research in both hematologic malignancies and solid tumours. Breast CSCs from a solid tumour was first identified by Al-Hajj et al., using CD44 and CD24 markers [25]. Since then, CSCs have been identified in a variety of solid tumours, including lung cancer [26, 27]. Common characteristics from these different tumour types are shared between the isolated CSCs. Characteristics include drug resistance, propagation of tumours, and asymmetric division. CSCs can be isolated and characterised by means of the following methodologies: isolation using CSC-specific cell surface markers by flow cytometry [28]; detection of side-population (SP) phenotypes by Hoechst 33,342 exclusion [29]; assessment of aldehyde dehydrogenase (ALDH) activity [30]; characterisation by tumourigenicity evaluation [31] and stem-ness gene expression and transcriptional factors [32].

3.3. Lung CSCs

Lung cancer's ability to recur, regardless of putative treatment, proposes that a small population of the disease contain the capacity for self-renewal and regeneration. This sub/side population (SP) of CSCs portray tumorigenic potential. With therapeutic targeting, treatments may have the potential to eliminate tumour recurrence [8].

The lung being highly compartmentalised, have led to various epithelial cell types being labelled as presumed lung precursors due to their stem/progenitor cell-like responses to injury. The behaviours and characteristics of these cells also include repopulation of injured tissue. Cell type AEC2 have been characterised as a limited, epithelial progenitor for the alveolus, as they are said to be the progenitor of AEC1, which is involved in gas exchange in the alveolus. Studies have indicated that the bronchio-alveolar stem cell (BASC) a less differentiated cell located in the bronchio-alveolar duct junction act as an injury-responsive, limited progenitor for the distal airway-alveolar epithelium. BASCs have been implicated in lung cancer tumour genesis due to their overexpression of oncogenic K-ras and rapid proliferation by K-ras signalling. Clara cell and AEC2 markers are found in tumour formation of BASCs that have been expressing long term activation of K-ras, both Clara cell secretory protein (CCSP) and surfactant protein C (SP-C) have been identified respectively. Studies have indicated that cancer cells portraying a distinctive combination of the clara cell and AEC2 markers present in BASCs can be isolated from lung tumours. Supporting evidence shows that BASCs constituting of these double positive tumorigenic cells may be responsible for adenocarcinoma development. Along with BASCs and AEC2 being exceedingly receptive to proliferative stimuli, they show resistance to cell damage and injury by expanding within the epithelium following lung tissue damage and repair. These characteristics are critical for both normal tissue and CSCs. As injury resistance of these cells in lung cancer, could serve as a stem cell-like reservoir for generating additional tumours [19].

Lung CSCs can phenotypically be identified and characterised using CSC identification methods. One such method includes the SP phenotyping where efflux of Hoechst 33,342 dye is measured due to the differential ability of the cancer cells imparted by the ATP-binding cassette family of transporter proteins present on the cellular membrane [9]. Increased ALDH activity is connected to cellular drug resistance, through detoxification of cytotoxic agents and oxidation of retinol to retinoic acid. It is also involved in early SC development and can be used as a reliable CSC marker [8].

Lung CSCs can also be tested for up regulation of SC genes. In a study conducted by Zakaria et al. they investigated CSCs isolated from lung cancer cell lines expressing SC transcription factors Sox2, Oct 3/4, Nanog, c-Myc, and Klf4. Gene expression in the lung CSCs were compared to the expression levels in normal SCs (PHBEC). Sox2, Oct4, c-Myc, and Klf4 were all detected and up-regulated in the CSCs. Currently, specific cell surface markers derived from the surface markers known to be present on normal haematopoietic or embryonic SCs are used to identify and isolate CSCs. For lung CSCs, CD133, CD166, EpCAM, CD90, and CD44 have been used as markers [10].

4. Photodynamic therapy

4.1. Fundamentals of PDT

PDT is a low cost, clinically approved, minimally invasive therapeutic procedure that can exert selective cytotoxic activity toward malignant cells. The procedure involves administration of a photosensitizing agent followed by irradiation at a wavelength corresponding to an absorbance band of the PS. In the presence of oxygen, a series of events lead to direct tumour cell death, damage to the microvasculature and induction of a local inflammatory reaction [11].

Molecular oxygen (O_2) is the terminal electron acceptor of the mitochondrial electron transport chain performing aerobic respiration. In the mitochondrion oxygen serves as an electron acceptor [33]. During PDT a photochemical reaction uses the free O_2, generating a highly reactive product termed singlet oxygen ($^1O_2$) and reactive oxygen species (ROS) which can rapidly cause significant toxicity leading to cell death via apoptosis or necrosis. Ground state/molecular oxygen has two unpaired electrons residing separately in the outermost antibonding orbitals. Depending on the electron configuration there are three possible states for O_2, the ground state of oxygen is called a triplet state $^3O_2$. Singlet oxygen is produced when undergoing photo-oxygenation, by inverting the spin of one of the outermost electrons (**Figure 1**). This type of oxygen is highly reactive and is the predominant cytotoxic agent produced during PDT [34].

A PS or photosensitizing agent is a chemical compound that can be excited by monochromatic light having a specific wavelength matched to an absorption peak of the administered compound. The excited PS subsequently transfers energy to a chosen reactant. This is commonly molecular oxygen [35, 36]. PSs commonly used in cancer are based on the tetra-pyrrole backbone simulating protoporphyrin found in haemoglobin. Naturally occurring tetra-pyrrol structures are found in haem (porphyrins), chlorophyll and bacteriochlorophyll. Synthetically synthesised tetra-pyrroles include phthalocyanines. As pyrrole-ring double bonds are successively reduced starting in porphyrins and going to chlorins and bacteriochlorins, the Q-band

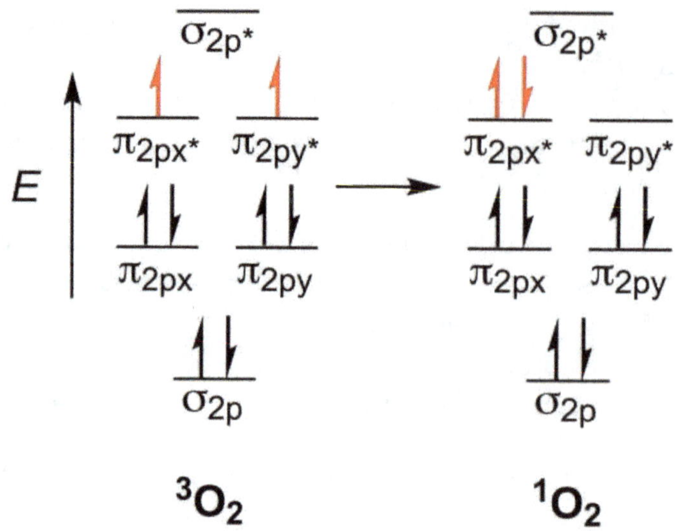

Figure 1. Molecular orbital diagrams showing the electron distribution in triplet and singlet oxygen [34].

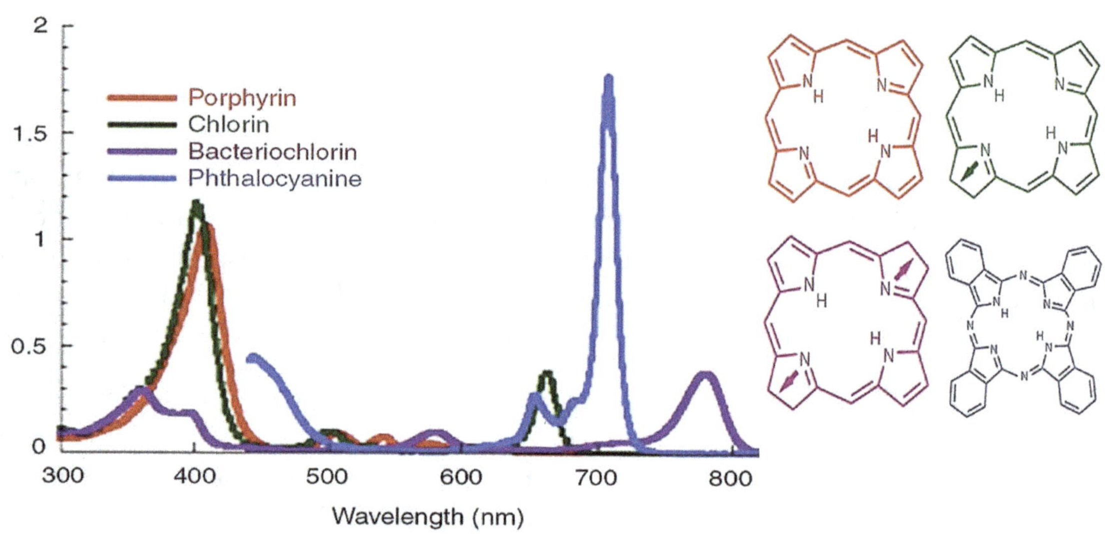

Figure 2. Tetrapyrrole absorption spectra showing porphyrins, chlorins, bacteriochlorins, and phthalocyanines [37].

moves to longer wavelengths and increases in size as seen in **Figure 2** [37]. Indicating that the structure of the PS has an influence on absorbance bands.

Efficient PSs should have a strong absorbance peak ranging from 600 to 800 nm in the deep-red to near-infrared (NIR) spectral region, which will allow for tissue penetration, as penetration tend to increase with wavelength. However, wavelengths longer than NIR are avoided, due to having a lower frequency and delivering too little energy for sufficient oxygen excitation. Ideally a PS should have suitable photo-physical characteristics. It should have a high-quantum yield of triplet formation ($\Phi T \geq 0.5$), a high singlet oxygen quantum yield ($\Phi\Delta \geq 0.5$), a relatively long triplet state lifetime (τT, μs range), and a high triplet-state energy (≥94 kJ mol^{-1}). Low dark toxicity and negligible cytotoxicity in the absence of light. Preferential accumulation in diseased/target tissue over healthy tissue. Rapid clearance from the body post-procedure, to decrease side effects. High chemical stability: single, well-characterised compounds, with a known and constant composition. Soluble in biological media as effective PSs tend to be relatively hydrophobic compounds that rapidly diffuse into tumour cells and localise in intracellular membrane structures such as mitochondria and endoplasmic reticulum (ER). It should produce a marked inflammatory response via apoptosis, causing an immunogenic effect against cancerous cells [36, 38].

Light source and light delivery are fundamental aspects in PDT. The light source depends on tumour location and the PS used. To date visible light ranging from 400 to 900 nm has been used in PDT. It has been noted that longer wavelengths in the visible red spectrum ranging between 600 and 810 nm are preferred due to optimum tissue penetration as well as PS structure mediating the use of red-shifted light. Historically PDT depended on low intensity lasers for a light source due to their valuable characteristics of monochromaticity, coherence, directionality and low power output (<100 mW), which removes the variable of heat that might have an influence on PDT. Lasers emit narrow beams of intense electromagnetic radiation that is monochromatic giving access to the wavelength region for excitation of PSs [37]. Coherence and directionality is correlated to the laser beams' divergence property. This is a qualitative measure of the laser irradiation to remain concentrated over a distance. Another important factor in choosing the light source is the fact that tissues have various optical properties depending on their bio-components. Tissue can both absorb and scatter visible light, this tend to decrease as the wavelength used increases [39].

4.2. Mechanisms of PDT

Three fundamental components act simultaneously in PDT (**Figure 3**): molecular oxygen, a light source and a PS. None of these is individually toxic.

During PDT, when a PS is absorbed it is still in its ground singlet state. A PS reaches its first excited singlet state through wavelength specific light activation. This first excited singlet state is unstable and can either deteriorate through energy loss by emitting fluorescence or, it can reach its excited triplet state accomplished through intersystem crossing of molecular oxygen, which is long lived and more stable [40] (**Figure 4**). In solution, intersystem crossing is increased by the probability of the presence of paramagnetic species such as molecular oxygen. When the PS reaches its excited triplet state it can follow two pathways. These pathways are named Type I and Type II reactions.

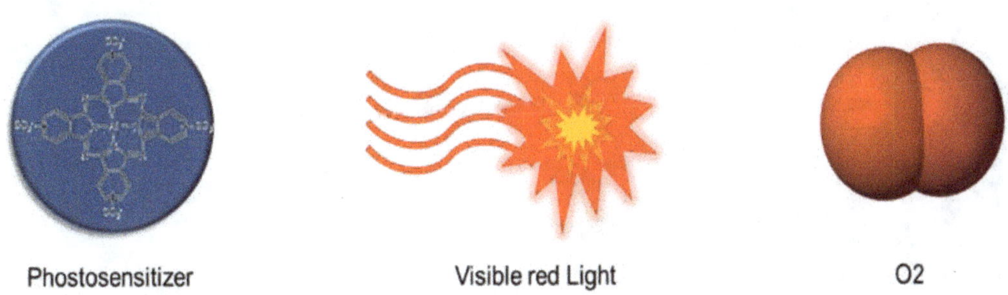

Figure 3. Fundamental components of PDT.

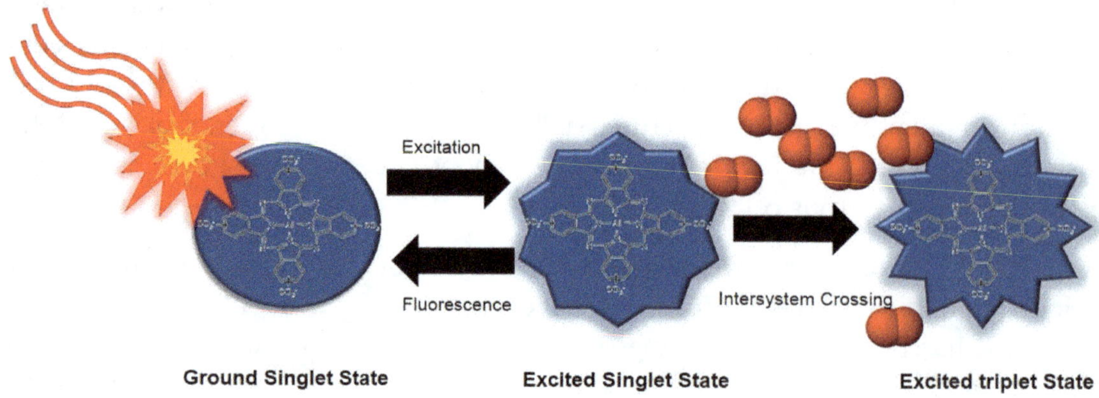

Figure 4. Activation of a PS in its ground singlet state to its excited triplet state via light activation and intersystem crossing with molecular oxygen.

Type I reactions generate ROS, whereby adjacent biomolecules (i.e. lipids, proteins, and nucleic acids) and the PS in its excited triplet state undergoes an acid-base reaction transferring hydrogen ions. Depending on the target molecule, i.e. lipids, proteins, or nucleic acids, free radicals and radical ions are generated that then react with oxygen forming ROS [41] (**Figure 5**).

Type II reactions are based on a phenomenon called triplet–triplet annihilation. This involves the production of highly reactive singlet oxygen which is also extremely cytotoxic. Singlet oxygen is generated through the PS in its excited triplet state reacting with ground state molecular oxygen [41] (**Figure 6**).

Type I and II reactions happen simultaneously. The oxygen species generated between the two reactions depend on the components, i.e., the PS and amount of oxygen available to react with as well as PS localization in the biomolecules. Type II is considered the primary mechanism of cell death due to singlet oxygen generation. ROS and singlet oxygen have a high reactivity and short half-life, affecting only the biomolecules the PS had localised in or are close to the region where these species are generated, usually within a 20 nm radius. PS localization promotes selective sensitization and is therefore a primary factor in drug release studies to target tissues [41].

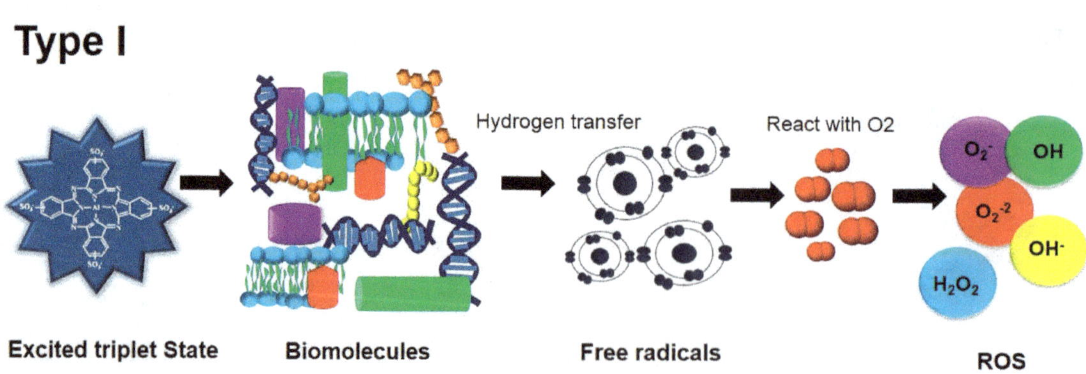

Figure 5. Type I reaction in PDT.

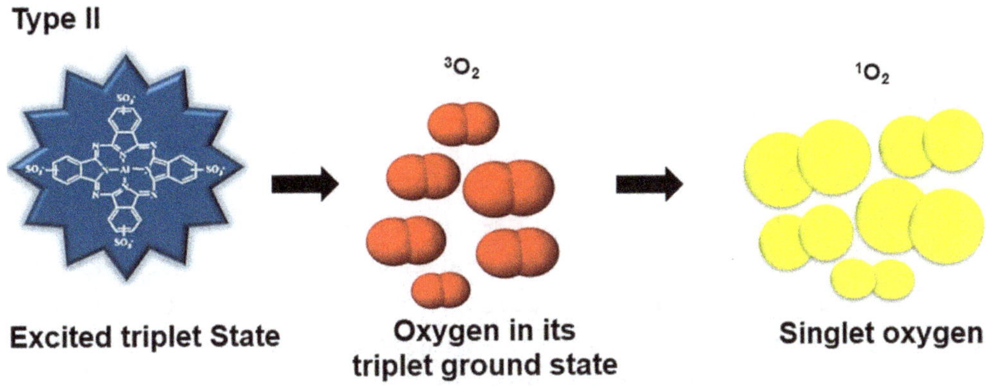

Figure 6. Type II reaction in PDT.

4.3. PDT and lung cancer

Currently PDT, alone or as an adjunct therapy is increasingly being used to treat thoracic malignancies. Effects exerted include both apoptosis and necrosis, damage to tumour vasculature as well as inducing an inflammatory reaction. It does not lose efficacy with repeated treatments and allow for combination treatment [42].

Porfimer sodium is the PS most commonly used to treat lung and other thoracic malignancies. It has been approved by the US Food and Drug Administration (FDA) for cases of NSCLC where standard therapies are not appropriate and to palliate symptoms from airway obstruction [43]. It is also reported to be a safe and effective neoadjuvant treatment, where it has been reported to significantly decrease tumour size, convert tumour operability and improve complete surgical resection [12]. Over the past decade, prospective clinical studies evaluated a variety of PSs, in treating early and advanced stage NSCLC. Early-stage disease had a complete response range from 72% to an impressive 94 and 100%. Advanced disease, local control and partial response ranged from 78 to 100%, respectively [12]. Key indications for the use of PDT to treat lung cancer include: Intraoperative PDT by transthoracic or thoracoscopic irradiation after tumour resection and complete removal of the macroscopic disease, where the margins in the surgical bed are illuminated before wound closure to treat undetected viable cancer cells, which could lead to a reduction in local recurrence [44]. Interstitial PDT, where intra-tumor light delivery is required to activate the PS, using image guidance and treatment planning, when the tumour is deep-seated and larger than 1 cm [45]. Definitive PDT treatment where indication includes early stage, superficial, and centrally located endobronchial NSCLC tumours, where the treatment option used is admittance of the PS and activation through bronchoscopic irradiation [12].

PDT has shown to be a safe and minimally invasive therapy designed as an anti-cancer drug, but still have room for improvement. Current PSs lack sufficient tumour selectivity which may result in uptake of the PS in non-cancerous tissue that can lead to adverse effects [46]. Another major trial in medicine today is drug delivery, this includes PDT. When administering a PS it is taken up by the blood and lymphatic systems, which can lead to photosensitivity [13].

5. Targeted PDT

5.1. Immunotherapy and PDT

Photoimmunotherapy (PIT) actively and specifically targets antigens via monoclonal antibodies (MAb) or antibody fragments (AbFs) used for drug delivery. PIT uses a PS conjugated to an Ab against a tumour, tumour associated (e.g. CSC) or tumour vasculature antigen [47]. Some of the advantages seen in PIT, compared to conventional cancer treatment such as chemotherapy/chemo-immunotherapy, is that during laser activation of the Ab-PS conjugate there is cell specific cytotoxicity of cancerous cells sparing the surrounding healthy tissue. Additionally PIT is neither immunosuppressive nor does it have an affinity for rapidly dividing cells, making it less likely to develop treatment induced resistance due to neoplastic cells up regulating alternative or circumventive pathways commonly seen in chemotherapy [48].

PIT has shown to be effective in various studies conducted on cancer using a variety of MAbs. This includes a study conducted by Savellano et al., where they conjugated a clinically approved benzoporphyrin derivative (verteporfin) to the anti-EGFR MAb cetuximab. Results showed that conjugated verteporfin had an affinity for EGFR-overexpressing A431 epidermal carcinoma and ovarian cancer cells, killing them via PDT mediated mechanisms, whereas free verteporfin exhibited no specificity [49]. In another PIT study they explored the effectiveness of PIT on metastatic lung carcinoma *in vitro* and *in vivo* using a mouse model. IRDye700DX is a silica-phthalocyanine dye that is extremely hydrophilic. It has an excitation wavelength of 690 nm which is NIR, allowing for enhanced tumour penetration of light. IR700 conjugated to MAbs showed *in vitro* results of target cell specificity with little to no toxic effects on non-target adjacent tissue. Targeted cells demonstrated cell membrane rupture within minutes of exposure to NIR-light activating the Ab-PS conjugate [50, 51]. *In vivo* experiments using trastuzumab-IR700 was used to treat early-stage lung metastases in a murine model. Results indicated specific binding, rapid induction of necrotic cell death, target specific cell death and prevented metastasis by target-specificity [52].

5.2. Nanomedicine and PDT

NPs are biomolecules synthesised for drug delivery and is used in nanomedicine today. Incorporating nanostructured drug delivery systems of PSs conjugated to NPs may have advantages that include improvement of transcytosis across epithelial and endothelial barriers, optimise delivery of low water soluble PSs and co-delivery of PSs into cells [41]. Other advantages of using PS-NP conjugates are defence against enzymatic degradation, controlled PS release into cancer cells, its small size allow for cellular penetration, NPs are biocompatible and photos table [53]. NPs can be classified according to their composition, morphology or structure [54]. Covalently binding the PS to the NP can enhance delivery of the PS to cancerous cells, as well as increase singlet oxygen production [37].

NPs are susceptible to engulfing by macrophages after intravenous administration. This can be overcome by polyethylene glycol (PEG) coating, enhancing bloodstream circulation time and allowing for tumour accumulation. Studies have showed encouraging results for the use of PS-NP conjugates, whereby different compositions of NPs have been proposed [55]. One such study indicated that the use of dendrimer phthalocyanine (DPc)-encapsulated non active polymeric micelles have been successfully used both *in vivo* and *in vitro* treating human and subcutaneous mouse lung adenocarcinoma A549. Both experimental systems had a significant increase in PS-NP conjugate PDT efficiency as compared to PDT alone, where mitochondrial localization was observed [56]. Another method of enhancing PDT is by improving on the conjugation methods for PSs and NPs. Instead of using PS-NP encapsulation, PS-NP conjugation can be achieved through covalent binding [57]. One NP in particular that can be applied by covalent bonding of PSs to its surface is gold-NPs (Au-NPs). Au-NPs has enhanced surface-plasmon resonance (SPR) effects due to the non-linear optical fields found in metal NPs being very close [58]. Au-NPs have good biocompatibility, versatile surfaces, and unique optical properties [59], whereby their optical field can be enhanced by the SPR by changing the shape of the NP specifically to a ring [60]. Studies have conjugated Au-NPs to Abs, for specific cell surface receptor targeting, in anti-cancer treatments whereby the use of NIR-light produced photo-thermal heat destruction. Results showed a significant increase in apoptosis induction as compared to unconjugated NPs [61]. A drawback in using Ab-NP conjugates alone for cancer treatment was that to induce photo-thermal heat destruction a high power density laser had to be used. This led to unselective damage of normal tissue in the laser path surrounding the target of interest [62]. However, cancer cell death induction using TPDT requires low power lasers that are efficient in activating the PS avoiding destruction of normal tissue. Coating the NP with polyethylene glycol (PEG) have also enhanced conventional methods of Ab conjugation to NPs that led to poor orientation of the functional group of the Ab. NP PEGylation allows for covalent attachment of an Ab to the outer end of the PEG chain, thus maintaining availability of Ab binding sites to cell surface receptors. Studies using this method of Ab conjugation showed efficient internalisation into cancerous cells [63, 64]. TPDT involves

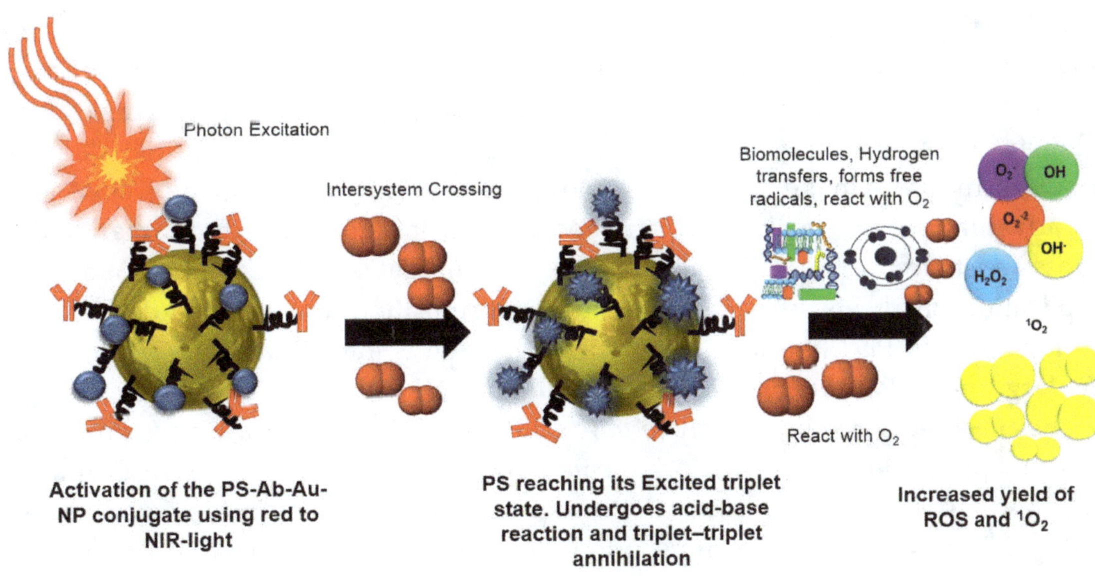

Figure 7. TPDT using a PS-Ab-Au-NP (PEG) conjugate.

the use of either/both an Ab or NP conjugated to a PS. The mechanisms still follow Type I and Type II reactions (**Figure 7**).

6. Conclusion

Despite intensive research and development of therapies, lung cancer still remains a primary contributor to cancer related deaths, with survival rates of patients diagnosed being dismal. Prompt diagnosis and effective treatment will radically improve patient outcome. Due to late diagnoses of lung cancer, conventional therapies show to be ineffective [18]. Lung cancer initiation and progression mechanisms have been identified that will be able to drive future research on molecular and biological targets. Conventional therapies are limited by drug resistance. Characterising and evaluating the mechanisms as well as lung CSCs leading to the acquisition of drug evasion, can aid in the development of therapies that will combat therapeutic resistance [65].

According to the CSC hypothesis, these cells are involved in tumorigenesis. This is because of their stem-cell like abilities that include indefinite self-renewal, slow replication, intrinsic resistance to chemotherapy and radiotherapy, and an ability to give rise to differentiated progeny. Studies have been able to identify CSCs in various cancers, including lung. Lung CSCs have been phenotypically identified using bio-markers typically expressed by normal SCs. Some of the markers include CD133, CD166, CD44 and ALDH1. Molecular pathways regulating SC proliferation, differentiation, and apoptosis are found to be active in CSCs as well, all giving rise to CSCs unique capability of drug evasion and metastasis or cancer relapse [66]. Due to conventional therapeutic strategies only targeting rapidly dividing cells destroying the bulk of the tumour, complete eradication of rare CSCs also need to be addressed. Therapies that aim to identify CSCs and overcome drug resistance due to CSCs having increased levels of efflux pumps need to be developed [27].

A potential therapy that can be advanced to treat CSCs is PDT. PDT involves the use of a nontoxic PS that localises in cellular organelles and when activated using light of a specific wavelength, reacts with oxygen to form free radicals leading to cell death. PSs have an affinity for malignant cells, inducing apoptosis via caspase reactions, mitochondrial damage and cytochrome c release. Unlike chemo and radiation inducing cell death via DNA damage. Another advantage of PDT is that cells that become resistant to chemo and radiation does not cause cross-resistance to PDT and there is no toxic accumulation [67]. Several modes of clinical PDT application has been defined, pertaining to localization and tumour density, as these factors play a role in PDT efficacy. One mode of concern is interstitial PDT, which is used on tumours larger than 1 cm in size [45]. This mode of PDT which is indicated for multicellular tumours has been explored previously *in vitro*. The efficacy of PDT concerning a monolayer as compared to multicellular spheroids indicated that spheroids are more resistant to PDT, however this can be overcome using a dose dependent manner of inducing cell death [68]. Although PDT has successfully been used to treat lung cancer a major pitfall still include low tumour selectivity, especially in a scenario where the lung cancer's genomics are predisposed to malignant metastatic tumours [42].

PIT uses a PS conjugated to and Ab allowing for cell specific cytotoxicity and does not develop treatment induced resistance. Interest has grown in the biomedical field for the use of NPs as a drug delivery vehicle specifically Au-NPs, due to their biocompatibility, high surface area and functionalized facile surface supporting self-assembly of thiolates [69]. Au-NPs can be synthesised to a structure supporting absorption in the far red to NIR wavelength. The combination of using an Ab-NP conjugate allows for all the significant contributions and advantages to be applied in one treatment, TPDT, having improved cell specific targeting as well as allowing significant accumulation of PS in the tumour site by using Abs to direct the PS to CSC specific markers for example, and NPs enhancing PS uptake that can increase singlet oxygen yield and effective cancer/ CSC death. Results indicate that TPDT might prove to be a promising treatment modality for lung cancer and targeting lung CSCs. As TPDT can be used as a primary or adjuvant therapy for lung cancer depending on the morphological state and tumour localization. Targeted PDT can lead to complete cancer eradication and prevent cancer relapse by destroying the bulk of the tumour as well as targeting the underlying CSCs. Improving the overall survival rate of patients diagnosed with lung cancer as well as increase quality of life through minimal side effects when receiving treatment.

Acknowledgements

This work is based on the research supported by the South African Research Chairs Initiative of the Department of Science and Technology and National Research Foundation of South Africa (Grant No 98337). The authors sincerely thank the University of Johannesburg, the National Laser Centre and the National Research Foundation of South Africa (CSIR-DST) for their financial grant support.

Conflict of interest

The material in this paper, submitted to *InTechOpen* is original work from the author and is not being considered elsewhere for publication. The authors indicate no potential conflict of interest.

Author details

Anine Crous and Heidi Abrahamse*

*Address all correspondence to: habrahamse@uj.ac.za

University of Johannesburg, Gauteng, South Africa

References

[1] CANSA. Research Findings. Global Cancer Statistics [Internet]. 2017. Available from: http://www.cansa.org.za/global-cancer-statistics/ [Accessed: March 13, 2018]

[2] Martinez JD, Parker MT, Fultz KE, Ignatenko NA, Gerner EW. Molecular biology of cancer. Chemotherapeutic agents. In: Abraham DJ, editor. Burger's Medicinal Chemistry and Drug Discovery. 6th ed. Hoboken, NJ: John Wiley & Son Inc; 2003. pp. 1-50

[3] SEER Training Modules. Cancer Classification. US National Institutes of Health. National Cancer Institute [Internet]. Available from: https://training.seer.cancer.gov/disease/categories/classification.html [Accessed: March 13, 2018]

[4] Zappa C, Mousa SA. Non-small cell lung cancer: Current treatment and future advances. Translational Lung Cancer Research. 2016;**5**(3):288-300. DOI: 10.21037/tlcr.2016.06.07

[5] American Cancer Society. Treating Non-Small Cell Lung Cancer [Internet]. 2016. Available from: https://www.cancer.org/cancer/non-small-cell-lung-cancer/treating/by-stage.html [Accessed: March 20, 2018]

[6] Brummendorf TH, Dragowska W, Zijlmans JMJM, Thornbury G, Lansdorp PM. Asymmetric cell divisions sustain long-term hematopoiesis from single-sorted human fetal liver cells. The Journal of Experimental Medicine. 1998;**188**(6):1117-1124

[7] Zhang PY, Yang YJ, Xue Y, Fu J, Zhang CX, Wang Y, Yang Y, Shi H. Cancer stem cells: Targeting tumors at the source. European Review for Medical and Pharmacological Sciences. 2015;**19**(10):1821-1828

[8] Alamgeer M, Peacock CD, Matsui W, Ganju V, Watkins DN. Cancer stem cells in lung cancer: Evidence and controversies. Respirology. 2013;**18**(5):757-764. DOI: 10.1111/resp.12094

[9] Goodell MA, Brose K, Paradis G, et al. Isolation and functional properties of murine hematopoietic stem cells that are replicating in vivo. The Journal of Experimental Medicine. 1996;**183**:1797-1806

[10] Zakaria N, Yusoff NM, Zakaria Z, Lim MN, Baharuddin PJ, Fakiruddin KS, Yahaya B. Human non-small cell lung cancer expresses putative cancer stem cell markers and exhibits the transcriptomic profile of multipotent cells. BMC Cancer. 2015;**15**:84. DOI: 10.1186/s12885-015-1086-3

[11] Agostinis P, Berg K, Cengel KA, Foster TH, Girotti AW, Gollnick SO, Hahn SM, Hamblin MR, Juzeniene A, Kessel D, Korbelik M, Moan J, Mroz P, Nowis D, Piette J, Wilson BC, Golab J. Photodynamic therapy of cancer: An update. CA: A Cancer Journal for Clinicians. 2011;**61**(4):250-281. DOI: 10.3322/caac.20114

[12] Shafirstein G, Battoo A, Harris K, Baumann H, Gollnick SO, Lindenmann J, Nwogu CE. Photodynamic therapy of non-small cell lung cancer. Narrative review and future directions. Annals of the American Thoracic Society. 2016;**13**(2):265-275. DOI: 10.1513/AnnalsATS.201509-650FR

[13] Bellnier DA, Greco WR, Nava H, Loewen GM, Oseroff AR, Dougherty TJ. Mild skin photosensitivity in cancer patients following injection of photochlor (2-[1-hexyloxyethyl]-2-devinyl pyropheophorbide-a; HPPH) for photodynamic therapy. Cancer Chemotherapy and Pharmacology. 2006;**57**:40-45

[14] NCI Dictionary of Cancer Terms. Malignancy [Internet]. Available from: https://www.cancer.gov/publications/dictionaries/cancer-terms/def/malignancy [Accessed: March 01, 2018]

[15] Bertram JS. The molecular biology of cancer. Molecular Aspects of Medicine. 2000;**21**(6): 167-223

[16] Willeit P, Willeit J, Mayr A, Weger S, Oberhollenzer F, Brandstätter A, Kronenberg F, Kiechl S. Telomere length and risk of incident cancer and cancer mortality. The Journal of the American Medical Association. 2010;**304**(1):69-75

[17] Dela Cruz CS, Tanoue LT, Matthay RA. Lung cancer: Epidemiology, etiology, and prevention. Clinics in Chest Medicine. 2011;**32**(4). DOI: 10.1016/j.ccm.2011.09.001

[18] Lemjabbar-Alaoui H, Hassan O, Yang Y-W, Buchanan P. Lung cancer: Biology and treatment options. Biochimica et Biophysica Acta. 2015;**1856**(2):189-210. DOI: 10.1016/j.bbcan.2015.08.002

[19] Lundin A, Driscoll B. Lung cancer stem cells: Progress and prospects. Cancer Letters. 2013; **338**(1):89-93. DOI: 10.1016/j.canlet.2012.08.014

[20] Gedaly R, Galuppo R, Daily MF, Shah M, Maynard E, Chen C, Zhang X, Esser KA, Cohen DA, Evers BM, Jiang J, Spear BT. Targeting the Wnt/β-catenin signaling pathway in liver cancer stem cells and hepatocellular carcinoma cell lines with FH535. PLoS One. 2014;**9**(6): e99272. DOI: 10.1371/journal.pone.0099272

[21] Chiang M, Shestova O, Xu L, Aster J, Pear W. Divergent effects of supraphysiologic notch signals on leukemia stem cells and hematopoietic stem cells. Blood. 2013;**121**:905-917

[22] Visvader JE, Lindeman GJ. Cancer stem cells: Current status and evolving complexities. Cell Stem Cell. 2012;**10**(6):717-728. DOI: 10.1016/j.stem.2012.05.007

[23] Tirino V, Desiderio V, Paino F, De Rosa A, Papaccio F, La Noce M, Laino L, De Francesco F, Papaccio G. Cancer stem cells in solid tumors: An overview and new approaches for their isolation and characterization. The FASEB Journal. 2013;**27**(1):13-24. DOI: 10.1096/fj.12-218222

[24] Bonnet D, Dick JE. Human acute myeloid leukemia is organized as a hierarchy that originates from a primitive hematopoietic cell. Nature Medicine. 1997;**3**(7):730-737

[25] Al-Hajj M, Wicha MS, Benito-Hernandez A, Morrison SJ, Clarke MF. Prospective identification of tumorigenic breast cancer cells. Proceedings of the National Academy of Sciences of the United States of America. 2003;**100**(7):3983-3988

[26] Eramo A, Lotti F, Sette G, Pilozzi E, Biffoni M, Di Virgilio A, Conticello C, Ruco L, Peschle C, De Maria R. Identification and expansion of the tumorigenic lung cancer stem cell population. Cell Death and Differentiation. 2008;**15**(3):504-514. DOI: 10.1038/sj.cdd.4402283

[27] Tirino V, Camerlingo R, Franco R, Malanga D, La Rocca A, Viglietto G, Rocco G, Pirozzi G. The role of CD133 in the identification and characterisation of tumour-initiating cells in non-small-cell lung cancer. European Journal of Cardio-Thoracic Surgery. 2009;**36**(3):446-453. DOI: 10.1016/j.ejcts.2009.03.063

[28] Tirino V, Desiderio V, d'Aquino R, De Francesco F, Pirozzi G, Graziano A, Galderisi U, Cavaliere C, De Rosa A, Papaccio G, Giordano A. Detection and characterization of CD133+ cancer stem cells in human solid tumours. PLoS One. 2008;**3**(10):e3469. DOI: 10.1371/journal.pone.0003469

[29] Moserle L, Indraccolo S, Ghisi M, Frasson C, Fortunato E, Canevari S, Miotti S, Tosello V, Zamarchi R, Corradin A, Minuzzo S, Rossi E, Basso G, Amadori A. The side population of ovarian cancer cells is a primary target of IFN-alpha antitumor effects. Cancer Research. 2008;**68**(14):5658-5668. DOI: 10.1158/0008-5472.CAN-07-6341

[30] Awad O, Yustein JT, Shah P, Gul N, Katuri V, O'Neill A, Kong Y, Brown ML, Toretsky JA, Loeb DM. High ALDH activity identifies chemotherapy-resistant Ewing's sarcoma stem cells that retain sensitivity to EWS-FLI1 inhibition. PLoS One. 2010;**5**(11):e13943. DOI: 10.1371/journal.pone.0013943

[31] Rosen JM, Jordan CT. The increasing complexity of the cancer stem cell paradigm. Science. 2009;**324**(5935):1670-1673. DOI: 10.1126/science.1171837

[32] Chambers I. The molecular basis of pluripotency in mouse embryonic stem cells. Cloning and Stem Cells. 2004;**6**:386-339

[33] van Boxel GI, Doherty WL, Parmar M. Cellular oxygen utilization in health and sepsis. Continuing Education in Anaesthesia Critical Care & Pain. 2012;**12**(4):207-212. DOI: 10.1093/bjaceaccp/mks023

[34] Macdonald IJ, Dougherty TJ. Basic principles of photodynamic therapy. Journal of Porphyrins and Phthalocyanines. 2001;**5**:105-129

[35] Chemical Entities of Biological Interest (ChEBI). Photosensitizing Agent [Internet]. 2016. Available from: https://www.ebi.ac.uk/chebi/chebiOntology.do?chebiId=CHEBI:47868 [Accessed: April 04, 2018]

[36] Bown SG. Photodynamic therapy for photochemists. Philosophical Transactions. Series A, Mathematical, Physical, and Engineering Sciences. 2013;**371**(1995):20120371. DOI: 10.1098/rsta.2012.0371

[37] Kashef N, Huang Y, Hamblin MR. Advances in antimicrobial photodynamic inactivation at the nanoscale. Nano. 2017;**6**(5):853-879. DOI: 10.1515/nanoph-2016-0189

[38] Abrahamse H, Hamblin MR. New photosensitizers for photodynamic therapy. Biochemical Journal. 2016;**473**(4):347-364. DOI: 10.1042/BJ20150942

[39] Jacques SL. Optical properties of biological tissues: A review. Physics in Medicine and Biology. 2013;**58**:R37-R61

[40] Muehlmann LA, Joanitti GA, Silva JR, Longo JP, Azevedo RB. Liposomal photosensitizers: Potential platforms for anticancer photodynamic therapy. Brazilian Journal of Medical and Biological Research. 2011;**44**(8):729-737

[41] Calixto GM, Bernegossi J, de Freitas LM, Fontana CR, Chorilli M. Nanotechnology-based drug delivery systems for photodynamic therapy of cancer: A review. Molecules. 2016; **21**(3):342. DOI: 10.3390/molecules21030342

[42] Simone CB II, Cengel KA. Photodynamic therapy for lung cancer and malignant pleural mesothelioma. Seminars in Oncology. 2014;**41**:820-830. DOI: 10.1053/j.seminoncol.2014.09.017

[43] Federal Drug Administration. Medical Devices. [Internet]. 2014. Available from: http://www.fda.gov/Medical Devices/default.htm [Accessed: May 04, 2018]

[44] Friedberg JS, Mick R, Stevenson JP, Zhu T, Busch TM, Shin D, Smith D, Culligan M, Dimofte A, Glatstein E, et al. Phase II trial of pleural photodynamic therapy and surgery for patients with nonsmall- cell lung cancer with pleural spread. Journal of Clinical Oncology. 2004;**22**:2192-2201

[45] Wilson BC, Patterson MS. The physics, biophysics and technology of photodynamic therapy. Physics in Medicine and Biology. 2008;**53**:R61-R109

[46] Shirasu N, Nam SO, Kuroki M. Tumor-targeted photodynamic therapy. Anticancer Research. 2013;**33**(7):2823-2831

[47] Wu AM, Senter PD. Arming antibodies: Prospects and challenges for immunoconjugates. Nature Biotechnology. 2005;**23**:1137-1146

[48] Pye H, Stamati L, Yahioglu G, Butt MA, Deonarain M. Antibody-directed phototherapy (ADP). Antibodies. 2013;**2**:270-305

[49] Savellano MD, Hasan T. Photochemical targeting of epidermal growth factor receptor: A mechanistic study. Clinical Cancer Research. 2005;**11**:1658-1668

[50] Sato K, Watanabe R, Hanaoka H, Harada T, Nakajima T, Kim I, Paik CH, Choyke PL, Kobayashi H. Photoimmunotherapy: Comparative effectiveness of two monoclonal antibodies targeting the epidermal growth factor receptor. Molecular Oncology. 2014;**8**:620-632. DOI: 10.1016/j.molonc.2014.01.006

[51] Sato K, Choyke PL, Kobayashi H. Photoimmunotherapy of gastric cancer peritoneal carcinomatosis in a mouse model. PLoS One. 2014;**9**:e113276. DOI: 10.1371/journal.pone.0113276

[52] Sato K, Nagaya T, Nakamura Y, Harada T, Choyke PL, Kobayashi H. Near infrared photoimmunotherapy prevents lung cancer metastases in a murine model. Oncotarget. 2015;**6**(23):19747-19758

[53] Calixto G, Bernegossi J, Fonseca-Santos B, Chorilli M. Nanotechnology-based drug delivery systems for treatment of oral cancer: A review. International Journal of Nanomedicine. 2014;**9**:3719-3735

[54] Allison RR, Mota HC, Bagnato VS, Sibata CH. Bio-nanotechnology and photodynamic therapy—State of the art review. Photodiagnosis and Photodynamic Therapy. 2008;**5**:19-28

[55] Konan YN, Gurny R, Allémann E. State of the art in the delivery of photosensitizers for photodynamic therapy. Journal of Photochemistry and Photobiology B. 2002;**66**(2):89-106

[56] Nishiyama N, Nakagishi Y, Morimoto Y, Lai PS, Miyazaki K, Urano K, Horie S, Kumagai M, Fukushima S, Cheng Y, Jang WD, Kikuchi M, Kataoka K. Enhanced photodynamic cancer treatment by supramolecular nanocarriers charged with dendrimer phthalocyanine. Journal of Controlled Release. 2009;**133**(3):245-251. DOI: 10.1016/j.jconrel.2008.10.010

[57] Perni S, Prokopovich P, Pratten J, Parkin IP, Wilson M. Nanoparticles: Their potential use in antibacterial photodynamic therapy. Photochemical & Photobiological Sciences. 2011; **10**:712-720

[58] Chu CK, Tu YC, Hsiao JH, et al. Combination of photothermal and photodynamic inactivation of cancer cells through surface plasmon resonance of a gold nanoring. Nanotechnology. 2016;**27**:115102

[59] Cheng Y, Meyers JD, Broome AM, Kenney ME, Basilion JP, Burda C. Deep penetration of a PDT drug into tumors by noncovalent drug-gold nanoparticle conjugates. Journal of the American Chemical Society. 2011;**133**:2583-2591

[60] Hu Y, Yang Y, Wang H, Du H. Synergistic integration of layerby-layer assembly of photosensitizer and gold nanorings for enhanced photodynamic therapy in the near infrared. ACS Nano. 2015;**9**:8744-8754

[61] Mukherjee P, Bhattacharya R, Bone N, Lee YK, Patra CR, Wang S, Lu L, Secreto C, Banerjee PC, Yaszemski MJ, Kay NE, Mukhopadhyay DJ. Potential therapeutic application of gold nanoparticles in B-chronic lymphocytic leukemia (BCLL): Enhancing apoptosis. NanoBiotechnology. 2007;**8**(5):4

[62] Huang X, Qian W, El-Sayed IH, El-Sayed MA. The potential use of the enhanced nonlinear properties of gold nanospheres in photothermal cancer therapy. Lasers in Surgery and Medicine. 2007;**39**(9):747-753

[63] Herrwerth S, Rosendahl T, Feng C, Fick J, Eck W, Himmelhaus M, Dahint R, Grunze M. Covalent coupling of antibodies to selfassembled monolayers of carboxy-functionalized poly(ethylene glycol): Protein resistance and specific binding of biomolecules. Langmuir. 2003;**19**:1880-1887

[64] Liu Y, Shipton MK, Ryan J, Kaufman ED, Franzen S, Feldheim DL. Synthesis, stability, and cellular internalization of gold nanoparticles containing mixed peptide-poly(ethylene glycol) monolayers. Analytical Chemistry. 2007;**79**:2221-2229

[65] MacKinnon AC, Kopatz J, Sethi T. The molecular and cellular biology of lung cancer: Identifying novel therapeutic strategies. British Medical Bulletin. 2010;**95**:47-61. DOI: 10.1093/bmb/ldq023

[66] O'Flaherty JD, Barr M, Fennell D, Richard D, Reynolds J, O'Leary J, O'Byrne K. The cancer stem-cell hypothesis: Its emerging role in lung cancer biology and its relevance for future therapy. Journal of Thoracic Oncology. 2012;**7**(12):1880-1890. DOI: 10.1097/JTO.0b013e31826bfbc6

[67] Castano AP, Demidova TN, Hamblin MR. Mechanisms in photodynamic therapy: Part two—Cellular signaling, cell metabolism and modes of cell death. Photodiagnosis and Photodynamic Therapy. 2005;**2**(1):1-23. DOI: 10.1016/S1572-1000(05)00030-X

[68] Manoto S, Houreld N, Abrahamse H. Resistance of lung cancer cells grown as multicellular tumour spheroids to zinc sulfophthalocyanine photosensitization. International Journal of Molecular Sciences. 2015;**16**:10185-10200. DOI: 10.3390/ijms160510185

[69] Stuchinskaya T, Moreno M, Cook MJ, Edwards DR, Russell DA. Targeted photodynamic therapy of breast cancer cells using antibody-phthalocyanine-gold nanoparticle conjugates. Photochemical & Photobiological Sciences. 2011;**10**(5):822-831. DOI: NNNNN10.1039/c1pp05014a

7

Pleural Effusions in Lung Cancer: Detection and Treatment

Milic Medenica, Miras Medenica and Danilo Cosovic

Abstract

In all cell types of lung cancer, pleural effusion is a possible complication of disease. Paramalignant pleural effusions [PMPE] are not a consequence of malignant disease spreading to pleura. The probability that an effusion is paramalignant is higher if the effusion is a transudative or parapneumonic effusion. Differentiating between paramalignant and malignant effusions has both therapeutic and prognostic significance. MPEs are a sign of metastatic dissemination of neoplastic disease. In pleural fluid or tissue, there are malignant cells. In PMPE, lung cancer had been previously diagnosed. Bronchoopstruction, atelectasis, infection, pulmonary emboli, air therapy, and heliotherapy result in effusion development. PMPEs equally appear in all pathohistological types of lung cancer, as MPEs are the most common in lung adenocarcinoma. Also, there are biochemical properties of PMPE and MPE. Therapeutic procedures depend on the presence of respiratory distress, biochemical properties of pleural fluid, type of primary tumour, and expected response to the therapy.

Keywords: paramalignant, malignant, effusion, thoracocentesis, pleurodesis

1. Introduction

Over 175,000 MPE [1] are diagnosed yearly in USA and 50,000 [2] in the UK. In 75% of cases, MPE are a consequence of metastatic dissemination of lung or breast cancer [3]. Pleural effusion in lung cancer is a complication of terminal or preterminal stage of disease. Lung cancer disturbs one or more mechanisms of normal fluid flow, which is followed by inevitable accumulation of fluid in pleural space. Pleural effusion is not always a sign of cancer metastasising, but it is evident that in most cases it is related to the primary disease.

Pleural effusion is a possible complication of disease in all cell types of lung cancer [4, 5]. At the first presentation, around 15% of patients with lung cancer have a pleural effusion [5]. For the duration of disease, approximately 50% of patients develop a pleural effusion. Depending on the presence of malignant cells in pleural fluid, pleural effusions are divided into two groups: paramalignant pleural effusions [PMPE] and malignant pleural effusions [MPE] [3]. Distinguishing between PME and MPE can be challenging. Analytical limitations do not allow the use of a single method to pursue the diagnosis and also can expose the patients to invasive procedures. PMPE are not a consequence of malignant disease spreading to the pleura. The probability that an effusion is paramalignant is higher if the effusion is a transudative or parapneumonic effusion. Differentiation between PMPE and MPE is important, so that appropriate decisions about treatment modalities can be made, and also due to different prognosis of the two conditions.

2. Clinical features of pleural effusion

In patients with lung cancer and pleural effusion, there is a mild to medium symptomatology of respiratory distress. Clinical history usually points to the diagnosis of lung, breast, ovarian cancer or lymphoma. At the time of diagnosis of malignant pleural effusion, 23% of patients are asymptomatic [4]. Pleural effusion followed by pleural pain indicates the inflammation of the parietal pleura. Dull pain in the chest wall stirs suspicion of pleural malignancy [6]. Nevertheless, pleuritic or dull pain in the chest wall indicates a distortion of the parietal pleura and a high probability of an exudative effusion developing. As a rule, pain is a consequence of pleural disease. Localisation of pain is correlated to the area of pleura that is affected (parietal pleura is innervated by intercostal nerves). Occasionally, pleuritic pain spreads into upper parts of stomach [intercostal nerves innervate the abdomen as well]. Exception in pain localisation and spreading of the pain are noted when the central parts of diaphragmatic pleura are affected by the disease. These parts of the pleura are innervated by phrenic nerves and consequently the pain localises to the ipsilateral shoulder. In over 70% of patients with MPE intrathoracic pain is a symptom of the disease [7]. Non-productive cough can also be a symptom of a pleural effusion. Mechanism of genesis of the cough is not clear and is probably related to pleural inflammation. Alternatively, compression of lungs and bronchial wall by fluid might stimulate the cough reflex [8]. Cough is present in over 50% of patients. A common symptom of pleural effusion is dyspnoea. Dyspnoea is present in around 70% of patients with MPE [7]. The severity of dyspnoea is often not proportional to the size of pleural effusion [4]. Dyspnoea is usually present in diaphragmatic dysfunction. In an inverted diaphragm, dyspnoea is disproportional to the size of the effusion. Mulvey [9] classified hemi-diaphragmatic alterations seen on chest radiographs and fluoroscopy into three groups. The three groups are: normal function of the hemidiaphragm, fixed hemidiaphragm, and hemidiaphragm with paradoxical movement. Patients with normal functioning diaphragm are usually asymptomatic, even with a large pleural effusion. The second group of patients are the patients with a fixed hemidiaphragm. Immobile diaphragm disables sufficient ventilation of the lungs. In the third patient group, hemidiaphragm exhibits paradoxical movement which results in severe dyspnoea. Paradoxical movement of the right hemidiaphragm is rarely seen, probably due to proximity of the liver. The severity of respiratory insufficiency depends on the size of the effusion and previous lung function. Pleural effusion reduces the thoracic space and lung volumes or in turn the thoracic cavity enlarges as the ipsilateral hemidiaphragm descends. Therefore, fluid in the pleural space causes restrictive ventilator defect. Small to moderate pleural effusions cause dislocation rather than lung compression and they have a little consequential effect on the lung function [6]. In massive pleural effusions, the most common symptoms are the ones that are a direct consequence of lung function compromise. Improvement of lung function after therapeutic thoracocentesis is less than expected [10]. Explanation of inadequate improvement of lung function probably lays in the fact that usually, besides pleural effusion, there are also changes in the lung parenchyma. In massive pleural effusions, the mechanism of dyspnoea is closely related to the reduction of chest wall compliance, counter lateral mediastinum movement, and loss of the ipsilateral lung volume with additional action of neurogenic factors of the pulmonary parenchyma [11].

In 26 patients, spirometry was performed before thoracocentesis and 24 hours after thoracocentesis. Average amount of evacuated fluid was 1740 ml [12]. After thoracocentesis, vital capacity increased for 410 ± 390 ml. Estenne et al. [13] examined respiratory mechanics in nine patients, before and 2 hours after evacuation of 600–2750 ml (average amount = 1818 ml) of pleural fluid. Before thoracocentesis, forced vital capacity (FVC) was between 22 and 51% of predicted values. After thoracocentesis, the average value of FVC has increased only by 300–460 ml. Estenne interprets reduction in dyspnoea by reduction in the size of the thoracic volume. Reduction of the thoracic cavum enables inspiratory muscles to function in much more favourable length-tension relationship. Before thoracocentesis, maximum inspiratory pressure at TLC (total lung capacity) was −16 cm H_2O, and after thoracentesis, the pressure fell to −25 cm H_2O. Explanation of these phenomena probably lays in the fact that hemidiaphragm is released from the pressure of pleural fluid. In pleural effusion, PaO_2 is usually low, as alveolar-arterial gradient is increased.

Patients with pleural effusion complain of intolerance to exertion. Exertional intolerance was examined in 24 patients, before and after thoracocentesis. There were no significant changes in hypoxia and hypercapnia level. A number of patients had malignant effusions and it is possible that the given results are the consequence of primary disease rather than lung function being compromised by pleural effusion [14].

Systemic symptoms are a consequence of cancer development. The most common systemic symptoms are weight loss, general weakness, haemoptysis, fever, cyanosis, and dysphagia [4]. Over 40% of patients had systemic symptoms, general weakness, and loss of weight. Eighteen percent of patients had fevers, and 9% of patients had haemoptysis [13]. Similar data were found by Chernow, Sahn [4] and Baburao and assoc. [15]. The patients with MPE had chest pain in 32% cases, compared to 11% of patients with benign effusions, while the patients with benign effusions were more commonly found to have pleuritic pain [51 versus 24%]. Fever was more common in the patients with benign effusion (73 versus 37%) [8].

Massive pleural effusion can compromise cardiac function. It has been proven that massive pleural effusion can lead to the right ventricular diastolic collapse with consequential reduction of cardiac output. In artificial bilateral pleural effusions, right ventricular diastolic collapse appears at the pressure of about 4 mmHg [16]. This value of pleural pressure is also seen with the patients with massive pleural effusion [17]. Arterial-blood gases usually have clinically acceptable values.

On examining the patient, the absence of the pectoral fremitus, shortened and dull percussion sound, and weakened respiratory sounds are usually found. By auscultation above the fluid level, the change of breathing pattern (area of the compromised lung), that is, aegophony is heard. Conversing through auscultation of the affected side, increased resonance of voice can be heard. Experienced doctors think that dullness to percussion and aegophony are two most common findings that are present in over 90% of patients with pleural effusion. Above the area of dullness to percussion, humid sounds are heard ausculatorily [18]. Contralateral displacement of the trachea could be found in massive effusion.

3. Paramalignant pleural effusion

The main characteristic of PMPE is that the lung cancer had been previously diagnosed, and that malignant cells had not been identified in the effusion either cytologically or pathohistologically. These effusions are not a sign of malignant disease spreading to the pleura [3].

PMPEs are a direct consequence of local or systemic effect of tumour. Pulmonary infection distally from partial or complete obstruction of bronchi could be a cause of parapneumonic effusions. Obstruction of main or lobar bronchi by neoplasm leads to consequential atelectasis of the corresponding part of the lung. In order to compensate for the lost volume, the remainder of the lung must additionally expand or the hemithorax must be contracted. This sequence of events results in lower intrapleural pressure. Low intrapleural pressure is an additional factor of more intensive fluid accumulation.

Furthermore, the incidence of pulmonary emboli in malignant disease is not negligible, and pulmonary embolus can also be one of the causes for pleural effusion development. Additionally, certain chemotherapeutic protocols are a cause of increased retention of fluid in pleural space. Lymphatic obstruction is a common property of lung cancer and lymphoma and at the same time is a possible complication of radiotherapy which is a contributing factor of fluid accumulation in pleural space.

A considerable number of patients with malignant disease are malnurtured. Hypoproteinemia can in rare cases lead to transudative pleural effusion. In malignant disease, metastatic changes on the pericardium can be found. Pericardial effusion leads to the increase of hydrostatic pressure in systemic and pulmonary circulation which leads to transudative pleural effusion development [19].

In around 5% of patients with lung cancer, PMPEs are diagnosed. Frequency of PMPE in squamous cell carcinoma is 4.5%, in adenocarcinoma 6.2% and in SCLC 6.5%, so they are equally present in all pathohistological types of lung cancer [7, 21].

In 67% of patients, PMPEs are moderate or massive. They are mostly serous or cloudy (60%), and haemorrhagic effusions represent 21.3% of all PMPEs [7, 20].

3.1. Pleural fluid analysis

Compared to the MPE ratio of LDH—E/S (effusion/serum) is higher in PMPE, but not significantly higher. This can be interpreted with the help of the fact that in PMPE, parapneumonic effusion (inflammation is followed by high values of LDH in effusion) is diagnosed in 18.3% of patients. Significant differences in other biochemical characteristics (glucose, proteins, and cholesterol) were not found either [7].

Compared to MPE, total number of cells, eosinophils, and PMN [polymorphonuclear cells] is higher in the group of patients with PMPE, but not significantly. Lymphocytes and PMN dominate in the differential picture in PMPE. Percentage of PMN is usually below 25%, but cases when they dominate are not rare, for example, in secondary pleural inflammation. In PMPE, eosinophils are found in 51% of patients diagnosed with PMPE. The percentage range of eosinophils in pleural fluid ranged from 1 to 24% [7].

3.2. Management of paramalignant pleural effusion

PMPEs are not an absolute contraindication for operative treatment. It is a therapeutic challenge to establish the optimal therapeutic protocol for the patients who are diagnosed with lung cancer and ipsilateral pleural effusion in which no malignant cells are found cytologically. Rodriguez-Panadero [21] performed thoracoscopy on 21 patients with lung cancer and paramalignant effusion. After thoracoscopy, thoracotomy was indicated in five patients. Invasion of mediastinal lymph nodes was found in all five patients. In another study, five patients out of 73 with PMPE have survived long term after surgery [22]. It can be concluded that in the patients with PMPE, thoracoscopy and CT of the thorax should be firstly done for the evaluation of mediastinal lymph nodes. In the case of enlarged lymph nodes, mediastinoscopy is indicated. In the patients with negative thoracoscopy, even if lymphatics are not enlarged, explorative thoracotomy is recommended. Before resection, lavage of pleural space with cytological analysis of the obtained material should be performed. One study that encompassed more than 1200 patients found that in patients with lung cancer without an effusion undergoing surgical resection with curative intent, 5.3% of patients had positive cytological findings of the pleural fluid lavage at the time of thoracotomy before surgical resection took place [23]. In PMPE, most commonly performed therapeutic procedures are thoracocentesis (51%) and pleurodesis (39%). Thoracotomy was done in two (6%) patients [7].

4. Malignant pleural effusion

Malignancy is the most common cause of massive pleural effusions opacifying the entire hemithorax and of large pleural effusions opacifying two thirds of a hemithorax. MPE is an end-stage sign of malignant disease. Sometimes MPE can be the first clinical sign of a tumour, given that often lung cancer are not detected in the beginning of disease development. In a retrospective series of 766 patients, carcinoma was the cause of 55% of massive and large pleural effusions [24]; other causes included tuberculosis effusion and pleural empyema.

In older age groups (>60 years old), malignant pleural effusions are the most common cause of exudative effusions and they are often the first clinical manifestation of disease (**Figure 1**) [3, 5]. Diagnosis of malignant effusion is established by the identification of malignant cells in effusion or pleural tissue. Pathohistological and/or cytological investigations are not of credible diagnostic significance until malignant cells are defined.

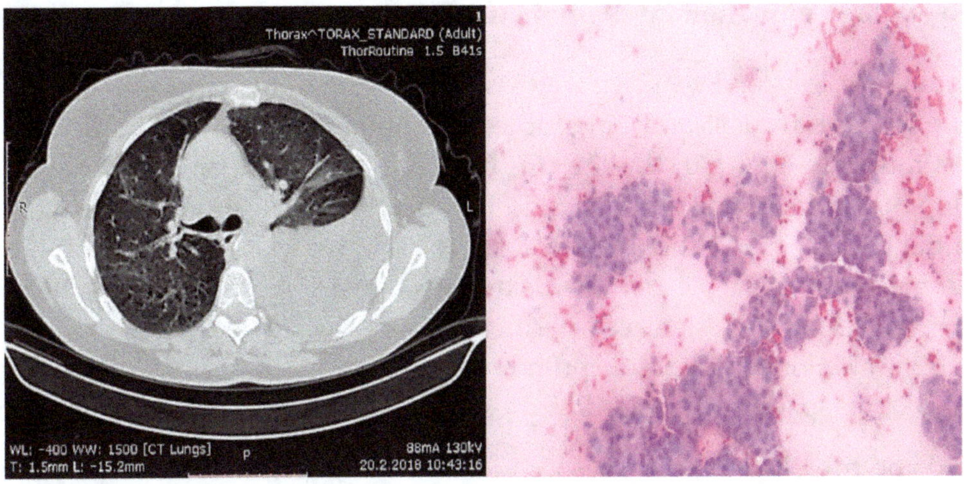

Figure 1. Pleural fluid sample containing cells of adenocarcinoma. N.B.—Origin of the primary tumour is unknown.

In over a half of MPE in men, the effusion is caused by lung cancer. MPEs appear in all cell types of lung cancer [3]. Incidence of MPE in lung adenocarcinoma is significantly higher in comparison to other pathohistological types of cancer. Thirty one percent of patients (out of 96) with lung adenocarcinoma developed a MPE, while 8.6% of patients (out of 404) with squamous cell carcinoma and between 7 and 10% with patients with small-cell carcinoma developed a MPE [7, 25–27].

The next most common causatives of malignant effusions are lymphoma and leukaemias (20%). Seven percent of MPE are a result of spread of gastrointestinal system cancer, 6% of genitourinary system and 11% of tumour are of unknown primary source [28]. Incidence of MPE in regards to primary tumour localisation is given in **Table 1**.

In women, around 40% of MPE is a direct consequence of spread of breast cancer. In about 50% of patients with breast cancer, pleural effusion is developed during evolution of disease [29]. Twenty percent of effusions are the consequence of genital tract tumour spread, 15% of lung malignoma, 8% of lymphoma or leukaemia, 3% of melanoma, and 9% of tumours of unknown primary source.

Primary tumour localisation	Incidence %
Breast	26–49
Lung	10–24
Lymphoma	Up to 24
Non-Hodgkin lymphoma	13–24
Ovary	6–17
Hodgkin's disease	Up to 13

Table 1. Causes of malignant pleural effusions.

4.1. Pathophysiology of malignant pleural effusions

Malignant tumours can lead to pleural effusion development either by direct or indirect spread of the disease. In post-mortem studies, malignant disease of the pleura without an effusion was found in 40% [30] to 45% [6] of cases. Pleural effusions in malignancy most likely develop due to increased entry of fluid into pleural space and decreased evacuation of liquid from the pleural space. Increased transport of liquid into pleural space occurs due to increased permeability of the pleural vessels by direct invasion of the tumour cells, vasoactive and inflammatory cytokines. Increased permeability of pleural vessels can also be caused by injury, infection, pulmonary embolus, pulmonary infarction that causes movement of liquid from lung to pleural space by increased hydrostatic forces caused by venous obstruction [31].

Pleural liquid and protein are largely resorbed by the lymphatic system of the parietal pleura. The exit of fluid from pleural space could be decreased by several mechanisms that reduce lymphatic drainage. Lymphatic obstruction at any point, from the stomata of parietal pleura to mediastinal lymph nodes is a dominant cause of increased accumulation of pleural fluid [3, 20]. Insufficiency of lymphatic drainage appears for two reasons. The first one is that the transport of liquid from pleural space through stomata and lymphatic vessels of parietal pleura is disabled because of the presence of metastases and other reason, as the lymphatic vessels of parietal pleura are mostly drained by mediastinal lymph nodes. So, neoplastically changed mediastinal lymph nodes decrease the clearance of pleural cavum thus contributing to additional accumulation of fluid [32]. Obstruction of thoracal ductus by malignant tumour can also be a cause of pleural effusion development. In these cases, a chylothorax develops. Chylothorax is the most common complication of mediastinal tumours, mostly lymphoma (in 50%). Furthermore, chylothorax is a complication of surgery (20%) and trauma to the thorax (<5%) [33].

In atelectasis pleural pressure is lower due to bronchial obstruction and therefore the exit of fluid from pleural space is reduced. In superior vena cava syndrome, pleural liquid drainage is reduced due to elevated central venous pressure.

Cellular and molecular mechanisms of localisation of pleural metastases are still mostly unclear. From visceral pleura malignant cells spread to parietal pleura, where they multiply [20]. Pleural metastases are also found on visceral and parietal pleura, while isolated metastases of parietal pleura have never been identified. From visceral pleura, malignant cells spread on parietal pleura [3]. In the process of pleural metastase development, several steps are necessary. First, malignant cells must leave the primary tumour. For this step, deregulation of cellular adhesion is necessary. Deregulation of cellular adhesion depends on the changes in the extracellular matrix and the change of expression degree of integrin with simultaneous increase of cell motility. By leaving the primary tumour, tumour cells via vascular or lymphatic structures (they can cause different haemodynamic and immunological changes in these structures) find their way towards distant organs or lymph nodes. With the help of video microscopy, it has been shown that a great number of circulating tumour cells (80%) stay alive even up to 3 days after their entry, both into circulation and/or extravascular space. Only small subgroups of cells (0.07%) can form metastases [34].

Control of extravascular cell growth is crucial in forming of metastases. Formation of pleural metastases is probably mediated by the interaction of mesothelial and neoplastic cells. Tumour activated mediators (VEGF, ligand for CC-sequence of chemokines CCL2 and TNF) stimulate the accumulation of inflammatory cells [35, 36]. IL-5 stimulates the development of MPE, accumulation of Eo as well as myeloid suppressor tumour-activating cells [37]. On the other hand, tumour cells activate proinflammatory and proangiogenic transcription programs controlled by nuclear transcription factor (NF)-kB [38] and signal transduction of transcription activator (STAT)3 [39]. Tumour necrosis factor (TNF), interleukin 6([IL-6), and osteopontin (OPN) participate in positive reverse coupling (povratna sprega) regulating the activation of tumour NF-kB/STAT3. The end result of these events is the formation of MPE [35]. Furthermore, stimulated mesothelial cells secrete different factors, such as chemoattractants, chemokines, and platelet-derived growth factor (PDGF). These products facilitate the appearance of metastases. Simultaneously, the production of adhesion molecules is increased, such as intracellular adhesive molecules [ICAM-1] and vascular molecules of cell adhesion (VCAM-1) which, in vitro, in contact with cancer cells secrete metalloproteinase [40].

And finally, continuous growth of metastatic foci depends on angiogenesis. Vascular endothelial growth factor (VEGF) stimulates proliferation and migration of endothelial cells. At the same time, invasion of pleural space by malignant cells and VEGF expression from tumour cells is necessary for the formation of pleural liquid [41]. Angiogenesis is the primary process that disables the growth and progression of tumour [42]. Yano et al. [41] used human cells of pulmonary adenocarcinoma and squamous cell cancer, with different invasive properties and different levels of VEGF expression, and they have proven that invasion of pleural space by malignant cells and VEGF expression from tumour cells is necessary for the formation of pleural fluid. VEGF is one of the most powerful known chemokines that directly affect the increase of vascular permeability [42]. In comparison to tuberculosis effusions and transudative effusions, the concentration of VEGF is significantly higher in malignant effusion [42, 43]. The average value of VEGF in malignant pleural effusion is significantly higher than in pleural effusions that are a consequence of congestive cardiac failure [41].

Malignant effusion in comparison to benign incidence of CD4+ cells is significantly increased [44]. Accumulation of immunosuppression and protumour CD4+ lymphocytes contributes to weakening of the immune response and simultaneous growth of tumour cells [45].

On development of pleural metastases, tumour cells disseminate onto the mesothelial surface or malignant cells penetrate the subserosa. When the mesothelium is encompassed by the tumour, 'excess' of tumour cells appears in the pleural fluid. However, when only submesothelium is infiltrated by the tumour, there is a small number of malignant cells in pleural liquid. In these cases, malignant cells are rarely identified in pleural fluid, that is, thoracocentesis does not have any diagnostic significance [46, 47]. Infiltration of pleura by tumour results in reactive changes of mesothelium, that is, fibrosis. In advanced stage of disease, disposal of collagen into submesothelial pleural tissue is increased, which is at least a part of the cause of low values of pH and glucose in the effusion.

Another, and less likely mechanism of metastases development is by direct invasion of pleura by tumour, whether it is lung or breast cancer. In some cases, spread of tumour to the pleura is evident, and in spite of this, the effusion does not develop. For example, effusion rarely appears when pleura is invaded by sarcoma. One of the properties of sarcoma is the absence of lymphogenic metastases [20].

Bilateral metastases in lung cancer are usually indirect evidence of the primary neoplasm spreading to the liver and of subsequent disease dissemination to the lungs. However, if the lungs are not the primary source of carcinoma, this implies that the changes on pleura are a tertiary consequence of metastasis spreading from the liver [4, 19].

4.2. Pleural fluid analysis

Pleural effusions in lung cancer are usually classified as exudates [4, 48]. In 5–10% of cases, the pleural effusion is a transudate [4, 54]. Transudative effusions are more likely when the lymphatic drainage is obstructed by the tumour and in atelectasis caused by bronchial obstruction or congestive cardiac failure [31]. Malignant cells can be found in transudative effusions as well. Macroscopic MPEs can be serous, serosanguinous, and haemorrhagic. Erythrocyte count in pleural fluid is often between 30,000 and 50,000/μl [48]. Erythrocyte count over 100,000/μl, in the absence of trauma, indicates a probable diagnosis of malignant disease. Direct invasion of blood vessels, occlusion of venules, increased permeability of capillaries due to vasoactive chemokines and cytokines, occlusion of venules usually result in a bloody, malignant pleural effusion.

In more than half of malignant effusions, lymphocytes are present in 50–70% range, but are typically present in lesser amount than they occur with tuberculosis pleurisy (usually ≥80%) [12, 49]. In TBCPE, the number of lymphocytes was 153,696 × 10^4 versus 95,414 × 10^4/ml in MPE [7]. In order to differentiate between tuberculosis and malignant effusions, determining adenosine deaminase (ADA) presence in the effusion is of significance. The level of ADA greater than 70 U/l in effusion indicates to tuberculosis aetiology, while the ADA level below 40 U/l excludes the tuberculosis aetiology [50, 51]. Although the cause of lymphocytosis is unclear, the lymphocytes that are most prevalent are T lymphocytes that have a role in local defence systems against tumour invasion of the pleural cavity. In vitro, lymphocytes of malignant pleural effusions spontaneously secrete lymphokines [52]. Mesothelial cell percentage in malignant effusion varies ranging from few percent to a large percentage of total cells. Mesothelial cell abundance occurs early in the course of infiltration of the pleura, well before pleural fibrosis and marked tumour infiltration. Fewer mesothelial cells are seen in advanced stages of pleural metastases due to pleural fibrosis.

The percentage of PMN is usually below 25%, even though often PMN can dominate the percentage, as in secondary inflammation of pleura. Eosinophils are present in up to 36% of malignant effusions [7]. The percentage in which eosinophils are a significant finding in pleural liquid is considered to be higher than 10%. In MPE, eosinophil percentage ranges from 1 to 52% [7]. Eosinophilic pleural effusion is the most common in malignant disease (34, 8%) [24], which is then followed by infections (19, 2%), effusions of unknown aetiology (14, 1%), post-traumatic effusions (8, 9%), and effusions (23%) in other diseases.

Usually, eosinophilia is related to the presence of blood or air in pleural space. Eosinophilic effusions reappear even after repeated thoracocentesis [53]. Good correlation was found between IL-5 levels and the number of eosinophils in pleural fluid [54]. In MPE, compared to other cells, malignant cells are rarely found. Significant concentrations of proteins are found in pleural fluid. Nevertheless, the total amount of protein transported from pleural space is lesser than the amount of protein transported in tuberculosis effusions, effusions in pulmonary embolism, and congestive cardiac failure.

Chronic pleural effusions (CPE) are very rarely found to be transudates. Characteristic biochemical property of CPEs is that they have low pH and low glucose concentration, while they have a large protein concentration. The ratio of pleural protein to serum protein can found to be low, and nevertheless, the effusion would still be classified as an exudate. If in exudative effusion only the LDH criterium is positive, this points to the diagnosis of malignancy [48, 55, 56].

In one third of MPE, pH is less than 7.30 (ranging from 6.95 to 7.29) [57]. Effusions with low pH value have a high concentration of glucose (<60 mg/dl) and pO_2, and additionally a high concentration of lactate and pCO_2. Glucose concentration can be rarely reduced to the value of 5 mg/dl and it usually ranges from 30 to 55 mg/dl [55]. Malignant effusions with low values of pH and glucose characteristically have a longer evolution of up to several months and they usually follow the fast tumour and pleural fibrosis [54]. Pathologically altered pleura reduce glucose entry into the pleural space and at the same time disable the transport of metabolic products. The end result of this disorder is local acidosis [56]. Low level of LDH in effusion indicates a higher possibility of negative pathohistological results. In effusions with high LDH level, the percentage of positive biopsies is higher [58].

Pleural fluid amylase concentration is found to be elevated in 10% of patients diagnosed with a MPE. However, the origin of amylase in pleural fluid is not pancreatic but is found to be salivary instead. In a series of consecutive effusions, a very high amylase level in malignant pleural fluid (>600 IU/L) was found to be a poor prognostic factor [59].

4.3. Tumour markers in pleural liquid

Biological markers of malignancy are yet to be identified, but may be identified in the future as the molecular biology of cancer is better understood. Pleural fluid biomarkers could potentially assist the cytological diagnosis. Unfortunately, biomarkers have been found to have indeterminate specificity and sensitivity which has led to overlap between malignant and benign conditions. An approach that has been used is to combine the tumour markers to improve the diagnostic yield. However, the diagnosis of malignancy can also be reached by using the clinical characteristics—duration of symptoms for more than a month, absence of fever, CT thorax findings of malignancy, and serosanguinous fluid [60].

4.3.1. Carcinoembryonic antigen

It has been concluded in several reports that determining the CEA level in pleural fluid is useful in establishing the diagnosis of malignant pleural effusion [61, 62]. CEA level below 10 ng/ml is usually found in lymphoma, sarcoma, and mesothelioma. CEA higher than 10 ng/ml could indicate a malignant disease; however, it does not have diagnostic significance, and routine measuring of CEA is not recommended.

4.3.2. Carbohydrate antigen

It is known that three different carbohydrate antigens (Ca 15-3, CA 19-9, and CA 72-4) are present in malignant disease. These antigens have been studied in order to differentiate malignant and benign effusions [63]. Comparing the levels of these three antigens in malignant and benign effusions, there is a significant overlap of the obtained results. Hence, this test is not sensitive enough and it is not used in routine diagnostics.

4.3.3. Sialyl stage-specific antigen-1

Sialyi stage-specific antigen-1 is a carbohydrate antigen present in malignant disease. Patients with positive cytological findings of pleural fluid to adenocarcinoma cells have higher values of this antigen in effusion in comparison to effusions of other aetiologies [64]. However, simultaneously, significant overlap of value levels of this marker was recorded, and therefore sialyl stage-specific antigen-1 in effusions of unclear aetiology does not bare a diagnostic significance.

4.3.4. Cytokeratin-19 fragments

Cytokeratin 19 (CYFRA 21-1) is the main component of cytoskeletal filaments of epithelial cells. It is significantly increased in malignant diseases. The level of CYFRA-21 higher than 100 ng/ml is present in around 60% of patients with carcinoma and mesothelioma [65]. A significant overlap has been found in CYFRE levels in both malignant and benign effusions, and therefore this test is not recommended in routine work.

4.3.5. Enolase

Enolase is a glycolytic enzyme present in extracts of neuroendocrine tumours. In pleural effusions in small cell lung cancer, higher levels of enolase are found when compared to pleural effusions in non-small cell lung cancer and benign effusions [66], but as there is a significant overlap in measured enolase values establishing its presence has no diagnostic significance.

4.3.6. Squamous cell carcinoma antigens

Squamous cell carcinoma antigen (SCC) has been used as a serum marker for squamous cell carcinoma. In the greatest number of patients with pleural effusion in malignant disease, a low level of this marker was found. This marker was positive in 7 out of 11 patients (64%) with squamous cell carcinoma. However, SCC values are very high in some benign effusions as well; thus, SCC is not used in squamous cell carcinoma diagnostics [66].

4.3.7. Oncogenes

Oncogenes are closely related to the development of malignancy, and one of the hypotheses has suggested that in the pleural fluid of patients with pleural malignancy cells containing oncogenes are present. In 11 (34%) of malignant effusions, protein p53 has been detected, and should be noted that it has not been found in any non-malignant effusion [67].

There is no significant difference in CMYC oncogene expression between malignant and benign effusions [68]. CHARAS oncogene has been detected in 21 out of 24 malignant effusions, but it has also been found in 6 out of 16 benign effusions (37%), and therefore its diagnostic utility is limited [69].

4.3.8. *Hyaluronic acid*

Pleural fluid of patients with mesothelioma is sometimes extremely viscous. Increased viscosity of liquid is a consequence of hyaluronate, that is, hyaluronic acid presence. Hyaluronic acid level higher than 1 mg/ml indicates mesothelioma diagnosis. In no other aetiology of pleural effusion, hyaluronate level higher than 0.8 mg/ml was found. Sensitivity of this test for malignant mesothelioma is 56% [70]. Average values of hyaluronic acid in mesothelioma are comparable to values of hyaluronic acid present in pleural effusions in adenocarcinoma [71].

4.3.9. *Lectins binding*

Lectins are a class of glycoproteins of non-immune origin which bind specifically to the carbohydrate group in different biological products. Lectin binds much easier to adenocarcinoma cells compared to reactive mesothelial cells or mesothelioma cells [72]. These authors could not find significant differences in lectin binding between mesothelioma cells and reactive mesothelial cells.

4.3.10. *Flow cytometry*

Flow cytometry is a method of quick measuring of nuclear DNA. It has been postulated that this method would enable differentiation of benign from malignant cells, taking into account that malignant cells have numerous chromosomal abnormalities (aneuploidy) and consequentially abnormal DNA content (DNA aneuploidy). However, aneuploidy is present in benign effusions as well [73]. Flow cytometry is used in the identification of superficial lymphocyte markers and it has found the use in diagnosis of lymphoma [68].

4.3.11. *Chromosomal analysis*

Malignant cells have a higher number of chromosomes with structural abnormalities, such as translocation, ascension, dissension, discention, inversion, and isochromosomy [70]. The place of chromosome analysis in routine examination of pleural effusions remains to be established.

4.3.12. *Association of mRNA expression in metastatic malignant effusions*

Alternative diagnostic methods are still needed to assist in the diagnosis of pleural effusions. The supernatant of samples of pleural effusion might contain useful information such as nucleic acids and proteins. MicroRNAs that are circulating and cell free have been identified as potential biomarkers of cancer. MicroRNAs are heavily involved in processes of development, cell survival, carcinogenesis, and apoptosis. Hence, it is likely that they play a considerable role in modulating sensitivity and resistance to anticancer medications [74].

However, potential applications and the existence of cell-free microRNA in pleural effusion samples are uncertain. MicroRNA (miRNA) is a group of short RNAs that regulate expression of proteins post-transcriptionally by binding to the 3′UTRs target mRNAs. As MicroRNAs are involved in cancer development, the expression of a specific miRNA profile may suggest the disease status, prognosis, and response to chemotherapy agents.

Wang et al. [75] have used real-time quantitative PCR to analyse related gene expression in 46 patients with malignant effusion. Data were prospectively collected from gastric cancer, non-small cell lung cancer, and gynaecological cancer patients. Cancer cells that are viable and obtained from malignant effusions are tested for sensitivity to docetaxel and cisplatin using ATP-TCA assay. The authors have concluded that BRCA1 (breast cancer susceptibility gene 1) and ERCC1 (excision repair cross-complementing group 1) miRNA expression levels are in correlation with in vitro chemosensitivity to docetaxel and/or cisplatin in malignant effusions of gastric cancer and non-small cell lung cancer patients. Additionally, combining ERCC1 and BRCA1 may produce better results predicting the sensitivity to cisplatin than when only a single agent is considered.

4.4. Prognosis of malignant pleural effusion

By diagnosing a malignant effusion, prognostic information is obtained simultaneously [57]. Mean survival time of patients with lung cancer and MPE is between 3 and 4 months [76]. Multivariable analysis has demonstrated that shorter survival time was found in patients with a high level of serum CRP, low values of albumins, serum proteins, distant metastases and those patients who did not have chemotherapy [77]. Disease progression and poor prognosis can be related to the immunosuppressant effect of tumour and functional damage of the immune system.

In non-small cell carcinoma, mean survival time in patients with stage IIIb, IIIb with pleural effusion and stage IV was 15.3, 7.7, and 5.5 months, respectively [78].

From the time malignant, effusion is diagnosed, patients with lung, stomach, and ovarian cancer survive for only several months, while survival time in patients with breast cancer is longer—several months or years, depending on the response to chemotherapy [4, 55]. Survival time of the patients with lymphomatoid effusion is between the survival time of patients with breast cancer and cancers of different organs.

Prognosis of malignant effusion depends on the stage of the disease and contributing factors (**Table 2**) [55], which is of crucial importance for choosing the treatment modality. LDH criterium and pleural fluid pH in malignant effusions are important prognostic indicators. Poor prognosis is indicated by high LDH effusion/serum ratio, high level of LDH in effusion, and low pH of pleural fluid [55]. When pH and glucose levels are found to be low in a malignant pleural effusion (below 7.30 and 60 mg/dl, respectively), the survival time is found to be less for an average of 2 months when compared to those patients who have normal values of glucose and pH-average of 10-month survival time [76].

The only true predictive marker of mortality might be the performance status at the time of diagnosis. A Karnofsky score of more than 70 is associated with a median survival time of 13.2 months, while a Karnofsky score of less than 30 is associated with a median survival time of 1.1 months.

Tumour related	Non-tumour related
Extensive invasion of mediastinal lymph nodes	Tuberculosis or fungal infection
Parapneumonic effusion (obstructive pneumonia)	Immunological disorders: rheumatic, allergic, etc.
Pericardial effusion as a consequence of malignant disease	Pulmonary embolism
Previous mediastinal radiotherapy	Congestive cardiac failure
Malignant ascites	Parapneumonic effusion as a consequence of an unrelated pneumonia
Pulmonary embolus	Organ failure that is not a consequence of cancer or cancer treatment

Table 2. Factors contributing to the spread of pleural effusion.

4.5. Imaging

4.5.1. Chest radiographs

For documenting the presence of pleural fluid in pleural space, the most practical diagnostic test is conventional chest radiography [79]. Pathological changes of the pleura are commonly easily diagnosed by appropriate radiological modalities.

The distribution of fluid in pleural space is completely dependent on the laws of gravity. Fluid is firstly accumulated in basal parts of the hemithorax, that is, between the lower surface of the lung and diaphragm. When a large amount of fluid accumulates, the fluid starts spreading to anterior, posterior, and lateral costophrenic sinuses. The thickness of the fluid is greater laterally. The line of the border discretely fades on moving medially and ends in the mediastinum with a meniscus shaped line. On lateral radiographs, upper border of pleural fluid is semicircular, that is, the upper border is higher both anteriorly and posteriorly, while it gently descends in the middle part. A small amount of fluid seen on the chest radiograph is not indicative of a pleural effusion, as the diaphragmatic configuration is unchanged. During accumulation of a larger amount of pleural fluid, costophrenic angles are the first to be filled. Costophrenic angles are filled only after the quantity of fluid in sub-pulmonary space exceeds 175 ml s.

'Middle lobe step sign' can be often seen on a lateral view. The 'middle lobe step sign' is explained by the fact that the fluid firstly accumulates in the lower lobe, as it is the lowest of the pulmonary lobes. The middle lobe remains unchanged and its volume is preserved. Pleural fluid is most commonly evident in the posterior parts of the chest.

In massive pleural effusion, the sheer weight of the fluid can be a cause of inverted diaphragm, so much so that the normal convex appearance becomes concave. Inversion of the hemidiaphragm is more commonly seen on the left side. On diascopy of the inverted diaphragm, paradoxical movements are evident, that is, it rises on inspiration and descends on expiration [9].

It is common practice for the chest radiographs to be performed while the patient is standing. However, in critically ill patients, the chest radiographs can be only performed while the patient is lying down, and this could lead to the pleural effusion not being diagnosed. This is due to the fact that pleural fluid is being pulled by gravity and consequently localises in the posterior parts of the thoracic cavity.

Characteristic signs of a pleural effusion on chest radiograph when the patient is lying down are: blunting of the costophrenic angle, increased density of the part of the lung, loss of diaphragmatic silhouette, the presence of apical cap, elevation of a hemidiaphragm, difficulty in spotting vascular structures of the lower lobe, and accentuated small fissure [80]. These signs are not present in patients with a small or moderate pleural effusion.

Serial radiographs of the chest while the patient is lying down after moving the patient from one side to the other side can indicate a presence of mobile fluid and absence of loculations which in malignant pleural effusions enables the determination of a possible pleurodesis site [81].

Using the above mentioned radiological signs, it is possible to differentiate increased density of a pleural effusion from infiltrates for example. First, if the cause of increased density is a pleural effusion vascular structures of the lung will be visible on the radiograph. Any other intra-pulmonary process would cause an obliteration of vascular structures—'the silhouette effect'. Second, if pleural effusion is the cause of increased density, the visible change will be entirely homogenous. Infiltrates caused by an intrapulmonary process are usually less homogenous. Third, air bronchogram is only present when the increased density is a consequence of parenchymal infiltration.

Typical localization of fluid in pleural space of healthy lungs depends on the reverse action of elastic forces. Compared to other parts of the lung, the parts of the lung that are below the effusion exhibit different characteristics of elastic forces. Part of the lung above which the fluid is accumulated has a higher intensity of action reverse elastic forces. Accordingly, atypical localisation of fluid in the pleural space indicates that the part of the pulmonary parenchyma below the effusion is altered. Encapsulated fluid usually produces an image of a bi-convex lens or adopts a lenticular shape. For instance, if lower lobe pathology increases the intensity of action of reverse elastic forces, the fluid will accumulate posteriomedially. Characteristically, the opacity is higher in the axillary line. In some cases, a pleural effusion can mimic middle or lower lobe atelectasis. On the lateral radiographs, the upper border of the density is parallel to the main fissure and is higher in the posterior segments of the thorax, and on moving anteriorly, it descends into the costophrenic sulcus. Lobar or segmental lung collapse can be a cause of pleural effusion development. In these cases, the effusion can mimic pleural adhesion [82].

When the whole hemithorax is opacified, the first priority should be to determine the position of the mediastinum, as the position of the mediastinum depends on the intrapleural pressure. Lower intrapleural pressure will shift the mediastinum to the ipsilateral side of the effusion, (**Figure 2**) while if the pressure is higher on the side of the effusion mediastinum will shift contralaterally, (**Figure 3**) assuming that the mediastinum is not infiltrated by a tumour or an infiltrative process, that is, that it is not fixed. When the mediastinum is fixed, there is no mediastinal

Figure 2. Atelectasis of the left lung with ipsilateral shifting of the mediastinum.

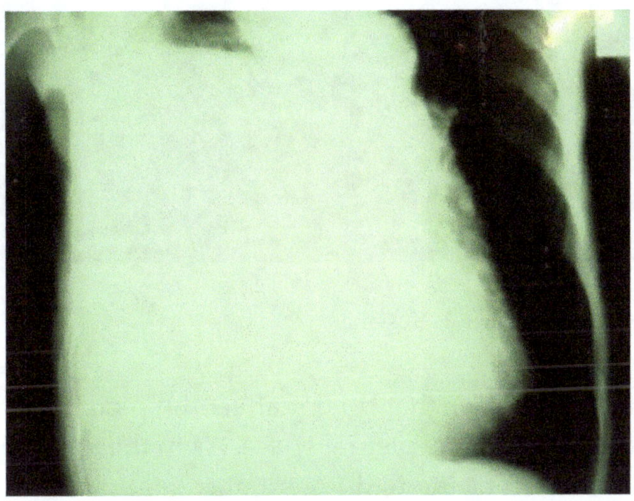

Figure 3. Massive pleural effusion with contralateral shifting of mediastinum.

shift seen. If the mediastinum shifts to the ipsilateral side of the effusion, it can be concluded that the underlying process is an expansive lung disease. Occasionally, in complete atelectasis contralateral lung is a cause of increased retrosternal light, which is clearly seen on a lateral radiograph. This radiological picture corresponds to complete obstruction of the ipsilateral bronchus by a neoplasm. In obstruction of a bronchus, thoracocentesis is not indicated as it is not necessary for diagnostic work up and as it carries a risk of additional increase of the negative intrapleural pressure. Possible complications include pneumothorax and re-expansive pulmonary oedema. In an obstructive lesion, evacuation of a large amount of fluid [more than 1000 ml] is only recommended if a simultaneous measuring if intrapleural pressure is possible [17].

4.5.2. Computed tomography [CT]

CT is efficient in diagnosing pathological alterations of the pulmonary parenchyma and changes that belong to pleural diseases (**Figure 4**). In comparison to standard radiography, pleural alterations are diagnosed much easier on the CT scan and are easily distinguished from the

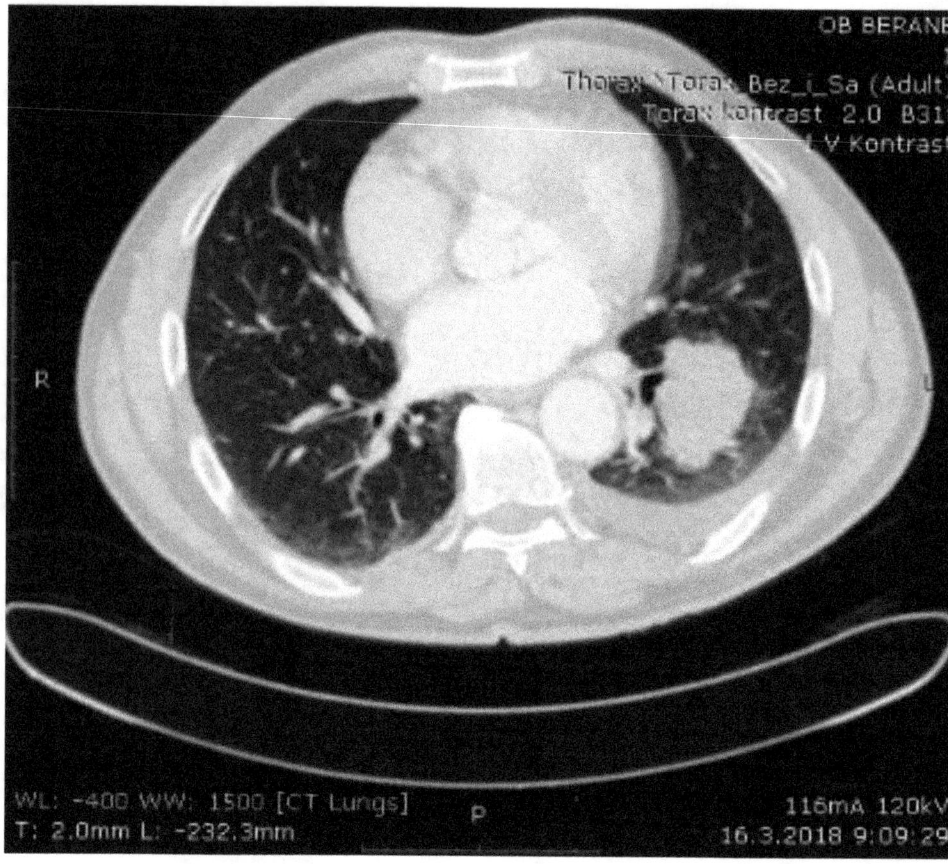

Figure 4. Lung cancer followed by an ipsilateral effusion.

pulmonary parenchyma and diseases that do not affect the pleura [83]. Collections of fluid or masses have a tendency to adjust to the pleural space. As in the radiograph, the angle between the lesion and thorax helps when trying to differentiate a pleural from a parenchymal change. If the angle between the lesion and thorax wall is sharp, then the change is likely to be a part of the lung parenchyma, while if the angle is blunt, then the lesion is more likely to be of pleural origin. Nevertheless, CT can also be inconclusive. The findings can be similar to the chest radiograph findings, especially when atelectasis or pneumonia are in question, or when a pleural collection forms a sharp angle with thorax wall. Free pleural fluid can form sickle-like opacities in the lowest and posterior parts of the thorax. Fluid collection that is loculated can be seen as a fixed, lenticular opacity. Thickening of the pleura almost invariably points to an exudative effusion [83]. Unreliable signs of pleural invasion are: absence of border area between pleura and primary lesion, blunt angle between the tumour and chest wall, and the presence of a pleural effusion. A probable sign of pleural invasion is if in addition to rib destruction simultaneously the distance between the surface of the tumour and wall of the thorax is less than 3 cm.

The typical features of malignant pleural disease are nodules, irregularity, and pleural thickening >1 cm. It was found that these pleural characteristics discriminated well between malignant and benign disease in a prospective chest radiograph study of 40 patients with suspected malignant effusions, with a sensitivity of 84% and specificity of 100% for malignancy [84]. However, pleural thickening alone was not found to be specific as it was found in malignancy as well as in empyema. Albeit, the presence of pleural nodules was found to be highly specific, it was found to have only 17% sensitivity—17% of patients with malignant effusion had associated pleural nodules. It is interesting that the half of the patient with malignant effusion had no pleural abnormalities on CT in this study [85]. In patients with lung cancer, even minimal pleural effusions can represent malignant involvement [86]. CT density coefficient is not specific enough to differentiate parenchymal lesion from a solid pleural mass or a serous effusion from blood or pus [87]. In these cases, ultrasound is the investigation of choice and has an edge over CT.

4.5.3. Magnetic resonance imaging [MRI]

Pleural effusion can be identified on an MRI scan; however, MRI is not advised for routine evaluation of malignant effusions.

Collections of pleural fluid are visible as areas of low intensity signal on T1 images, while signal is intensified on T2 images. MRI can sometimes enable the classification of a pleural effusion to transudate, chylothorax, empyema, but in essence, the information gained by MRI is usually insufficient to be of diagnostic use. However, its ability to produce excellent soft-tissue contrast can be useful for detailed evaluation of tumour invasion [88]. MRI is superior to CT in identification of solitary foci on the chest wall, changes of the endothoracic fascia and identifying the invasion of diaphragmatic muscles. MRI can be especially useful in evaluating apices of both hemithoraces.

4.5.4. Positron emission tomography with F-18-fluorodexyglucosae [PET]

PET-FDG imaging accurately detected malignant pleural involvement and the presence of malignant pleural effusion in 16 out of 18 patients and excluded pleural metastatic involvement or malignant effusion in 16 of 17 patients—sensitivity of 88.8%, specificity 94.1%, and accuracy of 91.4%. PET-FDG imaging is a highly reliable and accurate non-invasive test that can differentiate benign from malignant pleural effusions and/or pleural involvement in lung cancer patients and CT findings of suspected malignant pleural effusion [89]. Nonetheless, this form of imaging may not be able to differentiate pleural malignancy from benign inflammation of the pleura, for example, caused by talc pleurodesis [90].

4.5.5. Ultrasound

Thoracic ultrasound can be done with any modern ultrasound machine. Curved ultrasound probe 5–7.5 MHz enables the examination of deep structures of the chest wall. Intercostal spaces are utilised as an acoustic window [91]. When using high frequency probe of 7.5–10 MHz, parietal and visceral pleura are usually seen as echogenic lines, not thicker than 2 mm (**Figure 5**). Diaphragm is visualised as a bright curved line moving upwards or downwards, depending on the respiration phase. High frequency probes improve the resolution in the fields close to source of the echo, enabling differentiation of cystic lesions from solid masses. Ultrasound properties of pleural fluid are best evaluated by changing the form of the fluid during respiration [10]. Ultrasound discovers the presence of fluid in pleural space with an accuracy varying between 87 and 94% [92]. An amount of liquid present in pleural space can be quantified by ultrasonographic examination. Calculated amount of liquid is in better correlation with real amount of fluid present if it is defined by ultrasonographic examination. Amount of liquid

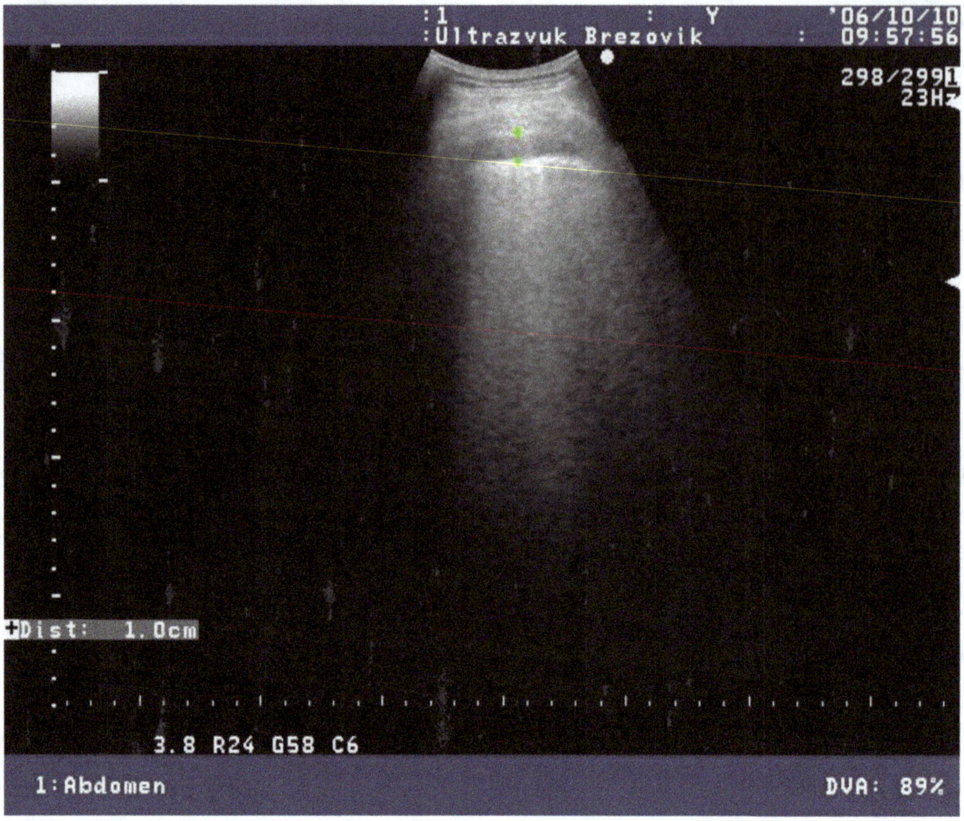

Figure 5. 'Comet tail' sign.

of 1000 ml on radiograms in lateral decubitus correlates to a 30-mm layer of liquid, while the same amount of fluid correlates to ultrasonographic thickness of 40 mm [93].

Ultrasound diagnostics is useful in determining a suitable spot for thoracocentesis, especially in loculated and small effusions [92, 94, 95]. Ultrasound is also helpful in therapeutic thoracocentesis for measuring effusion the depth of an effusion which makes this procedure safer. At thoracocentesis, the thickness of pleural liquid must not be less than 10 mm. Complications of ultrasound guided thoracocentesis are minimal [94].

Pleural thickenings are presented as constant regions of weak echogenicity. Differentiation of pleural thickening from effusion, tumour, and mesothelioma is uncertain. Respiratory dependent configuration change of identified lesion favours a pleural effusion, regular borders favour pleural thickening, and irregular borders favour a diagnosis of a tumour [96]. Plaques produce the image of focal zones of intensive reflection with dense posterior acoustic shadow and usually surrounding non-calcified pleural thickening.

Pleural masses are sonographically presented as masses of unclear limitation, weakly echogenic, nodal or linearly disseminated along the pleura. Malignant tumour of pleura can infiltrate the chest wall and it leads to poorly visible demarcation of pleural mass from the thoracic wall [97]. Pleural thickening over 1 cm brings forward justified suspicion of a malignant tumour. Accompanying pleural effusion is usually visible in a big field which spreads locally and is especially emphasised. The effusion is helpful in tumour identification and it enables differentiation of parietal from visceral pleura. Visceral pleural thickening is rarely seen. In pleural mass, respiratory motions of lungs during the respiratory cycle are reduced. Very clear echogenic and irregular reflexes are visible on passing towards the ventilated area of lungs.

Metastases might appear as diffuse parietal pleural thickenings. These can be seen as weakly echogenic and moderately echogenic structures; they are oval and easily nodal.

4.6. Cytological and pathohistological examination of pleural fluid and pleural tissue

The percentage of positive cytological results has a wide range, which depends on the type and location of the primary neoplasm, the number of samples being examined, methods and way of sample processing. Results of cytological examination depend on pathohistological type of tumour, number of prepared samples, length of time sample is kept, and interest of cytopathologist.

Malignant cells have several characteristic properties which differentiate them from other cells. They can significantly vary in form and size. They are usually large. The diameter of the nucleus ranges up to 50 μm and their diameter is significantly bigger than, for example, the nucleus of mesothelial cells that are rarely bigger than 20 μm (**Figure 6**). For comparison, small lymphocytes have diameter up to 10 μm. Nucleoli of malignant cells are up to 5 μm in size. Nucleoli of non-malignant cells do not exceed 3 μm. Malignant cells have a high nucleo-cytoplasmic ratio. Morphological analysis itself is not sufficient for differentiation of adeno-carcinoma cells from, for example, mesothelioma cells. Mesothelioma cells have a tendency to make papillary groups, and they are multinuclear, with atypia and cell to cell position. Adenocarcinoma cells have a greater tendency to form acini of similar structures. They can form big group of cells. Balloon-like cytoplasmic vacuolization is expressed [98].

Groups of 20 or more benign mesothelial cells can sometimes appear bizarre. Large, vacu-olated cells of adenocarcinoma enable differentiation between these two entities. A small number of mitotic figures are often present in benign effusions and the presence of such pic-ture does not point to malignant disease.

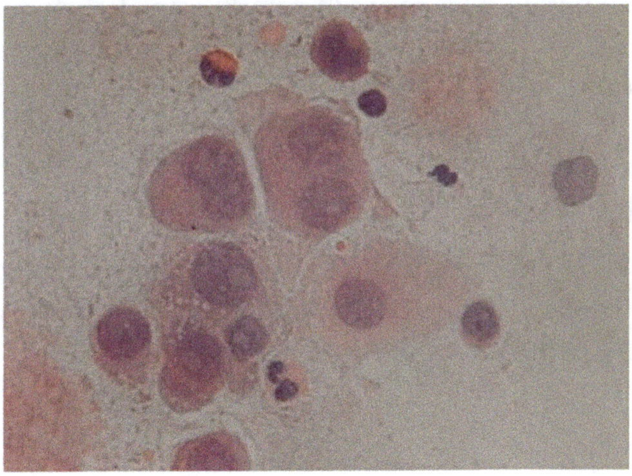

Figure 6. Atypical giant cells in pleural effusion.

Two most important histochemical tests commonly used are alcian blue staining and periodic acid-Schiff. Alcian blue staining enables the detection of acid mucins, which is a specific finding for mesothelioma. Alcian blue staining was positive in 14 out of 19 (73%) patients with mesothelioma, while it was negative in all the patients with adenocarcinoma [99]. Periodic acid-Schiff staining, after diastasis digestion (PAS-D), enables the detection of neutral mucins that have a diagnostic value for adenocarcinoma. PAS-D staining was positive in 27 out of 44 (61%) patients for adenocarcinoma, while it was negative in all patients with mesothelioma [100].

In differentiation of adenocarcinoma from mesothelioma, a whole palette of monoclonal antibodies is used. The same antibodies are found in the presence of benign mesothelial cells, adenocarcinoma, and malignant mesothelioma.

Immunohistochemical staining can be a useful diagnostic tool. Specific markers such as thyroid transcription factor 1 exhibit a high specificity for a primary lung carcinoma, whereas GATA3 has been advocated as a sensitive and specific immunostain for diagnosis breast cancer [101]. Cytological specimens are used for sequencing of mutations of epidermal growth factor receptor (EGFR), [102] and with the use of highly sensitive sequencing such as next-generation sequencing, these markers can be detected even when cytological examination affirms a low percentage of malignant cells or even no malignant cells [103].

Pathologist's challenge can be differentiating mesothelioma from both metastatic adenocarcinoma and non-malignant reactive mesothelium. Using a panel of immunohistochemical stains is now the standard for diagnosing mesothelioma, including using antibodies that stain positively for mesothelioma (WT1, cytokeratin 5/6, calretinin) and those that stain negatively (e.g. adenocarcinoma specific stains such as MOC- 31, CEA, Ber-EP4, and B72.3) [104, 105]. However, it is of note that pleural liquid mesothelin levels can be elevated in a significant number of patients with malignant effusions other than mesothelioma, while mesothelin levels are not elevated in benign effusions. Hence, a high mesothelin level strongly suggests a presence of some form of malignancy [106]. The future of diagnosis might include genetic analysis—either for microarray characteristic of tumours or for characteristics of malignancy (microsatellite, aneuploidy, telomerase DNA methylation, and mutations) [107, 108]. As explained earlier, pleural cells genetic testing may lead to therapeutic choices; for example, establishing an EGFR mutation in malignant pleural cells can the predict response to pertinent EGFR tyrosine kinase inhibitors, like gefitinib or erlotinib [102, 103, 109]. High throughput sequencing technology—a by-product of the Human Genome Project, enables rapid sequencing of either a small percentage of the genome that codes for expressed genes (the exome), or the whole genome. As all cancers are unique, the hope is that this could lead to patient-specific markers and subsequent therapies—for example, designing specific vaccines that 'drive' the immune system of the host to attack that patient's cancer [110].

In previously diagnosed neoplasms, pleural effusion cytology is positive in 50–90% of cases [112]. Falsely positive results range from 0 to 3% [111]. The absence of malignant cells in pleural effusion does not exclude malignancy and this infers the necessity of repeating the cytological investigations.

If repeated cytological analysis is negative, clinical observations and laboratory examinations do not point towards a probable aetiology of pleural effusion, and percutaneous blind biopsy is indicated (**Figure 7**).

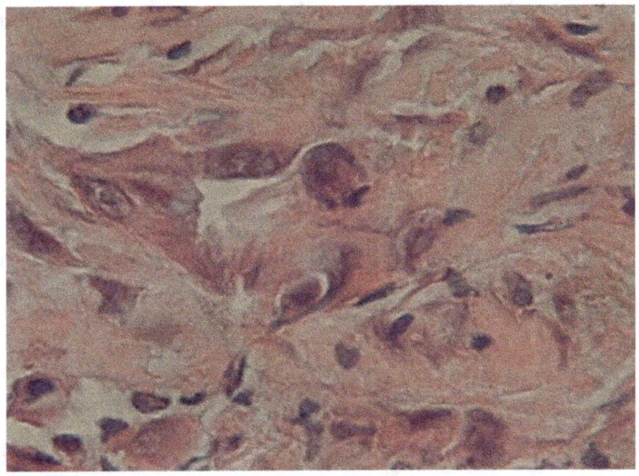

Figure 7. Adenocarcinoma invasivum pleurae HG2, NG3 (EMA × 400).

In seven series of malignant pleural effusions published and analysed in the literature (over 500 recorded cases), cytological analysis of pleural fluid sample had a diagnostic significance ranging from 66 [47] to 76% [57]. Pleural biopsy had positive predictive value of 46% [8]. Combining of these two procedures, cytological and pathohistological analysis, disease was diagnosed in 73% of patients. These data indicate that cytology is the more specific method compared to pleural biopsy, while they also suggest that these tests are complementary and that small samples given by pleural biopsy can be falsely negative.

In a randomised study that compared CT-guided biopsy with closed pleural biopsy using an Abrams needle, CT-guided biopsy was notably more sensitive (87 versus 47%) with a superior negative predictive value (80 versus 44%) [113]. Thoracoscopy is a procedure that is well tolerated and at the same time allows excellent visualisation of the entire pleural surface.

Correct identification of metastatic disease of pleura in nearly 100% of cases is achieved by directed pleural biopsies [117]. This technique provides additional advantages, including the ability to provide the information about the tumour's gross appearance, to provide the information for staging, to drain the pleural space for talc pleurodesis, to lyse adhesions, and the ability to produce large biopsy specimens for genetic and immunohistochemical analysis for molecular markers (e.g. EGFR) if needed. In routine examination, pleural effusion analysis by electronic microscopy has a slight advantage over cytological examination [115].

5. Possible therapeutic modalities of malignant pleural effusions

Treatment of patients with malignant pleural effusion has to be in accordance with the disease prognosis. Asymptomatic patients do not warrant treatment; nevertheless, most patients will go on to develop progressive pleural effusions that will elicit symptoms and require treatment. However, some patients will reach a stable state of pleural fluid formation and removal and these patients not progress to a symptomatic stage.

According to therapeutic possibilities, the doctor's first step is to estimate the patient's performance status. In order to get a clear answer to the question of should the patient with malignant effusion be treated or not treated, the following questions must be answered. Do the current symptoms reduce the patient's quality of life? What was the response of primary tumour to radiotherapy or chemotherapy? What is the performance status? What is the expected survival time? What was the patient's response to initial thoracocentesis? What is the liquid reaccumulation rate after evacuating thoracocentesis? For how long was the patient asymptomatic after thoracocentesis? Did lungs re-expand after drainage? Is the patient in a condition to tolerate intrapleural sclerotherapy?

If one is to follow this line of thought and principle, cooperation with oncologist, cardio-thoracic surgeon, radiotherapist, and everyone involved in the patient's treatment is necessary.

After diagnostic thoracocentesis is performed, therapeutic thoracocentesis follows (without intrapleural medication) which probably will not result in long-term control of pleural effusion [79, 116]. Possible complications of repeated thoracocentesis are secondary infections, loss of proteins, artificial pneumothorax, effusion loculation, and trapped lung.

5.1. Significance of specific oncological treatment

One of the important principles of oncological treatment is primary implementation of radio and/or chemotherapy. In cancers which have a high probability of being highly sensitive to systemic chemotherapy, for example, lymphoma, chemotherapy is the treatment of choice [79]. Of course, thoracocentesis is necessary in the initial phase of diagnostics and treatment, for both cytological examination and alleviating symptoms of respiratory distress.

Patients with an effusion and a tumour that is refractory to chemotherapy should have thoracontesis performed every 3-4 days for symptomatic relief. In NSCLS, colon and pancreatic cancer, favourable effects of primary systemic chemotherapy and/or radiotherapy are not expected. Intrapleural therapy will probably be indicated for these patients.

5.2. Treatment modalities—therapeutic approach

Moribund patients and patients in the preterminal phase of disease, with the symptoms of respiratory distress thoracocentesis is an urgent therapeutic procedure for alleviating current symptomatology. Aggressive therapy is not recommended in such patients. In view of possible complications during repeated thoracocentesis, a certain number of doctors reserve thoracocentesis only for moribund patients as a type of a short-term symptomatic therapy.

Patients who have a good performance status and longer survival time is expected, chemotherapy and/or radiotherapy is administrated after thoracocentesis. Generally, systemic chemotherapy produces disappointing results when it comes to control of malignant pleural effusion. Since the adverse effects from radiation pneumonitis outweigh the possible benefits of therapy, hemithorax radiation is contraindicated in malignant pleural effusion from lung cancer as a rule (**Figure 8**).

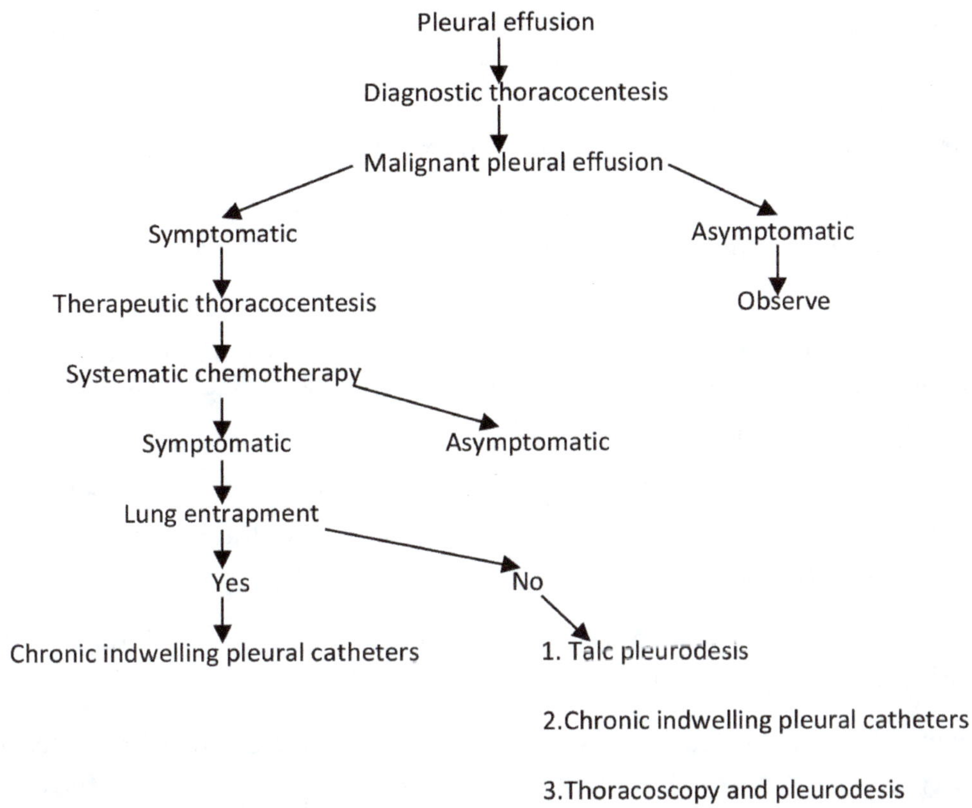

Figure 8. Diagnostic and therapeutic algorithm in malignant pleural effusions.

Drainage or intrapleural therapy is indicated if previous therapeutic protocols produce no results, that is, if they did not enable the control of pleural fluid production. Reaccumulation of larger amount of liquid leads to respiratory distress and/or worsening of clinical picture.

Pleurectomy, shunts, and other aggressive surgical interventions are reserved for patients refractive to intrapleural therapy. Pleurectomy and/or pleural abrasion are highly effective in obliteration of pleural space and in malignant pleural effusion control [117]. Therefore, this procedure is reserved for patients who have a reasonably long expected survival time and are in good general condition or who have failed a sclerosing agent therapeutic procedure. Pleuroperitoneal shunt has been demonstrated to be both safe and effective [118]. The shunt can be especially beneficial in refractory chylothorax where it allows recirculation of chyle [119]. Hyperthermic intrathoracic chemotherapy perfusion (HITHOC) combined with cytoreductive surgery can be performed in selected patients with acceptable mortality and morbidity rates [120].

5.3. Use of thoracic drain

Primary therapeutic task for treatment of patients with malignant effusion is alleviating dyspnoea. Reaccumulation of fluid sometimes can be controlled by intrapleural instillation of medication. In controlling the usual techniques of thoracocentesis, needle aspiration, and drainage are rarely efficient [79]. Treatment is basically palliative, disregarding the stage of disease and condition of the patient. Drainage postpones respiratory distress, but it does not prevent reaccumulation of liquid, dyspnoea, and pleural pain. Therefore, all patients with notable symptomatology, except moribund and those patients in preterminal stage of disease, are recommended to have drainage of pleural space with instillation of therapeutic solution. Intrapleural therapy often produces satisfactory outcomes with in regard of long term palliation of respiratory symptoms by reducing or eliminating pleural liquid formation.

In loculated effusions, drainage is not successful. This is due to the fact that the lung never re-expands sufficiently so that visceral and parietal pleura are in contact. In this case, intrapleural therapy is not recommended.

Instillation of thoracic drain is a safe and successful surgical procedure enabling at the same time diagnostics and treatment of malignant pleural effusion. If it is performed correctly, the method is relatively painless.

After placing the drain, it is necessary to perform control radiographs in order to check the correct position of the drain, exclude pneumothorax, establish lung expansion, and amount of liquid that is possibly retained.

Lung expansion is necessary to achieve in order to close the space previously filled with liquid and to bring pleural surfaces into contact.

Failure of pleurodesis is associated with abnormal lung expansion that is detected with pleural manometry. A pleural space elastance greater than 19.0 cm H_2O/L during the evacuation of first 500 ml of pleural liquid was found to predict 100% pleurodesis failure at 1 month [121]. Lung expansion abnormalities detected during later stages are indicative of immediate or delayed pleurodesis outcomes.

Prerequisite for pleurodesis is that the effusion is not loculated, that patient has a good performance status and that expected survival time is longer than 4 weeks. After adequate evacuation of liquid, medicines are instilled into pleural space by bolus. Whether the procedure is done with or without active suction, fast decompression should be avoided. Consequences of fast decompression are severe pain, pulmonary shock, mediastinal shift, and pulmonary oedema of the re-expanded lung. If the effusion is massive, 1000–1500 ml can be evacuated. Drained should be intermittently clammed, especially in the early phase of suction. This way, hemodynamic stabilisation of patient is ensured. Drainage is continuous while daily amount of aspirated content is higher than 100 ml. By irritating pleura and lungs, every drain will produce around 50 ml of pleural liquid during 24 h. Drainage gives satisfactory results in less than 20% of patients [69, 116]. Nevertheless, pleurodesis in an outpatient setting using small-bore catheters can be successfully performed with decreased cost and morbidity.

The utilisation of indwelling catheters [Denver Biomaterials, Golden, PleurX, Colorado] has attained popularity due to it being an outpatient procedure, which allows the patient and family to manage the pleural effusion in a timely fashion at home. For symptomatic refractory or recurrent malignant pleural effusion, these catheters have grown to be the mainstay of treatment in most centres in the United States. This is due to their ability to successfully palliate the symptoms of dyspnoea regardless of the presence of lung entrapment. Spontaneous pleurodesis is developed by approximately 50% of patients by 2 months [122, 123].

5.4. Medicine choice for intrapleural therapy

It is presumed that medications such as tetracyclines, talc, and nitrogen mustard, etc. cause inflammation of pleural surfaces. Inflammation leads to obliteration of pleural space disabling reacummulation of liquid [pleurodesis]. The mechanism of action of 5-fluorouracil effect is even less clear. Agents like cisplatin and cytosine arabinoside locally achieve high concentrations; thus, they are assumed to have a direct cytoreductive effect [116].

Choice of medication for pleurodesis partly depends on clinical, and partly on non-clinical parameters.

5.4.1. Nitrogen mustard

Nitrogen mustard (mechlorethamine) has been used in intrapleural therapy since 1949 and it is one of the first medications used in control of malignant pleural effusions [124]. Medicine efficiency is different and is accompanied by a large number of side effects such as chest pain, nausea, and vomiting [124, 125].

5.4.2. Talc

Talc is one of the oldest and most efficient medicines [79, 125]. Talc is instilled into the pleural space as a suspension or powder (**Figure 9**). Insufflation of talc powder has proven to be more efficient than instillation of the suspension [125]. Following talc poudrage and slurry, fever is a common occurrence, occurring 16–69% of the time. Complications that have also been reported with talc usage include arrhythmia, empyema, respiratory failure including pneumonitis, and adult respiratory distress syndrome (ARDS).

5.4.3. Quinacrine

Quinacrine is an antimalarial medication which has been recommended in therapy of malignant effusions for a period of time. Its use is completely abandoned now [79].

5.4.4. Biological agent—corynebacterium parvum

Biological agent—corynebacterium parvum in dose from 5 to 10 mg was promising at first; however, randomised study which compared its efficiency with efficiency of tetracycline did not show a statistically significant efficiency [126, 127].

5.4.5. Tetracycline

Tetracycline is a very popular medicine in intrapleural therapy because of its efficiency, affordability, and ease of use. Recommended dose for instillation is between 500 mg and 3 g of diluted tetracycline in 50–100 ml of normal saline [114, 127]. The most common side effects, in about 30–40% patients, are fever and moderate to severe chest pain which requires premedication [79]. Tetracycline is efficient in prevention of pleural effusion recurrence as well. Crucial factor for treatment success is fast and complete dispersion of tetracycline in pleural space [125].

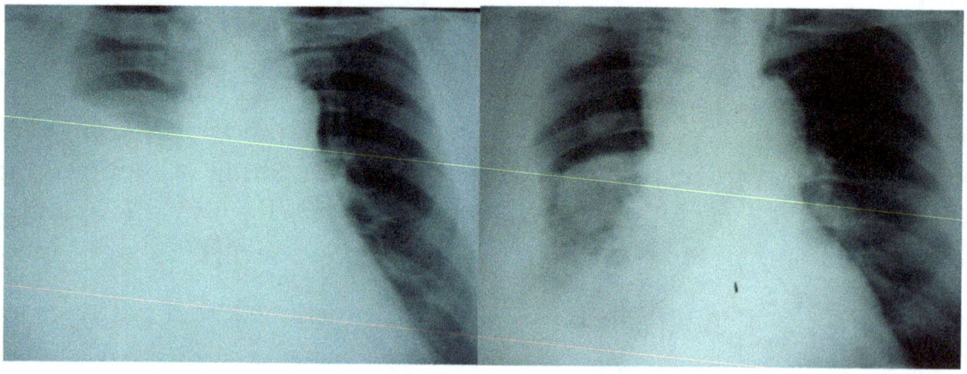

Figure 9. CXR before and after pleurodesis.

5.4.6. Bleomycin

Bleomycin is an antitumor, antibiotic producing significant results in prevention of pleural liquid reaccumulation [128]. Usual dose is 60 U in 100 ml D5W or normal saline [129, 130]. Systemic reabsorption is limited. About 40–45% of medicine is resorbed via pleura. This dose of medicine does not supress the bone marrow; thus, bleomycin can be used simultaneously with chemotherapy and radiotherapy and it can be used in patients that suffer from myelosuppresion [129].

In prevention of malignant pleural effusion, recurrence bleomycin is more efficient than tetracycline. Average time of effusion recurrence after tetracycline therapy (dose of 1 gram) was 32 days and 46 days for bleomycin (dose of 60 U) [129]. Series of three to four daily instillations of bleomycin is used in refractory effusions with a reduction in dosing from 60 to 30 U [131] is recommended.

5.4.7. Other medicines

Other medicines used for pleurodesis are thiotepa and 5-fluorouracyl, but they are less efficient than above mentioned medications. It is assumed that NaOH implementation achieves chemical pleuritis [132]. Doxorubicin has a similar effect to nitrogen mustard [121].

After pleurodesis, reaccumulation of liquid occurs in around 20–30% patients. If this is a small amount of fluid and is well tolerated by the patient, further treatment is usually not necessary.

The most efficacious methods in control of the effusion are pleural abrasion, chest tube drainage with sclerosing agent instillation, and pleurectomy. Mixed intravenous and intrapleural chemotherapy, with air therapy has produced response in 55% of patients, complete remission has resulted in 7%, partial remission in 48%, in 22% disease stabilisation has been achieved, and disease progression has been recorded in 22% of patients [133].

5.5. Therapy associated pain

After intrapleural administration of sclerotherapy, pain might occur. After drainage of 15–20 ml, 2% lidocaine is instilled via drain or catheter. The patient needs to breathe deeply and cough mildly for better distribution of anaesthetic over the surface of pleural space. Five to ten minutes before tetracycline is intravenously injected, 75–150 μg fentanyl is administrated, and

5–10 mg of morphine is given after that. Fentanyl acts very quickly, as morphine takes over the extended analgesic effect. Fentanyl is slowly injected, over 5–7 minutes. If an unwanted reaction to fentanyl is expected, naloxone is given. Doctor must make sure that drain or flexible catheter is vertical and that intrapleural agent from the drain interflows into pleural space. In the analgesic therapy, results are achieved with less strong medications; therefore, premedication with morphine 10 mg or meperidine 75–100 mg intramuscularly or subcutaneously is recommended. Just before tetracycline solution instillation, 20 ml of 2% lidocaine is given intrapleurally. Morphine, fentanyl as well as other analgesics can have a depressive effect on respiratory centre and therefore, these principles of pain therapy cannot be applied in elderly patients, patients who are predisposed to respiratory depression and those with a bad general condition.

6. Conclusion

PMPE were equally present in all pathohistological types of lung cancer, while MPE were most common in lung adenocarcinoma. The diagnostic yield of pleural fluid cytology and closed pleural biopsy combined was more than 90%. Most commonly used therapeutic procedures were thoracocentesis and pleurodesis. PMPE were not a contraindication for explorative thoracotomy.

Author details

Milic Medenica[1]*, Miras Medenica[2] and Danilo Cosovic[1]

*Address all correspondence to: milic.medenica@gmail.com

1 Hospital for Lung Diseases – Brezovik, Niksic, Montenegro

2 Wrightington, Wigan and Leigh NHS Foundation Trust, UK

References

[1] Taghizadeh N, Fortin M, Tremblay A. USA Hospitalizations for Malignant Pleural Effusions - Data from the National Inpatient Sample, 2012. Chest; Apr 2017;**151**(4):845-854

[2] Rahman NM, Ali NJ, Brown G, et al. Local anaestetic thorascopy: British thoracic society pleural disease guidline, 2010. Thorax. 2010;**65**(Suppl 2):ii54-ii60

[3] Johnston WW. The malignant pleural effusion: A review of cytopathlogical diagnoses of 584 specimens from 472 consecutive patients. Cancer. 1985;**56**:905-909

[4] Chernow B, Sahn SA. Carcinomatous involvment of the pleura of 96 patients. The American Journal of Medicine. 1977;**77**:507-513

[5] Naito T, Satoh H, Ishikawa H, et al. Pleural effusion as a significant prognostic factor in non small cell lung cancer. Anticancer Research. 1997;**17**:4743-4746

[6] Meyer PC. Metastatic carcinoma of the pleura. Thorax. 1966;**21**:437-443

[7] Medenica M. Pleural Effusion. Podgorica: University of Montenegro; 2015. [25, 26, 30, 35, 82, 83, 207, 209, 211]. ISBN 978-86-7664-131-4

[8] Marel M, Stastny B, Melinova L, et al. Diagnosis of pleral effusion: Experience with clinical studies, 1986-1990. Chest. 1995;**107**:1598-1603

[9] Mulvey RB. The effect of pleural fluid on the diaphragm. Radiology. 1965;**84**:1080-1086

[10] Marks WM, Filly RA, Callen PW. Real-time evaluation of pleural lesions: New observations regarding the probability of obtaining free fluid. Radiology. 1992;**142**:163-164

[11] Brown NE, Zamel N, Aberman A. Changes in pulmonary mechanics and gas excange following thoracentesis. Chest. 1978;**74**:540-542

[12] Light RW, Stansbury DW, Brown SE. The relationship between pleural pressures and changes in pulmonary function after therapeutic thoracentesis. The American Review of Respiratory Disease. 1986;**133**:658-661

[13] Estenne M, Yernault J-C, DeTroyer A. Mechanism of relief of dyspnea after thoracentesis in patients with large pleural effusions. The American Journal of Medicine. 1983; **74**:813-819

[14] Shinto R, Stansbury DW, Brown SE, et al. The effect of thoracocentesis improve the exercise capacity of patients with pleural effusion? The American Review of Respiratory Disease. 1987;**135**:A244

[15] Baburao A, Narayanswamy H. Clinico-pathological profile and haematological abnormalities associated with lung cancer in Bangalore, India. Asian Pacific Journal of Cancer Prevention. 2015;**16**(18):8235-8238

[16] Vaska K, Wan LS, Sagar K, et al. Pleural effusion as a cause of right ventricular diastolic collapse. Circulation. 1992;**86**:609-617

[17] Light RW, Jenkison SG, Minh V, et al. Obervation on pleural space pressures as fluid withdraw during thoracentesis. The American Review of Respiratory Disease. 1980;**121**: 799-804

[18] Gilbert VE. Shifting percussion dullness of the chest: A sign of pleural effusion. Southern Medical Journal. 1997;**90**:1255-1256

[19] Wong FM, Grace WJ, Rottino A. Pleural effusions, ascites, pericardial effusions and edema in Hodgkin's disease. The American Journal of the Medical Sciences. 1963;**246**:678-682

[20] Sahn SA. Pleural diseases related to metastatic maligancies. The European Respiratory Journal. 1997;**10**:1907-1913

[21] Rodriguez-Panadero F. Lung cancer and ipsilateral pleural effusion. Annals of Oncology. 1995;**6**(suppl 3):S25-S27

[22] Decker DA, Dines DE, Payne WS. The significance of a cytologically negative pleural effusion in bronchogenic carcinoma. Chest. 1978;**74**:640-642

[23] Shintani Y, Ohta M, Iwasaki T, et al. Intraoperative pleural lavage cytology after lung resection as an independent prognostic factor for staging lung cancer. The Journal of Thoracic and Cardiovascular Surgery. 2009;**137**(4):835-839

[24] Porcel JM, Vives M. Etiology and pleural fluid characteristics of large and massive effusions. Chest. 2003;**124**(3):978-983

[25] Herrstedt J, Clementsen P, Hansen OP. Increased myelosuppression during cytostatic treatmenst and pleural effusion in patients with small cell lung cancer. European Journal of Cancer. 1992;**28A**:1070-1073

[26] Livingston RB, JK MC, Trauth CJ. Isolated pleural effusions in small cell lung carcinoma: Favorable prognosis. Chest. 1982;**81**:208-211

[27] Hsu C. Cytolocig detection of malignancy in pleural effusion: A review of 5255 samples from 3811 patients. Diagnostic Cytopathology. 1987;**3**(1):8-12

[28] Antunes G, Neville E, Duffy J, Ali N. BTS guidelines for the management of malignant pleural effusions. Thorax. 2003;**58**:ii29-ii38

[29] Apffelstaedt JP, Van Zyl JA, Muller AG. Breast cancer complicated by pleural effusion: Patient characteristic and results of surgical management. Journal of Surgical Oncology. 1995;**58**:173-175

[30] Rodriguez-Panadero F, Borderas Naranjo F, Lopez Mejias J. Pleural metastatic tumours and effusions. Frequency and pathogenic mechanisms in a post-mortem series. The European Respiratory Journal. 1989;**2**:366-369

[31] Light RW, Hamm H. Malignant pleural effusion: Would the real cause please stand up? The European Respiratory Journal. 2007;**10**:1701-1702

[32] Wang NS. The preformed stomas connecting the pleural cavity and the lymhatics in the parietal pleura. The American Review of Respiratory Disease. 1975;**111**:12-20

[33] Staats BA, Ellefson RD, Badahn LL, Dines DE, Prakash UBS, Offord D. The lipoprotein profile of chylous and non-chylous pleural effusions. Mayo Clinic Proceedings. 1980;**55**: 700-704

[34] Sahn SA. Malignant pleural effusions. Clinics in Chest Medicine. 1985;**6**:113-125

[35] Stathopoulos GT, Kollintza A, Moschos C, et al. Tumor necrosis factor-alpha promotes malignant pleural effusion. Cancer Research. 2007;**67**:9825-9834

[36] Yano S, Shinohara H, Herbst RS, et al. Production of experimental malignant pleural effusions is dependent on invasion of the pleura and expression of vascular endothelial growth factor/vascular permeability factor by human lung cancer cells. The American Journal of Pathology. 2000;**157**:1893-1903

[37] Stathopoulos GT, Sherrill TP, Karabela SP, et al. Host-derived interleukin-5 promotes adenocarcinoma-induced malignant pleural effusion. American Journal of Respiratory and Critical Care Medicine. 2010;**182**:1273-1281

[38] Stathopoulos GT, Zhu Z, Everhart MB, et al. Nuclear factor-kappaB affects tumor progression in a mouse model of malignant pleural effusion. American Journal of Respiratory Cell and Molecular Biology. 2006;**34**:142-150

[39] Yeh HH, Lai WW, Chen HH, et al. Autocrine IL-6-induced Stat3 activation contributes to the pathogenesis of lung adenocarcinoma and malignant pleural effusion. Oncogene. 2006;**25**:4300-4309

[40] Cheng C-S, Rodriguez RM, Perkett EA, et al. Vascular endothelial growth factor in pleural fluid. Chest. 1999;**115**:760-765

[41] Yano S, Herbst SH, et al. Treatment for malignant pleural effusion of human lung adenocarcinoma by inhibition of vascular endothelial growth factor receptor tyrosine kinaze phosphorylation. Clinical Cancer Research. 2000;**6**:957-965

[42] Collins PO, Connolly DT, Williams TJ. Characterization of increase in vascular permeability induced by vascular permeability factor in vivo. British Journal of Pharmacology. 1993;**109**:195-199

[43] Jankowska R, Porebska I, Dyla T. Evaluation of vascular endothelial growth factor [VEGF] in neoplastic and tuberculosis effusions - preliminary results. Pneumonologia i Alergologia Polska. 2002;**70**:258-264

[44] J B, Ł S, M K, M F, J G-S, H B-G, J S. Regulatory T cells in malignant pleural effusions subsequent to lung carcinoma and their impact on the course of the disease. Immunobiology. 2016;**18**: 2985(16):30425-30429

[45] Ye ZJ, Zhou Q, Yin W, et al. Interleukin 22-producing CD4+ T cells in malignant pleural effusion. Cancer Letters. 2012;**326**:23-32

[46] Spriggs AI, Boddington MM. The Cytology of Effusionsss. 2nd ed. New York: Grune and Stratton; 1968

[47] Black LF. The pleural space and pleural fluid. Mayo Clinic Proceedings. 1972;**47**:493-506

[48] Light RW, MacGregor MI, Luchsinger PC, Ball WC. Pleural effusions: The diagnostic separation of transudates and exudates. Annals of Internal Medicine. 1972;**77**:507-513

[49] Bousfield LR, Greenberg ML, Pacey F. Cytogenetic diagnosis of cancer from body fluids. Acta Cytologica. 1985;**29**:768-774

[50] Ocana IM, Martinez-Vazquez JM, Seguna RM, et al. Adenosine deaminase in pleural fluids. Chest. 1983;**84**:51-53

[51] Perez-Rodriguez E, Walton IJ, Hernandez JJ, et al. ADA 1/ADAp ratio in pleural tuberculosis: an exelent diagnostic parameter in pleural fluid. Respiratory Medicine. 1999;**93**:816-821

[52] Yamagishi K, Tajima M, Suzuki A, Kimura K. Relation between cell composition of pleural effusions in patients with pulmonary carcinomas and their clinical courses. Acta Cytologica. 1976;**20**:537-541

[53] Mohamed KH, Abdel-Hamid AL, Lee YCG, et al. Pleural fluid levels of IL-5 and eosinophils are closley correlated. American Journal of Respiratory and Critical Care Medicine. 2001

[54] Schandene L, Namias B, Crusiaux A, et al. IL-5 in posttraumatic eosinophilic pleural effusion. Clinical and Experimental Immunology. 1993;**115**:115-119

[55] Clarkson B. Relationship between cell type, glucose concteracion, and response to treatment in neoplastic effusions. Cancer. 1964;**17**:914-928

[56] Good JT Jr, Taryle DA, Sahn SA. The pathogenesis of low glucose, low pH malignant effusions. The American Review of Respiratory Disease. 1985;**131**:734-741

[57] Sahn SA, Good JT Jr. Pleural fluid pH in malignant effusions. Diagnostic, prognostic and therapeutic implications. Annals of Internal Medicine. 1988;**108**:345-349

[58] Nusair S, Breuer R, Amir G. Closed needle biopsy: Predicting diagnostic yield examining pleural fluid parameters. Respiratory Medicine. 2002;**96**:890-894

[59] Villena V, Perez V, Pozo F. Amylase levels in pleural effusions: A consecutive unselected series of 841 patients. Chest. 2002;**121**:470-474

[60] Ferrer J, Roldan J, Teixidor J, et al. Predictors of pleural maliginancy in patients with pleural effusion undregoing thoracoscopy. Chest. 2005;**127**:1017-1022

[61] McKenna JM, Chandrasekhar AJ, Henkin RE. Diagnostic value of carcinoembryonic antigen in exudative pleural effusions. Chest. 1980;**78**:587-590

[62] Rittgers RA, Loewenstein MS, Feinerman AE, et al. Carcinoembryonic antigen levels in benign and malignant pleural effusions. Annals of Internal Medicine. 1978;**88**:631-634

[63] Miedouge M, Rouzaud P, Salama G, et al. Evaluation of seven tumour markers in pleural fluid for the diagnosis of malignant effusion. British Journal of Cancer. 1999;**81**:1059-1065

[64] Lee YC, Chern JH, Lai SL, et al. Sialyl stage-specific embryonic antigen-1 useful marker for differentiating the etiology of pleural effusion. Chest. 1998;**114**.1542-1545

[65] Lee YC, Knox BS, Garrett JE. Use of cytokratin fragments 19.1 and 19.21 [Cyrfa 21-1] in the differentiation of malignant and benign pleural effusion. Australian and New Zealand Journal of Medicine. **29**:765-769

[66] Tamura S, Nishigaki T, Moriwaki Y, et al. Tumor markers in pleural effusion diagnosis. Cancer. 1988;**61**:298-302

[67] Lai CL, Tsai CM, Tsai TT. Presence of serum anti-p53 antibodies is associated with pleural effusion and poor prognosis in lung cancer patients. Clinical Cancer Research. 1998;**4**:3025-3030

[68] Moriarty AT, Wiersema L, Snyder W, et al. Immunophenotyping of cytologic specimens by flow cytometry. Diagnostic Cytopathology. 1993;**9**:252-258. provjeriti

[69] Dewald G, Dines DE, Weiland LH, et al. Usefulness of chromosome examination in the diagnosis of malignant pleural effusions. The New England Journal of Medicine. 1976; **295**:1494-1500

[70] Nurminen M, Dejmek A, Martensson G, et al. Clinical utility of liquid-chronatographic analysis of effusions for hyaluronate content. Clinical Chemistry. 1994;**40**:777-780

[71] Hillerdal G, Lindqvist U. Hyaluronan in pleural effusions and serum. Cancer. 1991;**67**: 2410-2414

[72] Kawai T, Greenberg SD, Truong LD, et al. Differences in lectin binding of malignant pleural mesothelioma and adenocarcinoma of the lung. The American Journal of Pathology. 1988;**130**:401-410

[73] Rodriguez de Castro MT, Acosta O, et al. Value of DNA analysis in addition to cytological testing in the diagnosis of malignant pleural effusions. Thorax. 1994;**49**:692-694

[74] Xie L, Chen X, Wang L, et al. Cell-free miRNAs may indicate diagnosis and docetaxel sensitivity of tumor cells in malignant effusions. BMC Cancer. 2010;**10**:591

[75] Wang L, Wei J, Qian X, et al. ERCC1 and BRCA1 mRNA expression levels in metastatic malignant effusions is associated with chemosensitivity to cisplatin and/or docetaxel. BMC Cancer. 2008;**8**:97

[76] Heffner JE, Nietert PJ, Barbieri C. Pleural fluid pH as a predictor of survival for patients with malignant pleural effusions. Chest. 2000;**117**(1):79-86

[77] Kasapoglu US, Arınç S, Gungor S, et al. Prognostic factors affecting survival in non-small cell lung carcinoma patients with malignant pleural effusions. Immunobiology. 2016;**16**:30425-30429

[78] Sugiura S, Ando Y, Minami H, et al. Prognostic value of pleral effusion in patients with non-small cell lung cancer. Clinical Cancer Research. 1997;**3**:47-50

[79] Hausheer FH, Yarbo JW. Diagnosis and treatment of malignant pleural effusion. Cancer and Metastasis Reviews. 1987;**6**:23-40

[80] Ruskin JA, Gurney JW, Thorsen MK, et al. Detection of pleural effusions on supine chest radiographs. AJR. American Journal of Roentgenology. 1987;**148**:681-683

[81] Dhillon DP, Spiro SG. Malignant pleural effusions. British Journal of Hospital Medicine. 1983;**29**:506-510

[82] Rigby M, Zylak CJ, Wood LDH. The effect of lobar atelectasis on pleural fluid distribution in dogs. Radiology. 1980;**136**:603-607

[83] Henschke CI, Yankelevitz DF, Davis SD. Pleural diseases: Multimodality imaging and clinical management. Current Problems in Diagnostic Radiology. 1991;**20**:155-181

[84] Traill ZC, Davies RJ, Gleeson FV. Thoracic computed tomography in patients with suspected malignant pleural effusions. Clinical Radiology. 2000;**56**(3):193-196

[85] Arenas-Jimenez J, Alonso-Charterina S, Sanchez-Paya J, et al. Evaluation of CT fndings for diagnosis of pleural effusions. European Radiology. 2000;**10**(4):681-690

[86] Ryu JS, Ryu HJ, Lee SN, et al. Prognostic impact of minimal pleural effusion in non-small-cell lung cancer. Journal of Clinical Oncology. 2014;**32**(9):960-967

[87] Pugatch RD, Spirn PW. Radiology of the pleura. Clinics in Chest Medicine. 1985;**6**:17-32

[88] Knisely BL, Broderick LS, Kuhlman JE. MR imaging of the pleura and chest wall. Magnetic Resonance Imaging Clinics of North America. 2000;**8**(1):125-141

[89] Gupta NC, Rogers JS, Graeber GM. Clinical role of F-18 fluorodeoxyglucose poitron emission tomography imaging in patients with lung cancer and suspected malignant pleural effusions. Chest. 2002;**122**:1918-1924

[90] Weiss N, Solomon SB. Talc pleurodesis mimics pleural metastases: Differentiation with positron emission tomography/computed tomography. Clinical Nuclear Medicine. 2003; **28**(10):811-814

[91] Wernecke K. Sonographic features of pleural disease. AJR. American Journal of Roentgenology. 1997;**168**:1061-1066

[92] Kataoka H, Takada S. The role of thoracic ultrasonography for evaluation of patients with decompensated chronic heart failure. Journal of the American College of Cardiology. 2000;**35**:1638-1646

[93] Blackmore CC, Black WC, Dallas RV, et al. Pleural fluid volume estimation: a chest radiograph prediction rule. Academic Radiology. 1966;**3**:103-109

[94] Moyers JP, Starnes DL, Bienvenu GL, et al. Thoracentesis performed by radiologist using ultrasound guidance is safe regardless of the amount of fluid withdrawn. Chest. 1998;**114**:368S

[95] McLoud TC, Flower CD. Imaging the pleura: Sonography, CT, and MR imaging. AJR. American Journal of Roentgenology. 1991;**156**:1145-1153

[96] Lichtenstien DA, Menu Y. A bedside ultrasound sign ruling out pnemothorax in the critically ill. Lung sliding. Chest. 1995;**108**:1345-1348

[97] Mathis G. Thoraxsonography - part I: Chest wall and pleura. Ultrasound in Medicine & Biology. 1997;**23**:1131-1139

[98] Stevens MW, Leong AS, Fazzalari NL, et al. Cytopathology of malignant mesothelioma.: A stepwise logistic regression analysis. Diagnostic Cytopathology. 1992;**8**:333-342

[99] Ordonez NG. The immunohistochemical diagnosis of epithelial mesothelioma. Human Pathology. 1999;**30**:313-323

[100] Warnock ML, Stoloff A, Thor A. Differentation of adenocarcinoma of the lung from mesothelioma. Periodic acid-Schiff, monoclonal antibodies B 72.3, and Leu M1. The American Journal of Pathology. 1988;**133**:30-38

[101] Shield PW, Papadimos DJ, Walsh MD. GATA3: A promising marker for metastatic breast carcinoma in serous effusion specimens. Cancer Cytopathology. 2014;**122**(4):307-312

[102] Smouse JH, Cibas ES, Janne PA, et al. EGFR mutations are detected comparably in cytologic and surgical pathology specimens of nonsmall cell lung cancer. Cancer. 2009;**117**(1):67-72

[103] Buttitta F, Felicioni L, Del Grammastro M, et al. Effective assessment of *egfr* mutation status in bronchoalveolar lavage and pleural fluids by next-generation sequencing. Clinical Cancer Research. 2013;**19**(3):691-698

[104] Beasley MB. Immunohistochemistry of pulmonary and pleural neoplasia. Archives of Pathology & Laboratory Medicine. 2008;**132**:1062-1072

[105] Husain AN, Colby T, Ordonez N, et al. Guidelines for pathologic diagnosis of malignant mesothelioma: 2012 Update of the consensus statement from the international mesothelioma interest group. Archives of Pathology & Laboratory Medicine. 2013;**137**(5):647-667

[106] Creaney J, Yeoman D, Naumoff LK, et al. Soluble mesothelin in effusions: A useful tool for the diagnosis of malignant mesothelioma. Thorax. 2007;**62**(7):569-576

[107] Brock MV, Hooker CM, Yung R, et al. Can we improve the cytologic examination of malignant pleural effusions using molecular analysis? The Annals of Thoracic Surgery. 2005;**80**(4):1241-1247

[108] Holloway AJ, Diyagama DS, Opeskin K, et al. A molecular diagnostic test for distinguishing lung adenocarcinoma from malignant mesothelioma using cells collected from pleural effusions. Clinical Cancer Research. 2006;**12**(17):5129-5135

[109] Zhang X, Zhao Y, Wang M, et al. Detection and comparison of epidermal growth factor receptor mutations in cells and fluid of malignant pleural effusion in non-small cell lung cancer. Lung Cancer. 2007;**60**:175-182

[110] Kroemer G, Zitvogel L. Can the exome and the immunome converge on the design of effcient cancer vaccines? Oncoimmunology. 2012;**1**(5):579-580

[111] Grunze H. The comparative diagnostic accurancy, efficiency and specificity of cytologic techniques used in the diagnosis of malignant neoplasm in serous effusions of the pleural and pericardial cavities. Acta Cytologica. 1964;**8**:150-164

[112] Boutin C, Viallat JR, Cargnino P, Farisse P. Thoracoscopy in malignant effusion. The American Review of Respiratory Disease. 1981;**124**:588-592

[113] Maskell NA, Gleeson FV, Davies RJ. Standard pleural biopsy versus CT-guided cutting-needle biopsy for diagnosis of malignant disease in pleural effusions: A randomised controlled trial. Lancet. 2003;**366**:1326-1330

[114] Cardillo G, Facciolo F, Carbone L, et al. Long-term follow-up of videoassisted talc pleurodesis in malignant recurrent pleural effusions. European Journal of Cardio-Thoracic Surgery. 2002;**21**(2):302-305. discussion 305-306

[115] Gondos B, McIntosh KM, Renston RH, King EB. Application of electron microscopy in the definitive diagnosis of effusions. Acta Cytologica. 1978;**22**:297-304

[116] Ruckdeschel JC. Management of malignant pleural effusions: An overview. Seminars in Oncology. 1988;**15**(suppl):24-28

[117] Martini N, Bains MS, Beattie EJ Jr. Indications for pleurectomy in malignant effusion. Cancer. 1975;**35**:734-738

[118] Petrou M, Kaplan D, Goldstraw P. Management of recurrent malignant pleural effusions. Thecomplementary role of talc pleurodesis and pleuroperitoneal shunting. Cancer. 1995:801-805

[119] Murphy MC, Newman BM, Rodgers BM. Pleuroperitoneal shunt in the management of persistent chylothorax. The Annals of Thoracic Surgery. 1989;**48**:195-200

[120] Kerscher C, Ried M, Hofmann HS, Graf BM, Zausig YA. Anaesthetic management of cytoreductive surgery followed by hyperthermic intrathoracic chemotherapy perfusion. Journal of Cardiothoracic Surgery. 2014;**9**:125

[121] Rs L, Lo SK, Chuang NL, Yang CT, et al. Elastance of the pleural space: A predictor for the outcome of pleurodesis in patients with malignant pleural effusion. Annals of Internal Medicine. 1997;**126**:768-774

[122] Tremblay A, Michaud G. Single-center experience with 250 tunnelled pleural catheter insertions for malignant pleural effusion. Chest. 2006;**129**:362-368

[123] Putnam JB Jr, Walsh GL, Swisher SG, et al. Outpatient management of malignant pleural effusion by a chronic indwelling pleural catheter. The Annals of Thoracic Surgery. 2000;**69**:369-375

[124] Chahinian AP. Managment of pleural tumors and malignant pleural effusions. In: Chretein J, Bignon J, Hirsch A, editors. The Pleura in Haelth and Disease. New York, NY: Marcel Dekker Inc; 1985. pp. 571-584

[125] Anderson CB, Philpott GW, Ferguson TB. The treatment of malignant pleural effusions. Cancer. 1974;**33**:916-922

[126] Hausheer FH, Yarbo JW. Diagnosis and treatment of malignant pleural effusion. Seminars in Oncology. 1985;**12**:54-75

[127] Leahy BC, Honeybourne D, Brear SG. Treatment of malignant pleural effusions with intrapleural Corynebacterium parvum or tetracycline. European Journal of Respiratory Diseases. 1985;**56**:50-54

[128] Ostrowski MJ. Intracavitary therapy with bleomycin for the tretment of malignant pleural effusions. Journal of Surgical Oncology. 1989;(suppl):7-13

[129] Ruckdeshel JC, Moores D, Lee JZ. Intrapleural therapy for malignant pleural effusions: A randomized comparison of bleomycin and tetracycline. Chest. 1991;**100**:1535

[130] Rusch VW, Harper GR. Pleural effusions in patients with malinancy. In: Roth JA, Ruckdeschel JC, Weisseburger TH, editors. Thoracic Oncology. Philadelphia, PA: WB Co; 1989. pp. 594-605

[131] Hamed H, Fentimen IS, Chaudarz MA. Comparison of intracavitary bleomycin and talc for control of pleural effusions secondary to carcinoma of the breast. The British Journal of Surgery. 1989;**1266**:1266-1267

[132] Austin EH, Flye MW. The treatment of recurrent malignant pleural effusions. The Annals of Thoracic Surgery. 1979;**28**:190-203

[133] Su WC, Lai WW, Chen HH. Combined intrapleural and intravenous chemotherapy, and pulmonary irradiation, for treatment of patients with lung cancer presenting with malignant pleural effusion. A pilot study. Oncologia. 2003;**64**:18-24

8

Epigenetic Modifications and Potential Treatment Approaches in Lung Cancers

Metin Budak and Mustafa Yildiz

Abstract

Alteration of methylation is a process seen across a wide variety of species ranging from bacterial microorganisms to mammals, defined as the adaptation method the organism develops against environmental or intrinsic effects, or employs to switch off the genome regions which are no longer required through the evolutionary process. Scientific advancements have allowed detecting the regions that undergo different patterns of methylation. It has been demonstrated that the control on changes in gene expression is not guided by transcription factors alone and that epigenetic alterations are also involved in this process. Furthermore, epigenetic modifications have been shown to be considerably important in cancer development. This section focuses on epigenetic changes and potential treatment options in lung cancer.

Keywords: lung cancer, epigenetic, acetylation, methylation, treatment

1. Introduction

Lung cancer is one of the leading causes of death worldwide. The five-year survival rate is approximately 15% as the condition is often diagnosed at an advanced stage. Smoking is the underlying cause of about 90% of all lung cancers, and smokers constitute the major risk group for developing lung cancer. World Health Organisation (WHO) stratifies lung cancers into two histological groups: non-small cell lung cancer (NSCLC), accounting for 85% of the cases, and small cell lung cancer (SCLC), which constitutes the remaining 15%. The most valid hypothesis for the development of these cancers suggests that multi-phase genetic alterations and a series of epigenetic events result in lung cancer [1].

Owing to the technological advances of the twenty-first century, current practices offer personalised treatment alternatives by means of detailed diagnostics and a range of treatment approaches in lung cancer. While World Health Organisation classified lung cancers almost entirely under the category of adenomas until 1960s, the utility of advanced molecular tests has allowed convenient and thorough identification of subtypes. In addition with these developments, new molecular targets have emerged, leading to novel therapies [2]. During the last 20 years, studies on molecular mechanisms seeking to elucidate the development of cancers and the underlying mechanisms have shown the importance of epigenetic changes in these processes, leading to increasing interest and studies in this field.

Like all cancers, lung cancer develops with the deviation from a normal cell structure due to a number of problems that arise during cell cycle and differentiation. Deviations from normal state to tumour formation result from alterations in cell growth-signalling pathways and apoptosis mechanisms, including a series of epigenetic modifications, all of which are critical for the cell [3].

Epigenetic modifications usually occur in two forms: (1) acetylation, which occurs mainly in histone proteins at protein level and (2) methylation, which is often seen at DNA level.

2. Mutations in lung cancer

Small cell lung cancer (SCLC) accounts for approximately 16–20% of all lung cancers. Owing to the rapidly spreading pattern, SCLC is accepted as an aggressive and widespread disease; therefore, chemotherapy (CT) remains an important modality for the treatment of SCLC.

Non-small cell lung cancer (NSCLC) is responsible for about 85% of lung cancers. Postoperative adjuvant treatment approaches have become the standard of care in early stage tumours, and various systemic treatments are utilised in a metastatic setting. Although the systemic treatment approach in NSCLC according to the subtype has not changed profoundly through the years, the selection of a systemic treatment in metastatic cases has recently begun to differ based on molecular alterations and different histological subtypes of NSCLC. In addition to molecular changes that provide predictions for targeted therapies, separating NSCLC into two groups, that is, squamous and non-squamous, has been suggested to aid in selecting a more effective chemotherapy agent [4–6].

Lung cancer can be histologically divided into two main groups as NSCLC and SCLC. Mutations may be seen in genes such as EGFR, RET, PIK3CA, ALK, HER2, KRAS, BRAF, MET, NRS, MEK1 and ROS1, which are often referred to as signalling pathways and considered as drivers since they cause cancer development in NSCLCs. These mutations can be seen in current smokers, ex-smokers and non-smokers, whereas mutations in EGFR, ALK, HER2, ROS1 and RET genes are seen only in people who have never smoked. Such mutations may be observed in all histological subgroups of NSCLCs including adenocarcinomas, squamous cell carcinomas (SCCs) and large cell carcinomas [7–10].

Smoking causes chronic inflammatory stress on biological systems, thereby interfering with the cell cycle, cell development and differentiation. Long-term inflammation is associated with DNA methylation and contributes to lung cancer development via methylation mechanisms.

For example, genes such as APC, FHIT, RASSF1A and CCND2 are inactivated only in smokers due to promoter hypermethylation. Increased promoter hypermethylation of P161NK4A, MGMT, RASSF1A, FHIT and MTHFR, depending on the intensity of smoking, shows a strong correlation with NSCLCs compared to non-smokers [11, 12]. Promoter methylation of RARβ, FHIT, P161NK4A and RASSF1A increases as smoking intensifies.

Moreover, mutations in epigenetic regulator genes create a complicated situation owing to the fact that they prevent these genes from functioning properly, which is expected to impact cell cycle and cell development, thereby resulting in the development of cancer. However, these mechanisms may also offer certain advantages in favour of treatment as they may open new ways for cancer therapies (such as DNTM inhibitors) [13].

3. Acetylation of histones

Human genome, as that of any eukaryotic organism, is organised in a highly complicated manner. Except for the alterations in the genes effective in human development, the histone proteins that pack the genome serve to control the genome by undergoing various modifications. This is accomplished through various changes that occur during events such as DNA replication, repair and expression [14].

For instance, the amino terminal of the histone core is quite important as it contains a flexible and fairly simple tail domain, constituting a target region for several post-translational modifications. Histone modifications primarily occur in the form of addition of acetyl and methyl groups to lysine amino acids, addition of phosphorus to serine amino acids and methyl groups to arginines. These modifications play a critical role in the control of biological processes such as transcription [15].

Modifications in histone proteins develop by means of enzymatic pathways. Histone deacetylase inhibitors (HDACIs) also act as antagonists in cell differentiation by acetylating histones and non-histone proteins. Proteins in this group inhibit DNA repair, apoptosis and gene expression mechanisms. In addition, such proteins contain a zinc-binding group (ZBG) and a chain linking two proteins from these two groups referred to as the surface recognition polypeptide [16]. Therefore, molecules able to inhibit such proteins may be potential anti-cancer agents. For example, peptide-containing cyclic hydroxamic acids (CHAPs) may be suitable for therapeutic use as a group of potential anti-cancer agents. The molecule CHAP31, which acts on HDACIs, has been shown to have a highly effective anti-tumour effect on certain types of cancer such as lung, breast and gastric cancer as well as melanoma *in vivo* [17].

Fibrosis is one of the important factors contributing to cancer invasion and metastasis. Fibrosis results from fibroblast activation, which degrades and alters the physical structure of extracellular matrix (ECM). The fibrosis-induced increase in ECM fragility leads to pathological conditions such as epithelial-mesenchymal transition (EMT) with the transformation of normal cells into cancer. The change in the structure of collagen, one of the most important proteins in tissue structure, is another contributing factor. For this reason, collagen receptors are of particular importance regarding the progression of cancer. The discoidin domain receptors

(DDRs), DDR1 and DDR2, are overexpressed receptor proteins. DDRs mechanically increase the acetylation of c-Myb, the transcription factor of histone acetyltransferase (HAT) on rigid ECM, thereby leading to c-Myb binding to DDR2 promoter together with LEF1, and result in DDR2 upregulation in a rigid environment. Silenced c-Myb may cause DDR2 inhibition and invasion of lung cancer cells, and recovery of physical characteristics of the tissue has been shown when external interventions allow DDR2 expression [18].

Proteins in the Snail group, a zinc-binding superfamily of transcription factors, are responsible for cell migration and invasion during both the embryonic period and cancer process [19]. Snail proteins bind to the E-box sequence located in the promoter region of E-cadherin gene, which encodes the protein that is responsible for cell–cell adhesion. As a result, since E-cadherin synthesis is no longer possible, cell–cell adhesion cannot be achieved, and cancer cells gain metastatic properties [20]. Snail proteins are overexpressed in several types of cancer as they are strategically important for cancer cells. Rui et al. have emphasised that Snail, acetylated by P300, may be of value in terms of developing personalised treatments for lung cancer [21].

Furthermore, HDACs allow E-cadherin expression through non-coding RNAs. In addition, miRNAs serve to control EMT in lung cancer via TGF-β-, EGF- and HGF-signalling pathways. MiR200b and miR200c are effective on H3 acetylation in E-cadherin promoter (**Figure 1)** [22].

Epigenetic readers recognise modified histones by means of a group of polypeptides referred to as 'reader', and these polypeptides are involved both in normal cell growth and in cancer development by controlling several processes conducted together with chromatin [23].

Recently, Wenyi mi et al. identified the YEATS domain, defined as a novel acetyl-lysine-binding module. With regard to human cancers, the functional importance of proteins containing this domain remains unknown; however, the overexpression of the YEATS2 gene has been shown in non-small cell lung cancers. This domain is thought to decrease histone acetylation, thereby inactivating key genes [24, 25].

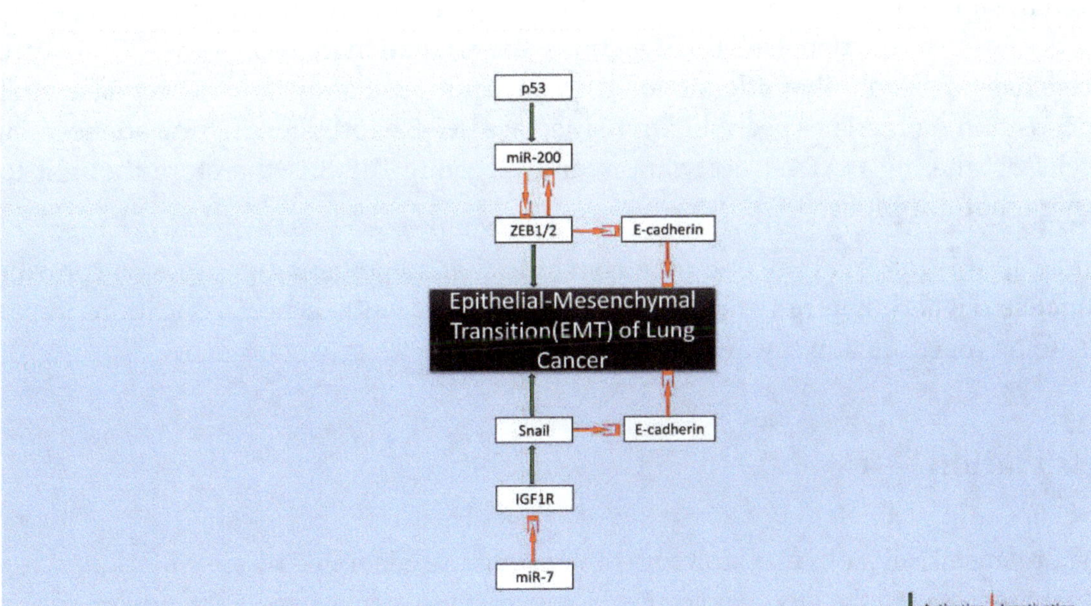

Figure 1. IGF and p53 pathways in lung cancer.

'Lunasin' is a soy protein consisting of 43 amino acids known to protect mammals against chemical carcinogens. In addition, it has been shown to be potentially beneficial in several conditions [26, 27]. A derivative of this protein originating from wheat has been reported to be effective even when taken orally and potentially effective in cancer prevention, regardless of the suppressed acetylation of core H3-H4 histone proteins [28].

As is the case in any intracellular event, the acetylation process occurs by means of enzymatic pathways. The removal of acetyl groups from histones is conducted by enzymes called histone deacetylases (HDACs). Cell viability continues normally as this is carried out in a balance of acetylation-deacetylation processes [29, 30]. Sometimes, hypoacetylation may occur when the process shifts towards deacetylation, and this is accompanied by cancer development. HDAC inhibitors are thought to possess the potential to reverse this process, leading to epigenetic reactivation of the suppressed anti-tumour genes [30]. This may help the suppression of certain tumours depending on which genes are expressed and which proteins are suitable.

Long Chen et al. believe that lysine acetyltransferase accelerates tumour formation due to the acetylation of histones and non-histone proteins despite the anti-tumour effect provided by acetylation-related HDAC inhibitors, and suggest that acetylation may shift to both sides (acetylation-deacetylation) depending on which genes are active at the time [30]. They highlighted the necessity to elucidate the relationship between lysine acetyltransferases (KAT) or HDAC and other proteins such as transcription factors in order to enhance the specificity.

Human MOF (hMOF and MYST1) is a member of the histone acetyltransferase (HAT) protein family. These proteins convert histone H4 acetylation to H4K16Ac, an epigenetic marker of active genes, in particular by adding an acetyl group to the lysine-16 amino acid. Irregularities in these epigenetic markers affect cell biology, potentially leading to cancer development. In correlation with H4K16Ac, hMOF has been shown to be overexpressed in non-small cell lung cancers. Investigators have indicated that this group of proteins may have potential oncological tasks and this may be a potential therapeutic target [31].

Although the interferon regulatory factor 3 (IRF-3), an important transcription factor for interferon genes, is often functional in viral infections, the regulation mechanism of IRF-3 expression in cancers has not been fully understood. The concurrent use of histone deacetylase inhibitors and Trichostatin A (TSA) has been shown to increase IRF-3 expression in lung adenocarcinoma A549 cells by altering GATA-1 acetylation, and targeting IRF-3 is therefore thought to be a novel therapeutic approach [32].

In light of all this information, one may conclude that some genes or proteins contribute to carcinogenesis when they function towards acetylation, while others contribute to carcinogenesis when they function towards deacetylation [22].

4. Methylation

In living organisms, all molecular structures and events are generated by specific sequences called genes that are found in the DNA molecule. However, these genes need to be governed and controlled so that they can participate in biological processes at the optimal time. Genes are actively controlled by specific genes and proteins referred to as transcription factors. However, there is a different mechanism that also determines gene expression, which can be transmitted from generation to generation and from cell to cell. This is called the epigenetic code [12]. DNA sequence does not undergo any changes during the formation of this code, but the relevant part of the DNA fragment becomes no longer meaningful. The most common epigenetic modifications are the changes in histone proteins and DNA methylation. The most widely studied and the most well-established epigenetic mechanism is DNA methylation. It is an enzymatic change where cytosines are converted to 5′-methylcytosine. The cytosine-end methylation seen in mammalian genome often occurs at the nucleotide pairs which are also called the CpG dinucleotides. Detection of these methylated gene segments on the genome is highly informative in terms of the effects of genes in several biological processes from carcinogenesis to ageing [33, 34].

Methylation-related changes may occur anywhere in the genetic material of a eukaryotic cell. In eukaryotic cells, genetic material is found in two organelles: the nucleus, which contains almost all of the genetic material, and mitochondrion, which has a very small genome compared to the nucleus. Certain methylations are specific to the genomes of these two organelles [1].

For several years since being discovered, the pattern of DNA hypomethylation in CpG dinucleotides has been shown to be highly important in cancer cells [35, 36].

A methylated gene becomes inactivated and therefore cannot synthesise the product, that is, the RNA or protein. Gene methylation occurs more commonly in promoter regions. Methylation in the promoters of tumour suppressor genes is mostly associated with carcinogenesis and often occurs in the form of hypermethylation [12].

Apart from global DNA hypomethylation reported in earlier stages, hypomethylation may also occur in the CpG islands in promoter regions of several specific genes or in the nucleotide pairs of genes that are activated by hypomethylation and silenced by hypermethylation. Methylation of a promoter region does not necessarily produce any protein or RNA [37]. The SHOX2 gene, a member of the Homeobox gene family, has been shown to be a specific biomarker with 60% sensitivity and 90% specificity when investigated by bisulphite modification-PCR in blood plasma samples during a case–control study of approximately 400 subjects with lung cancer. Also, in the same study, comparison against the results from another study conducted with bronchial aspiration samples revealed a higher level of sensitivity compared to results from blood plasma samples [38]. In bronchoalveolar lavage samples obtained from NSCLC patients, 24% methylation was observed in the promoter region of the CDKN2A gene, also known as P16INK4A, in addition to microsatellite instabilities and p53 mutations [39, 40].

The lungs are highly exposed to external factors owing to the nature of their functions. This constitutes a major risk factor in terms of epigenetic modifications as well as being associated with pulmonary diseases caused by environmental factors and smoking in particular. DNA methylation, histone modification and non-coding RNA have been shown to be increased in smokers [11].

Lung cancer develops upon the accumulation of numerous genetic and epigenetic alterations in the respiratory epithelium. Early promoter methylation and tumour suppressor gene inactivation are considered as signs of pulmonary carcinogenesis [12].

Defects in the apoptotic pathway are among the main reasons contributing to the high fatality of lung cancers. Apoptosis, also known as programmed cell death, has a wide range of physiological effects from embryonic stages to tumour formation. Inhibition of apoptosis is particularly detrimental in cancer treatments. The main reason of this is the fact that most treatments exert their effects by activating apoptotic mechanisms. Targeting the apoptotic pathway ensures the effectiveness of anti-cancer treatments [41, 42].

Survivin, one of the apoptosis inhibitor proteins, plays a critical role in cell division and in the continuation of cell survival [43, 44]. Since increased expression of survivin in human tumours leads to aggressive tumour development and resistance to main cancer treatments such as chemotherapy and radiotherapy, survivin gene and protein have been found to be important markers regarding the outcome of treatment [45, 46].

Computer analyses have shown a potential methylation region in exon 1 of the survivin gene; however, no methylation was found in lung cancer patients, and it has been shown that survivin gene expression in any cell may be effective not only with methylation but also through other transcription factors [47].

5. Importance of apoptosis

Apoptosis occurs during the normal development of multicellular organisms and continues throughout life. This mechanism is responsible for embryonic development and organ formation through cell differentiation. For example, toes are separated from one another by means of apoptosis.

Apoptosis also controls the immune system. T-lymphocytes are involved in the destruction of infected or damaged cells during cellular immunity. The T-lymphocytes produced in the thymus gland need to be active against foreign antigens before being released into bloodstream and should not show any activity against normal cells. Any inactive or semi-active T-cell is bound to be destroyed by apoptosis before they may begin their task.

Inhibitors of apoptosis proteins from the anti-apoptotic protein family have been identified in vertebrate and invertebrate species, and they are known to be negative regulators of programmed cell death. Some homologues identified in mammals include XIAP, cIAP1, cIAP2, NAIP, Bruce, Survivin and IAP. Most of these block cell death by directly binding to and inhibiting caspase-3, caspase-7 and caspase-9 [32].

Various diseases may arise in the event of any defect within the regulation of apoptosis. Among these, cancer is a condition characterised by little or no apoptosis. The mutations in cancer cells result in different cell-signalling and cell growth processes compared to normal cells. Under normal circumstances, when cells become damaged, they become apoptotic while cancer cells do not undergo apoptosis as a result of the cancerous mutations, which leads to uncontrolled cell differentiation and tumour formation. It is often difficult to eliminate such tumours with cell-damaging treatments such as chemotherapy and radiotherapy. In addition, some cancer cells develop resistance to treatments that target tumours with mutations in apoptotic pathways. Further understanding of the regulation of apoptosis in cancer cells is expected which allow developing novel therapies. While apoptosis is reduced in cancer, conditions with increased apoptosis lead to different problems. For example, neurodegenerative diseases such as Alzheimer's and Parkinson may be the result of increased cell death [43–46, 48].

6. Survivin and apoptosis

In early studies, caspase-3 suppression was suggested to be directly responsible for the anti-apoptotic mechanism of action of survivin. However, three-dimensional structural studies have shown that BIR (baculovirus IAP repeat domain) of survivin is not long enough to block the enzymatically active region of caspase-3. Survivin is thought to directly bind to caspase-9 as three-dimensional studies have revealed the similarity between the BIR domain of survivin and BIR domain of another IAP, XIAP, which directly binds to and inhibits caspase-9 *in vitro*. Another relevant mechanism is the inactivation of a pro-apoptotic molecule called SMAC/Diablo released together with cytochrome-c during mitochondrial apoptosis. SMAC/Diablo binds to IAPs and prevents their caspase-suppressing effect. Theoretically, survivin binds to SMAC/Diablo. Survivin bound to SMAC/Diablo protects other IAPs from the inhibitory effect of this protein. Thus, caspase suppression continues, leading to apoptosis blockade. There is evidence indicating that survivin plays an important role in p53-associated apoptosis. p53 blocks survivin transcription both through direct and indirect pathways. Conversely, overexpression of survivin inhibits p53-dependent apoptosis.

Phosphorylation of threonine-34 residues is necessary for survivin to bind to caspase-9. This is conducted by a kinase called p34cdc2-cyclin B1. Survivin-caspase interaction is shown in **Figure 2** [38].

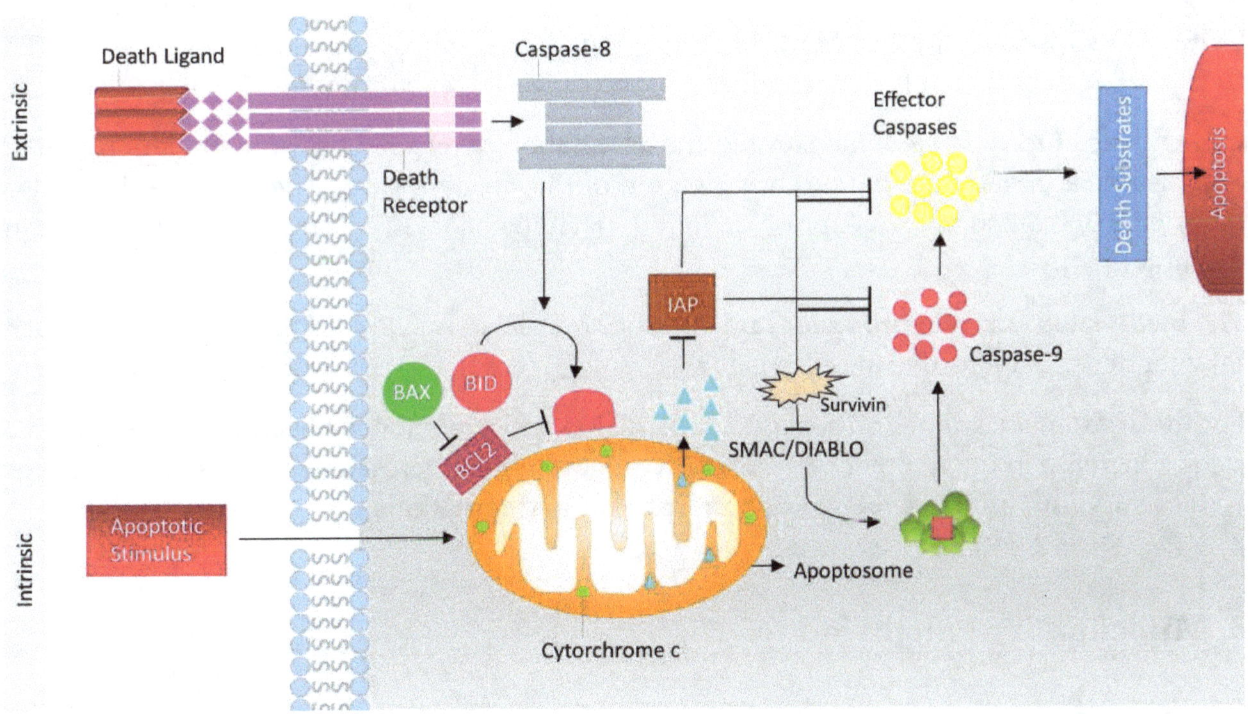

Figure 2. Apoptotic pathways.

7. Survivin gene and protein

Survivin molecule is expressed in special tissues and cells during certain phases of cell cycle. In humans, survivin expression occurs in the heart, liver, gastrointestinal tract and other foetal tissues from embryonic development until the end of foetal period, and in stem cells, epithelial cells and pancreatic endocrine cells during adulthood. Increased survivin expression has been shown in solid tumour tissues of adults, for example, lung, breast, brain, stomach, oesophagus, pancreas, liver, uterus and ovarian tumours. Increased survivin expression has also been reported in certain tumour tissues such as neuroblastoma, colorectal cancer and gastric cancer and has been associated with poor prognosis in these patients [49, 50]. Some studies have indicated the promotion of tumour development via survivin overexpression. There are numerous studies showing that survivin plays an important role not only in cell division and inhibition of apoptosis but also in cancer development [50, 51].

The human survivin gene is located on the telomeric position of chromosome 17 with a size of 14.7 kb. Survivin gene consists of four exons and three introns and encodes the survivin protein of 16.5 kD. While other IAPs contain more than one BIR in their structure, the survivin gene contains only one BIR region at the N-terminal domain and also contains an alpha-helix structure at the C-terminal domain. Survivin protein interacts with caspase-7 and caspase-9 via the BIR region while its alpha-helix structure interacts with tubulin subunits during mitosis [52, 53].

Survivin expression is suppressed during the G1 and S phases of the cell cycle but increases during G2/M. This control mechanism mostly functions at transcription level, occurring through cell cycle-dependent elements (CDEs) and cell cycle homology regions (CHRs). The CDE/CHR suppressor protein binds to this region, thereby suppressing gene expression. The CHR region is located at the proximal end of the survivin gene promoter [52, 53].

Cell-culture studies have demonstrated the association between SurKex methylation region and histone acetylation in the promoter region of the survivin gene. These studies have also reported a decreased mRNA expression in the survivin gene with the methylation of survivin promoter [54].

The methylated survivin promoter region has also been shown to inhibit p53 binding, which may render p53 ineffective in cell cycle [55].

For this reason, the studies on survivin gene region and protein have been intensified, with a steady increase in the number of studies investigating the expression analysis of survivin as well as survivin promoter-related polymorphisms and mutations.

8. Mitochondrial methylation

Mitochondrial functions provide several protein components synthesised from mitochondrial DNA (mtDNA) for the oxidative phosphorylation mechanism. In mammals, 12S and 16S rRNAs are encoded with 13 proteins from mtDNA. These genes are effective on cell homeostasis and apoptotic pathways [56].

Since mitochondria are dominant organelles regarding intracellular energy and because they have their own independent DNA genome, it is important to look at the genomic alterations of this organelle in certain diseases. These alterations are associated particularly with various pulmonary diseases and lung cancers [57, 58].

As mentioned earlier, mitochondrial methylation may also be affected in lung cells, which are considerably exposed to environmental effects. In their study dated 2013, Byun et al. have shown that mitochondrial RNA may undergo methylation [59].

9. Mechanisms of current therapies in lung cancer

Several treatment modalities are utilised in different subtypes and stages of lung cancer. Surgery is the first-choice treatment if tumour margins are well defined while adjuvant or neoadjuvant chemotherapy and hormone therapies are also applied with or after surgery. Treatment often continues in the form of chemotherapy, with practices that differ from country to country. The major chemotherapeutic agents approved for lung cancer include cyclophosphamide, doxorubicin, vincristine, cisplatin and mitomycin-C [60–62]. Almost all of these agents share the common feature that they induce apoptosis in the cell by triggering DNA damage in various ways.

Cyclophosphamide (Cytoxan, Neosar) is an immunosuppressant used for the treatment of lung cancer, and its metabolite, phosphoramide mustard, is the molecular structure form which exerts the actual effect. This agent alters DNA structure by forming irreversible cross-links between N-7 atoms of the guanine base in the DNA strand. This altered DNA structure stimulates intracellular apoptotic pathways, allowing the cell to undergo apoptosis [63].

Doxorubicin, sold under the commercial name Adriamycin, is another chemical agent that can be administered via intravascular route and interacts with DNA by intercalation. This agent prevents the biosynthesis of DNA macromolecules, inhibits DNA replication by stabilising topoisomerases and thereby shows the anti-cancer effect [64, 65].

Cisplatin is a platinum molecule with two chloride ions. This agent interferes with DNA, prevents replication and induces apoptosis in cells that are rapidly proliferating. Because of the different chloride concentration in intracellular and extracellular environment, cisplatin readily enters the cell and interacts with the water molecule to form a complex. This complex replaces the N-heterocyclic bases in DNA and has a particularly strong binding effect on guanine. This new structure forms the cis-[PtCl(NH3)2(N7-ACV)]$^{+}$ structure. In this situation, DNA repair mechanisms cannot work, and degradation of DNA is initiated in apoptotic cells [66, 67].

Mitomycin-C is another bactericidal chemotherapeutic agent. The mechanism of action of this agent is to generate DNA damage by alkylating the guanine nucleotide in 5′-CpG-3′ sequence via cross-links. Mitomycin-C exerts the anti-cancer effect by activating apoptotic pathways [68].

Another treatment modality employed for the treatment of lung cancers is radiation therapy. Radiotherapy is a radiation-based application that utilises ionised radiation, such as high-energy

X or gamma radiation. Radiotherapy can be applied before or after surgery and can also be combined with chemotherapy, depending on the localisation and stage of the tumours that are being treated. In this therapy, high-energy radiation beams cause DNA damage in the cell and result in apoptosis [69, 70].

The abovementioned therapeutic approaches share a common mechanism of action, in that almost all chemotherapeutic agents and radiotherapies induce DNA damage by activating apoptotic pathways and destroy the tumour with the help of apoptosis [71]. However, this requires the presence of intact apoptotic pathways; in other words, apoptotic pathways should not have been inhibited in order for these treatments to be effective. If anti-apoptotic mechanisms are activated, these treatments often fail, and drug resistance may develop. Specific targets of certain chemotherapeutic agents may be located in base sequences that undergo methylation, and motif changes may occur in the relevant DNA sequence due to methylation. In this case, chemotherapeutic agents may prove to be ineffective.

DNA methylations, chromosome acetylations and inhibited apoptotic pathways are among the reasons of resistance to therapeutic agents and radiotherapy. Studies have shown that epigenetic agents are highly promising in terms of overcoming the resistance to chemotherapy in various tumours [72]. A good understanding of acetylation, methylation and apoptosis mechanisms will allow developing more effective and targeted novel molecules.

10. Potential novel treatment approaches

Excision of the tumour tissue and the surrounding lymph nodes with the most recent surgical approach remains the optimal treatment in lung cancers. However, this may not always be possible owing to the anatomic location, spread pattern and metastasis status of the cancer. Chemotherapy or radiotherapy or both may be used in such cases. Response to treatment, however, is often not promising [73]. It is at this point where epigenetic alterations during cancer development emerge as therapeutic options. Due to their reversible characteristics, epigenetic modifications are therapeutic targets which may prove to have very good anti-cancer effects. For this reason, the US Food and Drug Administration (FDA) and European Medicines Evaluation Agency (EMEA) have started granting approval for certain drugs such as histone deacetylation inhibitors and DNA methyltransferase inhibitors. Among these, inhibitors of DNA methylation are the most effective treatment options and they appear to be effective in lung cancer as well [36].

DNA DNMTs are molecules that transfer methyl groups to cytosines via S-adenosyl methionine (SAM). Hypo- and hyper-methylation of DNA may occur in any cancer cell and silence tumour suppressor genes or inactivate T-cell recognition genes, which provide immune response, or affect the genes that trigger metastasis, angiogenesis and invasion [74]. The most important investigational DNA methyltransferase inhibitors and their analogues are presented in **Table 1** [74].

CI-994 is one of the candidate therapeutics in clinical testing phase. CI-994 is an orally bioavailable histone deacetylase (HDAC) inhibitor that causes histone hyperacetylation in viable cells. CI-994 shows inhibitory effects based on the concentration of HDAC1 and HDAC2.

DNA Methyltransferase Inhibitors Substance Group	Substance Name
Nucleoside analogs	Decitabine (5-aza-2'-deoxycytidine, Dacogen®, DAC)[1,2]
	Azacitidine (5-azacytidine, Vidaza®)[1,2]
	5-aza-fluoro-2'-deoxycytidine (FCdR)
	CC486 (oral azacitidine)
	Guadecitabine (SGI-110)
	Sinefungin
	Zebularine
Antisense oligonucleotide (ASO) inhibitors	DNMT1 ASO
	MG98
Others	1-Hydrazinophthalazine
	CBC12
	Epigallocatechin gallate (EGCG)
	Procainamide
	Psammaplin A
	RG-108
	SGI-1027
	Thioguanine

[1]Food and Drug Administration (FDA)-approve drugs. [2]European Medicine Agency (EMA)-approved drugs

Table 1. DNA methyltransferase inhibitors and their analogues [74].

Specifically, it mediates the arrest of cell cycle at G1, inhibits proliferation and induces apoptosis both *in vitro* and *in vivo* [75, 76].

FDA-approved epigenetic therapy agents are shown in **Table 2** together with their indications and year of approval [77].

Acetylation-based drug study is an early phase 2 trial of vorinostat (Zolinza®) [78]. Vorinostat is an HDAC inhibitor from the hydroxamate group. In this phase 2 study, vorinostat was

FDA-approved epigenetic therapy

Agent	Class	Approval Date	Indication
Azacitidine	DNMT Inhibitor	2004	Myelodysplastic syndrome
Decitabine	DNMT Inhibitor	2006	Myelodysplastic syndrome
Vorinostat	Pan-HDAC Inhibitor	2006	Cutaneous T-cell lymphoma
Romidepsin	Class I HDAC Inhibitor	2009	Cutaneous T-cell lymphoma
Bellnostat	Pan-HDAC Inhibitor	2014	Multiple myeloma
Panobinostat	Pan-HDAC Inhibitor	2015	Peripheral T-cell lymphoma

HDAC, Histone Deacetylase: DNMT, DNA methyltransferases.

Table 2. FDA-approved epigenetic therapy agents [77].

evaluated in breast, colorectal, and non-small lung cell cancers; however, adequate clinical response was not obtained, and authors reported that studies are to continue to determine appropriate doses [78]. While having a wide spectrum of tolerable side effects, it is a promising molecule in terms of chemotherapeutic utility [79].

In addition to survivin gene vaccines, a study has been conducted to target the methylated oligonucleotides of the survivin gene in non-small cell lung cancer. The study in question aimed to break down the apoptosis resistance of NSCLC by interfering with the survivin gene expression via oligonucleotides called SurKex1, which are specific to the promoter region of the methylated survivin gene. Data from this study were the first to show the utility of SurKex1 owing to its downregulating effects on survivin expression by means of DNMT1 activation [80, 81]. This study, although conducted in a cell-culture setting, is promising with regard to targeted survivin gene therapy in the near future.

Chemotherapy combined with immunotherapy may also be effective in treatment. High rates of response to treatment were demonstrated through PD-1 blockade via activated IFN signals by hypomethylation in treatments combined with IRF1/7 following treatment with decitabine (5-aza-2′-deoxycytidine or 5-Aza-Cdr or DAC), which was the first cytosine analogue synthesised by Pliml and Sorm in 1960. DAC, known to inhibit DNMT during cell division, is also a candidate for use in cancer therapy as an FDA-approved promoter hypomethylation inhibitor [82, 83].

Cystatin A (CSTA), a member of the type 1 cystatin superfamily, is essential to protect cells from cytoplasmic proteolysis and is mainly expressed in epithelial and lymphoid tissue. Furthermore, while cathepsins B, H and L, CSTA and cytoskeleton are known to be involved as tumour suppressors in oesophageal cancers, they have been found to exert such effects also in lung cancers. Histone methylation and acetylation play an important role in CSTA gene silencing in lung cancers. DAC treatments have an inhibitory effect on DNMT1, which is responsible for replicating DNA in a methylated form during replication. While limited CSTA expression is associated with high grades in squamous cell carcinoma (SCC), silencing in CSTA promoter region has also been demonstrated in the absence of CpG islands through epigenetic mechanisms such as partial methylation [84]. This renders DNMT1s a good target for novel treatment approaches.

In lung cancers, miR-9-3 hypermethylation occurs and the resulting downregulation of miR-9-3 expression leads to poor prognosis. Sulforaphane (SFN), a natural plant-derived molecule with anti-cancer properties, has been reported to decrease miR-9-3 methylation by attenuating DNMT activity in lung cancers and has a potential effect in improving the cancer prognosis [85].

It has been shown that Runx transcription factors (Runx1, Runx2 and Runx3), which play a critical role in organogenesis and cell differentiation pathways, are involved in lung cancers as they cause epigenetic silencing of a tumour growth inhibitor called BMP-3B. In this respect, downregulation of BMP-3B and lung cancers are closely related. Therefore, Runx transcription factors now appear to be a potential epigenetic target in lung cancers [86].

MARVELD1, a recently identified nuclear factor, is known to be extensively expressed in all human tissues and downregulated via promoter methylation in multiple cancer tissues. By working in combination with DNA methylation and histone acetylations, the epigenetic silencing of MARVELD1 leads to a decreased expression, causing unfavourable effects on histopathology and malignancy in lung cancers. This decreased MARVELD1 status in lung cancers eliminates the NMD complex-forming activity with UPF1/SMG1, resulting in premature termination codons and non-functional RNA. Epigenetic MARVELD1 silencing, which may serve as a diagnostic biomarker in lung cancers, appears to be a good target for anti-tumourigenesis [87].

Highly tumourigenic stem-like cells, which are thought to be tumour-initiating cells, cause the initiation, recurrence and drug resistance of cancers. Ca + 2/calmodulin-dependent protein kinase IIy (CaMKIIy), which is abnormally overexpressed in highly tumourigenic stem-like cells, is also associated with poor prognosis in lung cancers. Oct4 is one of the mRNA expression factors for pluripotent stem cells and regulates the differentiation of these cells by inhibiting CaMKIIy through epigenetic regulation. Therefore, Oct4 may be considered as a novel target approach in lung cancers [88].

The long non-coding RNAs are now also thought to offer a potential biomarker in non-small cell lung cancers. Studies have shown that they are particularly increased in non-small cell lung cancers. Because such RNAs occur mainly through methylation at DNA-gene level, long non-coding RNAs appear to be good markers and targets for novel treatment approaches in non-small cell lung cancers with regard to epigenetic mechanisms [89].

Among lung cancers, the metastatic risk is high in adenocarcinomas. In a study conducted to reveal possible biomarkers and therapeutic agent targets in these carcinomas, DNA methylation profile was downloaded from Gene Expression Omnibus (GEO) database, and DNA methylation profile of lung adenocarcinoma was investigated. This study concluded that methylated PTPRF, HOXD3, HOXD13 and CACNA1A genes may be potential biomarkers for the diagnosis and treatment of lung adenomas [90].

11. Conclusions

In light of all the information described earlier, one may conclude that acetylation at histone level and DNA methylations may be potential biomarkers and also good target molecules for treatment, particularly in lung cancers. Especially, the promoter regions of several tumour suppressor genes, and regions such as exon 1, although to a smaller extent, are inactivated through methylation. While the DNMT1 enzyme is in the position of a general target for inhibition to prevent these methylations, approaches such as inactivation of certain specific genes, oncogenes or apoptosis-inhibiting genes by means of methylated DNA oligo-primers appear to be a considerably good option. In the future, a combination of all these possibilities may allow treatments with significantly reduced side effects compared to current treatments as well as improved targeted approaches which destruct or prevent the progression of tumours.

Author details

Metin Budak* and Mustafa Yildiz

*Address all correspondence to: genomicdna2@yahoo.com

Biophysics Department, Faculty of Medicine, Trakya University, Edirne, Turkey

References

[1] Duruisseaux M, Esteller M. Lung Cancer Epigenetics: From Knowledge to Applications, Seminars in Cancer Biology. Elsevier; Sep 14. 2017 pii: S1044-579X(17)30166-9. [Epub ahead of print]

[2] Travis WD, Brambilla E, Nicholson AG, Yatabe Y, Austin JH, Beasley MB, Chirieac LR, Dacic S, Duhig E, Flieder DB. The 2015 World Health Organization classification of lung tumors: Impact of genetic, clinical and radiologic advances since the 2004 classification. Journal of Thoracic Oncology. 2015;**10**(9):1243-1260

[3] Larsen JE, Spinola M, Gazdar AF, Minna JD. An Overview of Molecular Biology of Lung Cancer. In: Pass HI, Carbone DP, Minna JD, Johnson DH, Scagliotti GV, Turrisi AT editors. Princibles and Practice of Lun Cancer, 4th editionPhiladelphia, USA: Lippincott Williams & Wilkins, a Wolters Kluwer business; 2010:59-75

[4] Demmy TL, Yendamuri S, D'Amico TA, Burfeind WR. Oncologic equivalence of minimally invasive lobectomy: The scientific and practical arguments. The Annals of Thoracic Surgery; 2018. DOI: 10.1016/j.athoracsur.2018.02.089 [Epub ahead of print]

[5] Hammerschmidt S, Wirtz H. Lung cancer: Current diagnosis and treatment. Deutsches Ärzteblatt International. 2009;**106**(49):809

[6] Inamura K. Lung cancer: Understanding its molecular pathology and the 2015 WHO classification. Frontiers in Oncology. 2017;**7**:193

[7] Raparia K, Villa C, DeCamp MM, Patel JD, Mehta MP. Molecular profiling in non–small cell lung cancer: A step toward personalized medicine. Archives of Pathology & Laboratory Medicine. 2013;**137**(4):481-491

[8] Bonaparte E, Pesenti C, Fontana L, Falcone R, Paganini L, Marzorati A, Ferrero S, Nosotti M, Mendogni P, Bareggi C. Molecular profiling of lung cancer specimens and liquid biopsies using MALDI-TOF mass spectrometry. Diagnostic Pathology. 2018;**13**(1):4

[9] Gibault L, Cazes A, Narjoz C, Blons H. Molecular profiling of non-small cell lung cancer. Revue de Pneumologie Clinique. 2014;**70**(1-2):47-62

[10] Khandekar MJ, Piotrowska Z, Willers H, Sequist LV. Role of epidermal growth factor receptor (EGFR) inhibitors and radiation in the management of brain metastases from EGFR mutant lung cancers. The Oncologist; 2018:2017-0557. DOI: 10.1634/theoncologist.2017-0557. [Epub ahead of print]

[11] Mari-Alexandre J, Diaz-Lagares A, Villalba M, Juan O, Crujeiras AB, Calvo A, Sandoval J. Translating cancer epigenomics into the clinic: Focus on lung cancer. Translational Research. 2017;**189**:76-92

[12] Langevin SM, Kratzke RA, Kelsey KT. Epigenetics of lung cancer. Translational Research. 2015;**165**(1):74-90

[13] Tang M, Xu W, Wang Q, Xiao W, Xu R. Potential of DNMT and its epigenetic regulation for lung cancer therapy. Current Genomics. 2009;**10**(5):336-352

[14] Verdone L, Caserta M, Mauro ED. Role of histone acetylation in the control of gene expression. Biochemistry and Cell Biology. 2005;**83**(3):344-353

[15] Verdone L, Agricola E, Caserta M, Di Mauro E. Histone acetylation in gene regulation. Briefings in Functional Genomics. 2006;**5**(3):209-221

[16] Abdul ASk, Adhikari N, Jha T. Structure-activity relationships of hdac8 inhibitors: Non-hydroxamates as anticancer agents. Pharmacological Research 2018;**131**:128-42. DOI: 10.1016/j.phrs.2018.03.001

[17] Furumai R, Komatsu Y, Nishino N, Khochbin S, Yoshida M, Horinouchi S. Potent histone deacetylase inhibitors built from trichostatin a and cyclic tetrapeptide antibiotics including trapoxin. Proceedings of the National Academy of Sciences. 2001;**98**(1):87-92

[18] Kim D, You E, Jeong J, Ko P, Kim J-W, Rhee S. DDR2 controls the epithelial-mesenchymal-transition-related gene expression via c-Myb acetylation upon matrix stiffening. Scientific Reports. 2017;**7**(1):6847

[19] Nieto MA. The snail superfamily of zinc-finger transcription factors. Nature Reviews Molecular Cell Biology. 2002;**3**(3):155

[20] Pećina-Šlaus N. Tumor suppressor gene E-cadherin and its role in normal and malignant cells. Cancer Cell International. 2003;**3**(1):17

[21] Chang R, Zhang Y, Zhang P, Zhou Q. Snail acetylation by histone acetyltransferase p300 in lung cancer. Thoracic cancer. 2017;**8**(3):131-137

[22] Dong N, Shi L, Wang DC, Chen C, Wang X. Role of epigenetics in lung cancer heterogeneity and clinical implication. Seminars in Cell & Developmental Biology: Elsevier; 2017;**64**:18-25

[23] Milosevich N, Gignac MC, McFarlane J, Simhadri C, Horvath S, Daze KD, Croft CS, Dheri A, Quon TT, Douglas SF. Selective inhibition of CBX6: A methyllysine reader protein in the polycomb family. ACS Medicinal Chemistry Letters. 2015;**7**(2):139-144

[24] Li Y, Wen H, Xi Y, Tanaka K, Wang H, Peng D, Ren Y, Jin Q, Dent SY, Li W. AF9 YEATS domain links histone acetylation to DOT1L-mediated H3K79 methylation. Cell. 2014;**159**(3):558-571

[25] Mi W, Guan H, Lyu J, Zhao D, Xi Y, Jiang S, Andrews FH, Wang X, Gagea M, Wen H. YEATS2 links histone acetylation to tumorigenesis of non-small cell lung cancer. Nature Communications. 2017;**8**(1):1088

[26] Lule VK, Garg S, Pophaly SD, Tomar SK. Potential health benefits of Lunasin: A multifaceted soy-derived bioactive peptide. Journal of Food Science. 2015;**80**(3):R485-R494

[27] Group TA. ALSUntangled update 1: Investigating a bug (Lyme disease) and a drug (Iplex) on behalf of people with ALS. Amyotrophic Lateral Sclerosis. 2009;**10**(4):248-250

[28] Jeong HJ, Jeong JB, Kim DS, Park JH, Lee JB, Kweon D-H, Chung GY, Seo EW, Ben O. The cancer preventive peptide lunasin from wheat inhibits core histone acetylation. Cancer Letters. 2007;**255**(1):42-48

[29] Dokmanovic M, Clarke C, Marks PA. Histone deacetylase inhibitors: Overview and perspectives. Molecular Cancer Research. 2007;**5**(10):981-989

[30] Chen L, Wei T, Si X, Wang Q, Li Y, Leng Y, Deng A, Chen J, Wang G, Zhu S. Lysine acetyltransferase GCN5 potentiates the growth of non-small cell lung cancer via promotion of E2F1, cyclin D1, and cyclin E1 expression. Journal of Biological Chemistry. 2013;**288**(20): 14510-14521

[31] Song JS, Chun S-M, Lee JY, Kim DK, Kim YH, Jang SJ. The histone acetyltransferase hMOF is overexpressed in non-small cell lung carcinoma. The Korean Journal of Pathology. 2011;**45**(4):386-396

[32] Wang L-L, Zhou L-B, Shu J, Li N-N, Zhang H-W, Jin R, Zhuang L-L, Zhou G-P. Up-regulation of IRF-3 expression through GATA-1 acetylation by histone deacetylase inhibitor in lung adenocarcinoma A549 cells. Oncotarget. 2017;**8**(44):75943

[33] Song K, Li L, Zhang G. The association between DNA methylation and exon expression in the Pacific oyster Crassostrea gigas. PLoS One. 2017;**12**(9):e0185224

[34] Tompkins JD, Jung M, C-y Chen Z, Lin J, Ye S, Godatha E, Lizhar XW, Hsu D, Couture LA. Mapping human pluripotent-to-cardiomyocyte differentiation: Methylomes, transcriptomes, and exon DNA methylation "memories". eBioMedicine. 2016;**4**:74-85

[35] Feinberg AP, Vogelstein B. Hypomethylation distinguishes genes of some human cancers from their normal counterparts. Nature. 1983;**301**(5895):89

[36] Mehta A, Dobersch S, Romero-Olmedo AJ, Barreto G. Epigenetics in lung cancer diagnosis and therapy. Cancer and Metastasis Reviews. 2015;**34**(2):229-241

[37] Lujambio A, Portela A, Liz J, Melo S, Rossi S, Spizzo R, Croce C, Calin G, Esteller M. CpG island hypermethylation-associated silencing of non-coding RNAs transcribed from ultraconserved regions in human cancer. Oncogene. 2010;**29**(48):6390

[38] Kneip C, Schmidt B, Seegebarth A, Weickmann S, Fleischhacker M, Liebenberg V, Field JK, Dietrich D. SHOX2 DNA methylation is a biomarker for the diagnosis of lung cancer in plasma. Journal of Thoracic Oncology. 2011;**6**(10):1632-1638

[39] Ahrendt SA, Chow JT, Xu L-H, Yang SC, Eisenberger CF, Esteller M, Herman JG, Wu L, Decker PA, Jen J. Molecular detection of tumor cells in bronchoalveolar lavage fluid from patients with early stage lung cancer. Journal of the National Cancer Institute. 1999; **91**(4):332-339

[40] Budak M, Yalcin O, Usta U, Tokuc B. Importance of p53, bcl-2, p21WAF1 and PCNA positivities in renal angiomyolipomas. Biomedical Research. 2017;**28**(10):4696-4702

[41] Mita AC, Mita MM, Nawrocki ST, Giles FJ. Survivin: Key regulator of mitosis and apoptosis and novel target for cancer therapeutics. Clinical Cancer Research. 2008;**14**(16): 5000-5005

[42] Budak M, Korpinar M, Kalkan T, Tuncel H. Mutation detection in the promoter region of survivin gene on N-methyl-N-nitrosourea induced colon tumor model in experiment. Bratislavske lekarske listy. 2014;**115**(9):554-556

[43] Kerr JF, Wyllie AH, Currie AR. Apoptosis: A basic biological phenomenon with wideranging implications in tissue kinetics. British Journal of Cancer. 1972;**26**(4):239

[44] Lechler P, Wu X, Bernhardt W, Campean V, Gastiger S, Hackenbeck T, Klanke B, Weidemann A, Warnecke C, Amann K. The tumor gene survivin is highly expressed in adult renal tubular cells: Implications for a pathophysiological role in the kidney. The American Journal of Pathology. 2007;**171**(5):1483-1498

[45] Jang JS, Kim KM, Kang KH, Choi JE, Lee WK, Kim CH, Kang YM, Kam S, Kim I-S, Jun JE. Polymorphisms in the survivin gene and the risk of lung cancer. Lung Cancer. 2008; **60**(1):31-39

[46] Chen X-Q, Yang S, Kang M-Q, Li Z-Y, Lu H-S, Lin T-Y. Survivin expression in human lung cancer and the influence of its downregulation on the biological behavior of human lung cancer cells. Experimental and Therapeutic Medicine. 2012;**3**(6):1010-1014

[47] Yalcin O, Budak M. Un-methylation of the survivin gene has no effect on immunohistochemical expression of survivin protein in lung cancer patients with squamous cell carcinoma. Bratislavske lekarske listy. 2017;**118**(3):160-163

[48] Dash PR, Cartwright JE, Baker PN, Johnstone AP, Whitley GSJ. Nitric oxide protects human extravillous trophoblast cells from apoptosis by a cyclic GMP-dependent mechanism and independently of caspase 3 nitrosylation. Experimental Cell Research. 2003;**287**(2): 314-324

[49] Wang T-T, Qian X-P, Liu B-R. Survivin: Potential role in diagnosis, prognosis and targeted therapy of gastric cancer. World Journal of Gastroenterology: WJG. 2007;**13**(20):2784

[50] Yagihashi A, Asanuma K, Nakamura M, Araya J, Mano Y, Torigoe T, Kobayashi D, Watanabe N. Detection of anti-survivin antibody in gastrointestinal cancer patients. Clinical Chemistry. 2001;**47**(9):1729-1731

[51] Song KY, Jung CK, Park WS, Park CH. Expression of the antiapoptosis gene survivin predicts poor prognosis of stage III gastric adenocarcinoma. Japanese Journal of Clinical Oncology. 2009;**39**(5):290-296

[52] Altieri DC. Survivin, cancer networks and pathway-directed drug discovery. Nature Reviews Cancer. 2008;**8**(1):61

[53] Zhu X-D, Lin G-J, Qian L-P, Chen Z-Q. Expression of survivin in human gastric carcinoma and gastric carcinoma model of rats. World Journal of Gastroenterology: WJG. 2003;**9**(7):1435

[54] Ma A-n, Lu J, Zhou X-j, Wang Y-x. Histone deacetylation directs DNA methylation in survivin gene silencing. Biochemical and Biophysical Research Communications. 2011; **404**(1):268-272

[55] Nabilsi N, Broaddus R, Loose D. DNA methylation inhibits p53-mediated survivin repression. Oncogene. 2009;**28**(19):2046

[56] Bogenhagen DF. Biochemical isolation of mtDNA nucleoids from animal cells. Methods in Molecular Biology. 2009;**554**:3-14

[57] Sun H, Shi W, Wang X. How Far Can Mitochondrial DNA Drive The Disease?, Mitochondrial DNA and Diseases. Springer; 2017. pp. 1-8

[58] van der Wijst MG, van Tilburg AY, Ruiters MH, Rots MG. Experimental mitochondria-targeted DNA methylation identifies GpC methylation, not CpG methylation, as potential regulator of mitochondrial gene expression. Scientific Reports. 2017;**7**(1):177

[59] Byun H-M, Panni T, Motta V, Hou L, Nordio F, Apostoli P, Bertazzi PA, Baccarelli AA. Effects of airborne pollutants on mitochondrial DNA methylation. Particle and Fibre Toxicology. 2013;**10**(1):18

[60] Fukuoka M, Furuse K, Saijo N, Nishiwaki Y, Ikegami H, Tamura T, Shimoyama M, Suemasu K. Randomized trial of cyclophosphamide, doxorubicin, and vincristine versus cisplatin and etoposide versus alternation of these regimens in small-cell lung cancer. JNCI: Journal of the National Cancer Institute. 1991;**83**(12):855-861

[61] Sundstrøm S, Bremnes RM, Kaasa S, Aasebø U, Hatlevoll R, Dahle R, Boye N, Wang M, Vigander T, Vilsvik J. Cisplatin and etoposide regimen is superior to cyclophosphamide, epirubicin, and vincristine regimen in small-cell lung cancer: Results from a randomized phase III trial with 5 years' follow-up. Journal of Clinical Oncology. 2002;**20**(24):4665-4672

[62] McGuire WP, Hoskins WJ, Brady MF, Kucera PR, Partridge EE, Look KY, Clarke-Pearson DL, Davidson M. Cyclophosphamide and cisplatin compared with paclitaxel and cisplatin in patients with stage III and stage IV ovarian cancer. New England Journal of Medicine. 1996;**334**(1):1-6

[63] Hall A, Tilby M. Mechanisms of action of, and modes of resistance to, alkylating agents used in the treatment of haematological malignancies. Blood Reviews. 1992;**6**(3):163-173

[64] Tacar O, Sriamornsak P, Dass CR. Doxorubicin: An update on anticancer molecular action, toxicity and novel drug delivery systems. Journal of Pharmacy and Pharmacology. 2013;**65**(2):157-170

[65] Pommier Y, Leo E, Zhang H, Marchand C. DNA topoisomerases and their poisoning by anticancer and antibacterial drugs. Chemistry & Biology. 2010;**17**(5):421-433

[66] Wang D, Lippard SJ. Cellular processing of platinum anticancer drugs. Nature Reviews Drug Discovery. 2005;**4**(4):307

[67] Johnstone TC, Suntharalingam K, Lippard SJ. The next generation of platinum drugs: Targeted Pt(II) agents, nanoparticle delivery, and Pt(IV) prodrugs. Chemical Reviews. 2016; **116**(5):3436-3486

[68] Tomasz M. Mitomycin C: Small, fast and deadly (but very selective). Chemistry & Biology. 1995;**2**(9):575-579

[69] Chang-Claude J, Popanda O, Tan X-L, Kropp S, Helmbold I, von Fournier D, Haase W, Sautter-Bihl ML, Wenz F, Schmezer P. Association between polymorphisms in the DNA repair genes, XRCC1, APE1, and XPD and acute side effects of radiotherapy in breast cancer patients. Clinical Cancer Research. 2005;**11**(13):4802-4809

[70] Stupp R, Hegi ME, Mason WP, van den Bent MJ, Taphoorn MJ, Janzer RC, Ludwin SK, Allgeier A, Fisher B, Belanger K. Effects of radiotherapy with concomitant and adjuvant temozolomide versus radiotherapy alone on survival in glioblastoma in a randomised phase III study: 5-year analysis of the EORTC-NCIC trial. The Lancet Oncology. 2009;**10**(5):459-466

[71] Baskar R, Dai J, Wenlong N, Yeo R, Yeoh K-W. Biological response of cancer cells to radiation treatment. Frontiers in Molecular Biosciences. 2014;**1**:24

[72] Strauss J, Figg WD. Using epigenetic therapy to overcome chemotherapy resistance. Anticancer Research. 2016;**36**(1):1-4

[73] Ettinger DS, Akerley W, Borghaei H, Chang AC, Cheney RT, Chirieac LR, D'amico TA, Demmy TL, Govindan R, Grannis FW. Non–small cell lung cancer, version 2.2013. Journal of the National Comprehensive Cancer Network. 2013;**11**(6):645-653

[74] Schiffmann I, Greve G, Jung M, Lübbert M. Epigenetic therapy approaches in non-small cell lung cancer: Update and perspectives. Epigenetics. 2016;**11**(12):858-870

[75] Kraker AJ, Mizzen CA, Hartl BG, Miin J, Allis CD, Merriman RL. Modulation of histone acetylation by [4-(acetylamino)-N-(2-amino-phenyl) benzamide] in HCT-8 colon carcinoma. Molecular Cancer Therapeutics. 2003;**2**(4):401-408

[76] Loprevite M, Tiseo M, Grossi F, Scolaro T, Semino C, Pandolfi A, Favoni R, Ardizzoni A. In vitro study of CI-994, a histone deacetylase inhibitor, in non-small cell lung cancer cell lines. Oncology Research Featuring Preclinical and Clinical Cancer Therapeutics. 2005;**15**(1):39-48

[77] Ansari J, Shackelford RE, El-Osta H. Epigenetics in non-small cell lung cancer: From basics to therapeutics. Translational Lung Cancer Research. 2016;**5**(2):155

[78] Vansteenkiste J, Van Cutsem E, Dumez H, Chen C, Ricker JL, Randolph SS, Schöffski P. Early phase II trial of oral vorinostat in relapsed or refractory breast, colorectal, or non-small cell lung cancer. Investigational New Drugs. 2008;**26**(5):483-488

[79] Bubna AK. Vorinostat—An overview. Indian Journal of Dermatology. 2015;**60**(4):419

[80] Li H, Ma A. Induction of apoptosis of non-small cell lung cancer by a methylated oligonucleotide targeting survivin gene. Cancer Gene Therapy. 2010;**17**(6):441

[81] Ciesielski MJ, Qiu J, Fenstermaker RA. Survivin as a Cancer Vaccine Target. J Vaccines Vaccin. 2014;**5**:230. DOI: 10.4172/2157-7560.1000230

[82] Lai Q, Wang H, Li A, Xu Y, Tang L, Chen Q, Zhang C, Gao Y, Song J, Du Z. Decitibine improve the efficiency of anti-PD-1 therapy via activating the response to IFN/PD-L1 signal of lung cancer cells. Oncogene. 2018;**37**(17):2302-2312

[83] Malik P, Cashen AF. Decitabine in the treatment of acute myeloid leukemia in elderly patients. Cancer Management and Research. 2014;**6**:53

[84] Ma Y, Chen Y, Li Y, Grün K, Berndt A, Zhou Z, Petersen I. Cystatin a suppresses tumor cell growth through inhibiting epithelial to mesenchymal transition in human lung cancer. Oncotarget. 2018;**9**(18):14084

[85] Gao L, Cheng D, Yang J, Wu R, Li W, Kong A-N. Sulforaphane epigenetically demethylates the CpG sites of the miR-9-3 promoter and reactivates miR-9-3 expression in human lung cancer A549 cells. The Journal of Nutritional Biochemistry. 2018;**56**:109-115

[86] Tandon M, Gokul K, Ali SA, Chen Z, Lian J, Stein GS, Pratap J. Runx2 mediates epigenetic silencing of the bone morphogenetic protein-3B (BMP-3B/GDF10) in lung cancer cells. Molecular Cancer. 2012;**11**(1):27

[87] Shi M, Wang S, Yao Y, Li Y, Zhang H, Han F, Nie H, Su J, Wang Z, Yue L. Biological and clinical significance of epigenetic silencing of MARVELD1 gene in lung cancer. Scientific Reports. 2014;**4**:7545

[88] Chai S, Xu X, Wang Y, Zhou Y, Zhang C, Yang Y, Yang Y, Xu H, Xu R, Wang K. Ca2+/calmodulin-dependent protein kinase IIγ enhances stem-like traits and tumorigenicity of lung cancer cells. Oncotarget. 2015;**6**(18):16069

[89] Osielska MA, Jagodziński PP. Long non-coding RNA as potential biomarkers in non-small-cell lung cancer: What do we know so far? Biomedicine & Pharmacotherapy. 2018;**101**: 322-333

[90] Han L, Xu G, Xu C, Liu B, Liu D. Potential prognostic biomarkers identified by DNA methylation profiling analysis for patients with lung adenocarcinoma. Oncology Letters. 2018;**15**(3):3552-3557

9

Diagnosis of Lung Cancer: What Metabolomics Can Contribute

Elien Derveaux, Evelyne Louis, Karolien Vanhove,
Liene Bervoets, Liesbet Mesotten,
Michiel Thomeer and Peter Adriaensens

Abstract

The reprogrammed metabolism of cancer cells reflects itself in an alteration of metabolite concentrations, which in turn can be used to define a specific metabolic phenotype or fingerprint for cancer. In this contribution, a metabolism-based discrimination between lung cancer patients and healthy controls, derived from an analysis of human blood plasma by proton nuclear magnetic resonance (^{1}H-NMR) spectroscopy, is described. This technique is becoming widely used in the field of metabolomics because of its ability to provide a highly informative spectrum, representing the relative metabolite concentrations. Cancer types are characterized by decreased or increased levels of specific plasma metabolites, such as glucose or lactate, compared to controls. Data analysis by multivariate statistics provides a classification model with high levels of sensitivity and specificity. Nuclear magnetic resonance (NMR) metabolomics might not only contribute to the diagnosis of lung cancer but also shows potential for treatment follow-up as well as for paving the way to a better understanding of disease-related diverting biochemical pathways.

Keywords: metabolomics, human blood plasma, metabolic phenotype, ^{1}H-NMR spectroscopy, metabolite spiking, multivariate OPLS-DA statistics, lung cancer, cancer cell metabolism, biomarker

1. Introduction

Metabolomics, or metabolite profiling, comprises the study of the entire spectrum of low-a large number of studies exploring the use of metabolomics in the field of disease diagnosis and prognosis, its application is also extended to other research areas such as toxicology [5], nutrition [6], microbiology [7], and drug discovery [8]. Together with high prevalence diseases such as diabetes [9], obesity [10–12], and neurological and cardiovascular disorders [13, 14], different types of malignant diseases including breast [15, 16], colorectal [17, 18], and lung cancer [19–24] are being extensively examined by using a metabolomics approach.

Nuclear magnetic resonance (NMR) spectroscopy and mass spectrometry (MS), which can possibly be connected to a gas- or liquid chromatography system (GC-MS/LC-MS), are the analytical techniques that are primarily used in the field of metabolomics [25–27]. While ^{13}C nuclei can be very useful in contribution to metabolite identification by NMR, the proton (^{1}H) nucleus is mostly studied in metabolomics NMR experiments [28]. The ^{1}H nucleus is omnipresent in metabolites, shows the highest relative sensitivity, and has a natural abundancy of 99.98%. ^{1}H-NMR spectroscopy is a noninvasive technique that needs no sample extractions and that enables the identification and quantification of metabolites in biofluids as well as in tissues and therefore is becoming widely used in the field of metabolomics [29]. Despite that ^{1}H-NMR is less sensitive compared to MS, it has many advantages: nondestructive, easy quantification, low cost per sample, minimal sample preparation requirements resulting subsequently in an excellent reproducibility and rapid high-throughput data acquirement [30]. In a single run of a few minutes, the ^{1}H-spectrum from one sample provides information regarding the relative concentrations of all present metabolites. The metabolic phenotype provides a representative snapshot of an individual's metabolic state and therefore enables the determination of cellular processes altered by disease [2].

Metabolites from a number of different diagnostic biofluids are already examined in multiple studies, mostly involving human blood plasma, serum, or urine [1, 22, 31, 32]. In parallel with biofluids, intact tumor tissues are frequently evaluated since intra-tumor heterogeneity is currently one of the major causes of treatment failure [33, 34]. To that end, high-resolution magic angle spinning NMR (HR-MAS NMR) as an analytical approach is gaining great attention [35–38].

This review intends to point out the results of ^{1}H-NMR metabolic profiling of lung cancer patients acquired by our research group and further explores the benefits which this method might deliver to contribute to an optimal treatment for lung cancer patients.

2. Methods

2.1. Sample collection and preparation

Experimental design focused on the analysis of fasting venous blood samples from lung cancer patients. Importantly, exclusion criteria were (i) not fasted for at least 6 h; (ii) fasting blood glucose concentration ≥ 200 mg/dl; (iii) medication intake in the morning of blood sampling, and (iv) treatment or history of cancer in the past 5 years, as described in the study of Louis et al. [20]. The blood samples were collected in lithium-heparin tubes and stored at 4°C within 5 min. Plasma aliquots were obtained after centrifugation at 1600 g for 15 min within 8 h after collection. Plasma sample preparation included a centrifugation step at 13,000 g for 4 min at 4°C and dilution of 200 μl of the supernatant with 600 μl deuterium oxide (D_2O) containing

0.3 μg/μl trimethylsilyl-2,2,3,3-tetradeuteropropionic acid (TSP) as a chemical shift reference of the spectra. After presaturation for water suppression, the Carr-Purcell-Meiboom-Gill (CPMG) pulse sequence was used to acquire slightly T2-weighted spectra on a 400 MHz (9.4 Tesla) NMR spectrometer [1].

2.2. Spectral processing

2.2.1. *Binning*

Before applying multivariate statistics, the data acquired by ^{1}H-NMR analysis should be preprocessed. Preprocessing of data usually includes phasing, baseline correction, alignment, and normalization. In addition, the spectrum has to be divided into regions of which the integration value (i.e., area under the peak) can be used as a variable for the statistical analysis. Binning or bucketing is a commonly used technique to produce such a reduced set of variables by segregating the spectrum [39]. In point-wise binning, the spectrum is divided into so-called equally-sized bins. An important limitation of this method is the possible splitting of peaks, resulting in a loss of differentiating power and possibly data misinterpretation. To overcome this, another methodology based on spiking of the plasma with known metabolites is proposed. This approach describes how the ^{1}H-NMR spectrum is divided into well-defined variable-sized integrations regions, being the variables for multivariate statistical analysis [40].

2.2.2. *Spiking methodology*

To obtain a correct signal assignment, ^{1}H-NMR spectra of reference plasma samples to which a known metabolite was spiked, were acquired. Hereto, stock solutions were prepared by dissolving a relevant concentration of a known metabolite in a reference plasma sample. Reference plasma can be obtained by pooling the plasma of several blood samples from a healthy person. Next, a small amount of stock solution can be added to a reference plasma NMR sample (e.g., 10 μl stock solution to 200 μl reference plasma and 600 μl D_2O containing the TSP reference). This procedure can be repeated for all metabolites of interest, using a fresh reference sample for each metabolite. The outcome of these spiking experiments allows an accurate identification of the chemical shifts and J-coupling patterns. On our 400 MHz (9.4 Tesla) NMR spectrometer, the described spiking method led to a segmentation of the spectra in 110 well-defined integration regions [40]. After integration and normalization (relative to the total integrated area, with exclusion of the contributions of TSP and water), these integration regions could be used as variables for multivariate statistical analyses.

2.3. Multivariate statistics

The statistics were carried out by using supervised orthogonal partial least squares discriminant analysis (OPLS-DA) to train and validate a classification model which enables optimal discrimination between lung cancer patients and a control population. The statistical classifier was constructed after detection and removal of outliers in the training data set via unsupervised principle component analysis (PCA). In addition, PCA was also conducted to visualize significant intrinsic clusters in the case–control data set upon which identification of possible confounders was based.

Model characteristics such as the total explained intra- (R^2X(Cum)) and intergroup (R^2Y(Cum)) variation were examined together with sensitivity and specificity values in order to evaluate strength performance of the OPLS-DA classifier. Predictive ability (Q^2(Cum)) of the model was demonstrated by cross-validation of the training set as well as by application of the model to an independent validation cohort.

3. Results

3.1. Detection of lung cancer

The assigned and normalized integration regions of the ^{1}H-NMR spectrum reflect the relative metabolite concentrations and thus represent the metabolic phenotype. Therefore, they can be used as variables for multivariate OPLS-DA statistics in order to discriminate between lung cancer patients and healthy controls. By applying this methodology on lung cancer plasma samples, a classification model that enables discrimination between those two groups was trained. Hereto, a large training cohort consisting out of 233 lung cancer patients and 226 controls was used. Characteristics of the subjects included in the training and validation cohort are summarized in **Table 1**. The trained OPLS-DA classifier resulted in a correct classification of 78% of the lung cancer patients and 92% of the control group (**Figure 1A**) [19]. To affirm that the discrimination was purely due to differences in plasma metabolite concentrations, PCA was conducted to exclude possible confounders. By means of PCA score plots, it was confirmed that gender, smoking status, disease, and chronic obstructive pulmonary disease (COPD) are no confounders [19].

While these results definitely support the applicability of this methodology for the detection of lung cancer, no clear differentiation between tumor stages or histological subtypes could be detected yet, that is, none of the trained OPLS-DA models already showed significant clustering of different tumor stages or histological subtypes. This probably is due to the limited number of lung cancer patients in the subgroups and the diffuse character of the subgroups formed on the basis of histology and clinical tumor stage. However, the ability of a constructed OPLS-DA model to discriminate between 76 stage I lung cancer patients and 76 randomly selected controls with 74% sensitivity and 78% specificity strongly suggests that plasma metabolite phenotyping reveals the presence of lung cancer already during early stadia of tumor development (**Figure 2**) [19].

3.2. Validation of the classification model

Importantly, after training of a promising classification model, confirmation of the validity of the model needs to be considered. When the metabolic fingerprint of a large cohort of patients and controls is available, this can be realized by applying the model on an independent validation cohort consisting out of an independent group of both lung cancer patients and controls. In this study, an independent cohort of 98 patients with lung cancer and 89 controls was used for validation of the trained model classifier. The trained model shows a high predictive accuracy with a sensitivity of 71% and a specificity of 81% (**Figure 1B** and **C**) [19].

	Training cohort		Validation cohort	
	C	LC	C	LC
Number of subjects, *N*	226	233	89	98
Gender, *N* (%)				
Male	119 (53)	160 (69)	44 (49)	66 (67)
Female	107 (47)	73 (31)	45 (51)	32 (33)
Age, yrs.	67 ± 11	68 ± 10	69 ± 10	64 ± 9
(range)	(38–88)	(36–88)	(47–89)	(45–83)
BMI, kg/m^2	28.3 ± 5.0	25.8 ± 4.5	28.4 ± 5.7	26.2 ± 4.7
(range)	(18.7–46.7)	(17.5–41.8)	(16.2–52.0)	(16.8–38.5)
COPD, *N* (%)	39 (17)	119 (51)	9 (10)	35 (36)
Taking lipid-lowering medication, *N* (%)	124 (55)	122 (52)	56 (63)	39 (40)
Diabetes, *N* (%)	23 (10)	40 (17)	20 (22)	12 (12)
Smoking habits				
Smoker, *N* (%)	47 (21)	113 (49)	15 (17)	48 (49)
Ex-smoker, *N* (%)	102 (45)	110 (47)	36 (40)	46 (47)
Non-smoker, *N* (%)	77 (34)	10 (4)	38 (43)	4 (4)
Pack years	16 ± 24	33 ± 21	13 ± 18	38 ± 21
(range)	(0–175)	(0–125)	(0–60)	(0–150)
Laterality				
Left, *N* (%)		103 (44)		40 (41)
Right, *N* (%)		119 (51)		54 (55)
Bilateral, *N* (%)		6 (3)		4 (4)
Unknown, *N* (%)		5 (2)		0 (0)
Amount of tumors, *N*		239		102
Histological subtype				
NSCLC-Adenocarcinoma, *N* (%)		91 (38)		46 (45)
NSCLC-Squamous carcinoma, *N* (%)		66 (28)		29 (28)
NSCLC-Adenosquamous carcinoma, *N* (%)		5 (2)		1 (1)
NSCLC-Carcinoid, *N* (%)		5 (2)		0 (0)
NSCLC-NOS, *N* (%)		8 (3)		6 (6)
SCLC, *N* (%)		30 (13)		15 (15)
Unknown, *N* (%)		34 (14)		5 (5)
Clinical stage according to 7th TNM edition				
IA, *N* (%)		55 (23)		12 (12)
IB, *N* (%)		21 (9)		5 (5)

	Training cohort		Validation cohort	
	C	LC	C	LC
IIA, *N* (%)		11 (5)		7 (7)
IIB, *N* (%)		15 (6)		4 (4)
IIIA, *N* (%)		48 (20)		17 (16)
IIIB, *N* (%)		26 (11)		12 (12)
IV, *N* (%)		63 (26)		45 (44)

BMI: Body mass index; C: controls; COPD: chronic obstructive pulmonary disease; LC: lung cancer patients; NOS: not otherwise specified; NSCLC: non-small cell lung cancer; SCLC: small cell lung cancer; and TNM: tumor, node, metastasis.

Table 1. Summary of the characteristics of the subjects included in the training and validation cohort.

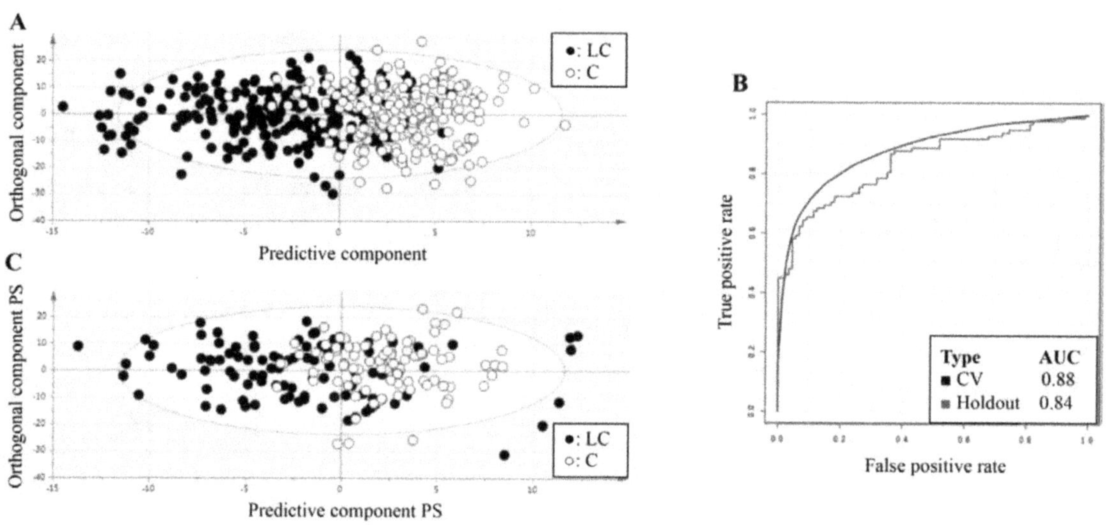

Figure 1. OPLS-DA score plots, resulting from the classification of the training cohort of 233 lung cancer patients and 226 controls (A) and the independent validation cohort of 98 lung cancer patients and 89 controls (C). The AUC of ROC curves confirms the predictive ability of the classification model by cross-validation of the training cohort and an independent validation model (B). AUC: Area under the curve; C: controls; CV: cross-validation; LC: lung cancer patients; PS: predicted scores; and ROC: receiver operating characteristic.

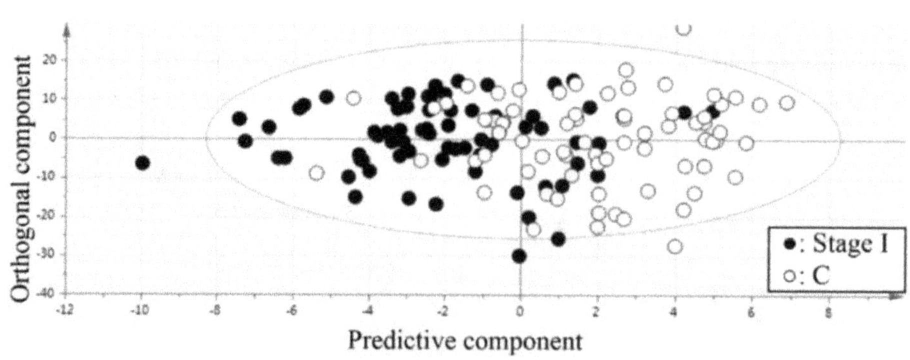

Figure 2. OPLS-DA score plot, resulting from the classification of 76 stage-I lung cancer patients and 76 randomly selected controls of the training cohort. C: Controls.

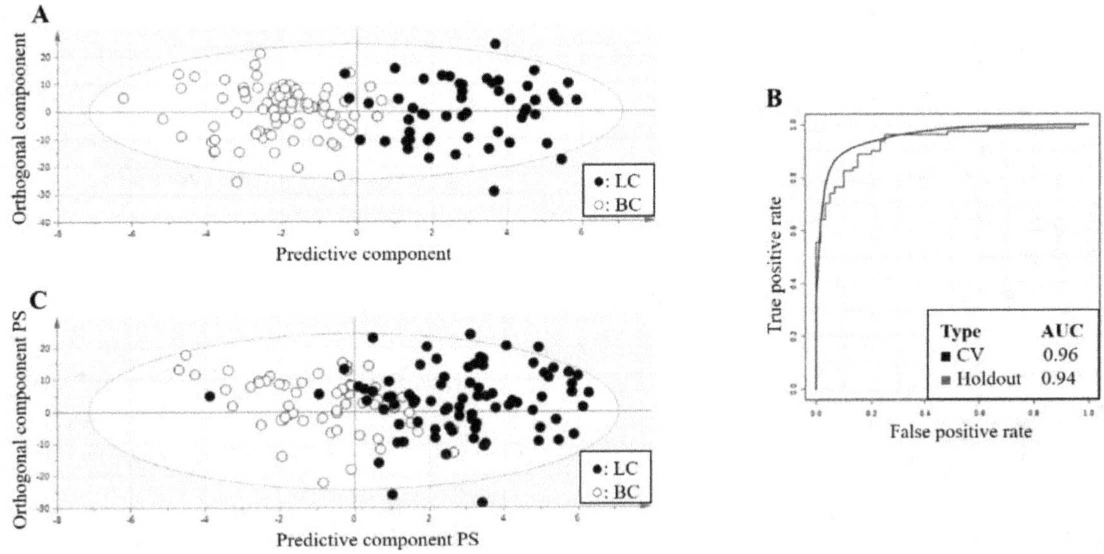

Figure 3. OPLS-DA score plots, resulting from the classification of the training cohort of 54 lung cancer patients and 80 breast cancer patients (A) and the independent validation cohort of 81 lung cancer patients and 60 breast cancer patients (C). The AUC of ROC curves confirms the predictive ability of the classification model by cross-validation of the training cohort and an independent validation model (B). AUC: Area under the curve; BC: breast cancer patients; LC: Lung cancer patients; PS: predicted scores; and ROC: receiver operating characteristic.

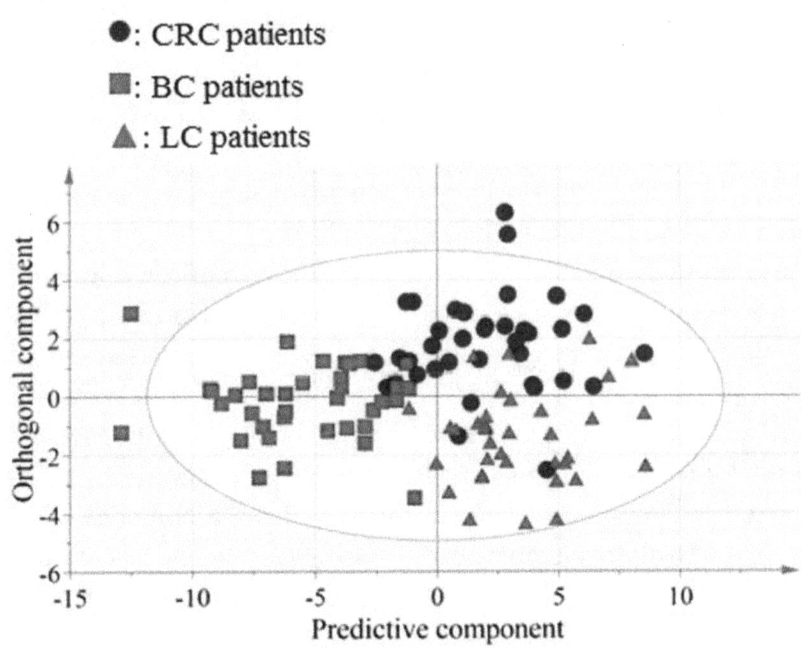

Figure 4. OPLS-DA score plot, resulting from the classification of a population of lung-, breast- and colorectal cancer patients, each group consisting of 37 individuals. CRC: Colorectal cancer patients; BC: breast cancer patients; and LC: lung cancer patients.

3.3. Differentiation between cancer types

To further illustrate the potential of the methodology described above, the following paragraph demonstrates that different cancer types are characterized by a specific metabolite profile. Hereto, the same workflow was applied on a data set of 54 lung cancer patients and

80 breast cancer patients. Again, the segmentation of the spectrum was based on metabolite spiking and OPLS-DA statistics were used to train a classification model, this time in discriminating lung cancer from breast cancer. The resulting model allows a correct classification of both cancer types with a sensitivity of 93% (93% of the 54 lung cancer patients were correctly classified) and a specificity of 99% (99% of the 80 breast cancer patients were correctly classified) (**Figure 3A**). Validation of the model by applying it on an independent cohort of 81 lung cancer patients and 60 breast cancer patients confirmed these findings and shows a sensitivity of 89% and a specificity of 82% (**Figure 3B** and **C**) [20]. Another recent study explored these promising results by establishing an OPLS-DA classification model that allows discrimination between three different types of cancers, that is, lung, breast, and colorectal cancers. After ^{1}H-NMR measurements of 37 plasma samples of each patient group, multivariate statistics revealed that each type of cancer was represented by a specific metabolic signature (**Figure 4**) [41]. Since the metabolic phenotype allows a clear differentiation between different cancer types, it can be assumed that the metabolic profile should not be considered as a general cancer marker but rather as a distinguishing characteristic of a specific cancer type.

4. Reorganization of metabolic pathways

The metabolites that contributed the most to the differentiation between lung cancer patients and healthy controls were identified and selected based on their variable importance for projection (VIP) value by means of an S-plot. The variables on the wings of the S-plot are the ones with the strongest contribution to the model and the highest statistical reliability [42]. Metabolic phenotyping of blood plasma shows that lung cancer patients are characterized by elevated glucose and decreased lactate levels, which implies an increased gluconeogenesis. This enhanced gluconeogenesis reflects the reaction of the human body to the Warburg effect or aerobic glycolysis in which, even in normoxic conditions, cancer cells rely on fermentation, that is, glycolysis leading to lactate production via fermentation of pyruvate. The Warburg effect, which takes place in cancer cells, can be observed in tumor tissue by means of ^{1}H-NMR as shown by Rocha et al. They demonstrated that lung tumors of different histological subtypes are all characterized by lowered glucose whereas lactate levels are increased, which is supported by the significantly enhanced glycolytic activity of cancer cells compared to normal cells [23]. Moreover, lung cancer patients show decreased phospholipid plasma levels, pointing to an increased lipogenesis and enhanced membrane synthesis, which is correlated with increased proliferation of cancer cells [43–46]. Other metabolites with an increased concentration in lung cancer patients compared to controls are N-acetylated glycoproteins, β-hydroxybutyrate, leucine, lysine, tyrosine, threonine, glutamine, valine, and aspartate. Contrarily, metabolites showing a decreased concentration in lung cancer patients are alanine, sphingomyelin, citrate, chlorinated phospholipids (e.g., phosphatidylcholine), and other phospholipids [19].

5. Metabolomics in daily clinical practice

5.1. Effect of the NMR magnetic field strength

Evaluation of the advantages versus limitations of NMR spectrometers with higher magnetic field strength was accomplished by comparing the results obtained for the same plasma samples on both a medium-field (9.4 Tesla; 400 MHz) and high-field (21.1 Tesla; 900 MHz) NMR spectrometer. For a 900 MHz spectrum, an improved resolution as well as a higher signal to noise (S/N) ratio is observed as compared to a 400 MHz spectrum (**Figure 5**) [47]. Because of these improved characteristics, measurements with a high-field spectrometer enable to define the integration regions more accurately using spiking experiments, resulting in less signal overlap and therefore in a larger number of integration regions that are representative for a single metabolite. Yet, discriminative power of both high- and medium-field spectra is rather comparable. These findings are in line with the study of Bertram et al., who demonstrated that the prediction performance and thus obtained information out of the spectra meant for diagnosis strongly increases when shifting the magnetic field strength from 250 to 500 MHz, whereas the effect of further increasing the magnetic field strength from 500 to 800 MHz appeared less strong when group discrimination is concerned [48]. However, analysis with a high-field spectrometer can be the preferred choice for the detection and identification of new, low-concentration metabolites and therefore can contribute to a better understanding of the underlying disturbed biochemical pathways of disease [47]. A drawback is the high cost of high-field spectrometers, which raises strongly with the magnetic field strength. By comparison, the cost of a 400 MHz spectrometer is in the order of €300,000 while a 900 MHz spectrometer can reach the cost of €2,750,000. The need of a supplementary cryoprobe can raise these estimated amounts even more with €200,000 [47]. In addition, such instruments demand for an isolated building for its housing, which is less practical in a clinical setting. Taken all into account, medium-field (400–600 MHz) spectrometers will probably become the preferred instruments for future application in clinical metabolomics.

5.2. Precision medicine

The contribution of metabolic phenotyping toward the clinical environment, often referred to as pharmacometabolomics, can encompass the entire patient journey, starting from an improved screening selection and earlier diagnosis to a follow-up for treatment response prediction and enhanced personalized choice of therapy [49]. Despite several challenges that accompany the implementation of such a unique innovative technique, for example, biomarker validation and cost-effectiveness [49, 50], the authors are highly convinced that metabolism-based biomarkers carry the potential to significantly contribute to future daily standard clinical practice.

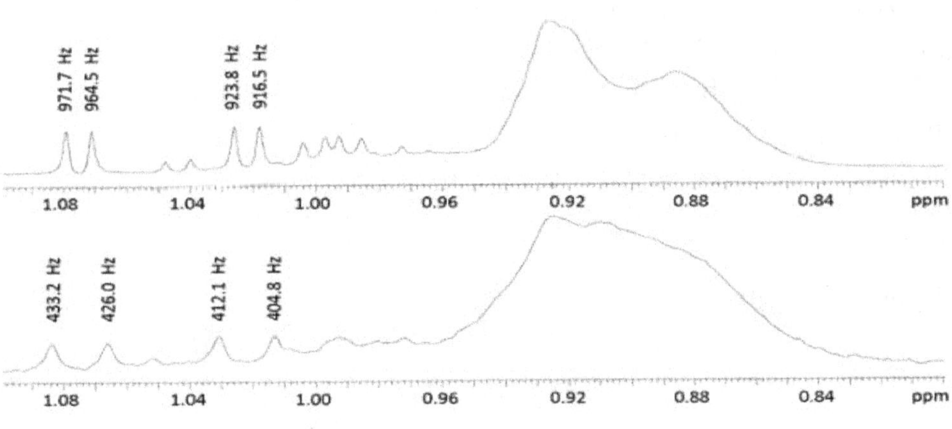

Figure 5. Comparison of the ^{1}H-NMR spectra of human blood plasma acquired at a high-field (900 MHz) (top) and medium-field (400 MHz) (bottom) spectrometer. Both spectra are zoomed-in between 0.80 and 1.10 ppm. The top spectrum shows an increased resolution and improved S/N ratio. The paired labeled peaks each represent a methyl group of the amino acid valine. ppm: Parts per million.

For lung cancer, metabolic phenotyping by means of ^{1}H-NMR can further be useful in preceding low-dose computed tomography (LDCT) scanning as a tool to deliver additional and complementary risk factors for a better selection of high-risk individuals. Currently, selection of those individuals is primarily based on age and smoking status/history [51]. As an outcome of the National Lung Screening Trial, it is stated that mortality is significantly reduced when screening with LDCT occurs [52]. Although sensitivity levels of LDCT screening are high and the number of diagnoses in early stadia increases, the positive predictive value of LDCT is currently still low [53]. Other drawbacks of LDCT screening are the high rate of false positive results, the high risk of overdiagnosis and consequently additional radiation exposure due to avoidable diagnostic tests [54]. In order to meet with the raising interest in improving the accuracy of risk prediction, promising clinically relevant diagnostic biomarkers which can add predictive value to existing models are indispensable [55, 56]. Therefore, a noninvasive blood-based screening test in complement with LDCT would be a valuable tool to reduce the number of individuals undergoing unnecessary and sometimes harmful follow-up treatments. Likewise, in a next phase, identification of prognostic biomarkers could assist in the tracing of early-stage lung cancer patients who would most likely benefit from current therapies, for example, surgery with curative intent or adjuvant chemotherapy [57].

Next to the discovery of diagnostic and prognostic biomarkers, metabolic profiling is being extensively examined for its use in prediction of individual therapy response [58–61]. Personalized treatment will contribute to a reduction of adverse reactions by (i) prediction of the patient's response and (ii) administration of the most efficient drug dose. Moreover, longitudinal monitoring of patients allows to track post-interventional outcome or deviations in response and therefore can assist in paving the way toward long-term personalized health [49].

6. Conclusion

Analysis of metabolic changes in blood plasma by ^{1}H-NMR spectroscopy allows to significantly discriminate between lung cancer patients and healthy controls. Additionally, metabolic phenotyping supports detection of lung cancer in all stages and enables differentiation between different cancer types such as breast and lung cancers. This indicates that a metabolomics approach can actively contribute to lung cancer diagnosis, even in early stages of tumor development. For daily clinical practice, where the main goal is to correctly classify patients, a medium-field (400–600 MHz) NMR spectrometer can provide sufficient discriminative power to perform clinical metabolomics. For research purposes, on the other hand, where disease-related disturbed pathways deserve a more extensive analysis, high-field NMR (e.g., 900 MHz) spectra are preferred. The ability of high-field NMR to observe a larger number of metabolites that are represented by a nonoverlapping signal, permits a deeper look into the underlying affected metabolic pathways. We show that increased glucose levels are observed while lactate levels are decreased in blood plasma of lung cancer patients. These aberrant metabolite concentrations indicate an increased gluconeogenesis as counteraction of the body to the Warburg effect in the cancer cells. Moreover, the fact that cancer cells manage an enhanced membrane synthesis can be confirmed by the lowered plasma levels of phospholipids.

Encouraged by all these promising results, the authors strongly believe that ^{1}H-NMR-based metabolic fingerprinting will become widely clinically implemented by serving as (i) an additional screening tool for lung cancer, (ii) a procedure to define complementary risk factors for current risk models toward an improved selection of lung cancer patients eligible for LDCT, and (iii) an innovative method to better characterize lung cancer patients in order to provide them with the best treatment strategies available.

Acknowledgements

This study is part of the Limburg Clinical Research Program (LCRP) UHasselt-ZOL-Jessa and supported by Kom op tegen Kanker (Stand up to Cancer), the Flemish Cancer Society. The authors like to thank Prof. Dr. Eric de Jonge and Prof. Dr. Philip Caenepeel for their support in sample recruitment.

Author details

Elien Derveaux[1], Evelyne Louis[2], Karolien Vanhove[1,3], Liene Bervoets[4], Liesbet Mesotten[1,5], Michiel Thomeer[1,6] and Peter Adriaensens[7]*

*Address all correspondence to: peter.adriaensens@uhasselt.be

1 Faculty of Medicine and Life Sciences, Hasselt University, Hasselt, Belgium

2 Department of Respiratory Oncology, University Hospitals KU Leuven, Leuven, Belgium

3 Department of Respiratory Medicine, Algemeen Ziekenhuis Vesalius, Tongeren, Belgium

4 Department of Medical Microbiology, Maastricht Universitair Medisch Centrum, Maastricht, The Netherlands

5 Department of Nuclear Medicine, Ziekenhuis Oost-Limburg, Genk, Belgium

6 Department of Respiratory Medicine, Ziekenhuis Oost-Limburg, Genk, Belgium

7 Applied and Analytical Chemistry, Institute for Materials Research, Hasselt University, Hasselt, Belgium

References

[1] Beckonert O, Keun HC, Ebbels TM, Bundy J, Holmes E, Lindon JC, et al. Metabolic profiling, metabolomic and metabonomic procedures for NMR spectroscopy of urine, plasma, serum and tissue extracts. Nature Protocols. 2007;**2**(11):2692-2703

[2] Holmes E, Wilson ID, Nicholson JK. Metabolic phenotyping in health and disease. Cell. 2008;**134**(5):714-717

[3] Duarte IF, Gil AM. Metabolic signatures of cancer unveiled by NMR spectroscopy of human biofluids. Progress in Nuclear Magnetic Resonance Spectroscopy. 2012;**62**:51-74

[4] Griffin JL, Shockcor JP. Metabolic profiles of cancer cells. Nature Reviews. Cancer. 2004; **4**(7):551-561

[5] Menon SS, Uppal M, Randhawa S, Cheema MS, Aghdam N, Usala RL, et al. Radiation metabolomics: Current status and future directions. Frontiers in Oncology. 2016;**6**:20

[6] Bondia-Pons I, Canellas N, Abete I, Rodriguez MA, Perez-Cornago A, Navas-Carretero S, et al. Nutri-metabolomics: Subtle serum metabolic differences in healthy subjects by NMR-based metabolomics after a short-term nutritional intervention with two tomato sauces. OMICS. 2013;**17**(12):611-618

[7] Tremaroli V, Workentine ML, Weljie AM, Vogel HJ, Ceri H, Viti C, et al. Metabolomic investigation of the bacterial response to a metal challenge. Applied and Environmental Microbiology. 2009;**75**(3):719-728

[8] Palmnas M, Vogel H. The future of NMR metabolomics in cancer therapy: Towards personalizing treatment and developing targeted drugs? Metabolites. 2013;**3**(2):373-396

[9] Bervoets L, Massa G, Guedens W, Louis E, Noben JP, Adriaensens P. Metabolic profiling of type 1 diabetes mellitus in children and adolescents: A case-control study. Diabetology and Metabolic Syndrome. 2017;**9**:48

[10] Elliott P, Posma JM, Chan Q, Garcia-Perez I, Wijeyesekera A, Bictash M, et al. Urinary metabolic signatures of human adiposity. Science Translational Medicine. 2015;**7**(285): 285ra62

[11] Newgard CB, An J, Bain JR, Muehlbauer MJ, Stevens RD, Lien LF, et al. A branched-chain amino acid-related metabolic signature that differentiates obese and lean humans and contributes to insulin resistance. Cell Metabolism. 2009;**9**(4):311-326

[12] Gralka E, Luchinat C, Tenori L, Ernst B, Thurnheer M, Schultes B. Metabolomic fingerprint of severe obesity is dynamically affected by bariatric surgery in a procedure-dependent manner. The American Journal of Clinical Nutrition. 2015;**102**(6):1313-1322

[13] Rhee EP, Gerszten RE. Metabolomics and cardiovascular biomarker discovery. Clinical Chemistry. 2012;**58**(1):139-147

[14] Botosoa EP, Zhu M, Marbeuf-Gueye C, Triba MN, Dutheil F, Duyckäerts C, et al. NMR metabolomic of frontal cortex extracts: First study comparing two neurodegenerative diseases, Alzheimer disease and amyotrophic lateral sclerosis. IRBM. 2012;**33**(5):281-286

[15] Singh A, Sharma RK, Chagtoo M, Agarwal G, George N, Sinha N, et al. ^{1}H NMR metabolomics reveals association of high expression of inositol 1, 4, 5 Trisphosphate receptor and metabolites in breast cancer patients. PLoS One. 2017;**12**(1):e0169330

[16] Hart CD, Vignoli A, Tenori L, Uy GL, Van To T, Adebamowo C, et al. Serum metabolomic profiles identify ER-positive early breast cancer patients at increased risk of disease recurrence in a multicenter population. Clinical Cancer Research. 2017;**23**(6):1422-1431

[17] Jimenez B, Mirnezami R, Kinross J, Cloarec O, Keun HC, Holmes E, et al. ^{1}H HR-MAS NMR spectroscopy of tumor-induced local metabolic "field-effects" enables colorectal cancer staging and prognostication. Journal of Proteome Research. 2013;**12**(2):959-968

[18] Chan EC, Koh PK, Mal M, Cheah PY, Eu KW, Backshall A, et al. Metabolic profiling of human colorectal cancer using high-resolution magic angle spinning nuclear magnetic resonance (HR-MAS NMR) spectroscopy and gas chromatography mass spectrometry (GC/MS). Journal of Proteome Research. 2009;**8**(1):352-361

[19] Louis E, Adriaensens P, Guedens W, Bigirumurame T, Baeten K, Vanhove K, et al. Detection of lung cancer through metabolic changes measured in blood plasma. Journal of Thoracic Oncology. 2016;**11**(4):516-523

[20] Louis E, Adriaensens P, Guedens W, Vanhove K, Vandeurzen K, Darquennes K, et al. Metabolic phenotyping of human blood plasma: A powerful tool to discriminate between cancer types? Annals of Oncology. 2016;**27**(1):178-184

[21] Duarte IF, Rocha CM, Barros AS, Gil AM, Goodfellow BJ, Carreira IM, et al. Can nuclear magnetic resonance (NMR) spectroscopy reveal different metabolic signatures for lung tumours? Virchows Archiv. 2010;**457**(6):715-725

[22] Carrola J, Rocha CM, Barros AS, Gil AM, Goodfellow BJ, Carreira IM, et al. Metabolic signatures of lung cancer in biofluids: NMR-based metabonomics of urine. Journal of Proteome Research. 2011;**10**(1):221-230

[23] Rocha CM, Barros AS, Goodfellow BJ, Carreira IM, Gomes A, Sousa V, et al. NMR metabolomics of human lung tumours reveals distinct metabolic signatures for adenocarcinoma and squamous cell carcinoma. Carcinogenesis. 2015;**36**(1):68-75

[24] Jordan KW, Adkins CB, Su L, Halpern EF, Mark EJ, Christiani DC, et al. Comparison of squamous cell carcinoma and adenocarcinoma of the lung by metabolomic analysis of tissue-serum pairs. Lung Cancer. 2010;**68**(1):44-50

[25] Alonso A, Marsal S, Julia A. Analytical methods in untargeted metabolomics: State of the art in 2015. Frontiers in Bioengineering and Biotechnology. 2015;**3**:23

[26] Barnes S, Benton HP, Casazza K, Cooper SJ, Cui X, Du X, et al. Training in metabolomics research. I. Designing the experiment, collecting and extracting samples and generating metabolomics data. Journal of Mass Spectrometry. 2016;**51**(7):461-475

[27] Stringer KA, McKay RT, Karnovsky A, Quemerais B, Lacy P. Metabolomics and its application to acute lung diseases. Frontiers in Immunology. 2016;**7**:44

[28] Dona AC, Kyriakides M, Scott F, Shephard EA, Varshavi D, Veselkov K, et al. A guide to the identification of metabolites in NMR-based metabonomics/metabolomics experiments. Computational and Structural Biotechnology Journal. 2016;**14**:135-153

[29] Nagana Gowda GA, Raftery D. Can NMR solve some significant challenges in metabolomics? Journal of Magnetic Resonance. 2015;**260**:144-160

[30] Collino S, Martin FP, Rezzi S. Clinical metabolomics paves the way towards future healthcare strategies. British Journal of Clinical Pharmacology. 2013;**75**(3):619-629

[31] Dona AC, Jimenez B, Schafer H, Humpfer E, Spraul M, Lewis MR, et al. Precision high-throughput proton NMR spectroscopy of human urine, serum, and plasma for large-scale metabolic phenotyping. Analytical Chemistry. 2014;**86**(19):9887-9894

[32] Suarez-Diez M, Adam J, Adamski J, Chasapi SA, Luchinat C, Peters A, et al. Plasma and serum metabolite association networks: Comparability within and between studies using NMR and MS profiling. Journal of Proteome Research. 2017;**16**(7):2547-2559

[33] Hiley C, de Bruin EC, McGranahan N, Swanton C. Deciphering intratumor heterogeneity and temporal acquisition of driver events to refine precision medicine. Genome Biology. 2014;**15**(8):453

[34] Bedard P, Hansen A, Ratain M, Siu L. Tumour heterogeneity in the clinic. Nature. 2013; **501**(7467):355-364

[35] Beckonert O, Coen M, Keun HC, Wang Y, Ebbels TM, Holmes E, et al. High-resolution magic-angle-spinning NMR spectroscopy for metabolic profiling of intact tissues. Nature Protocols. 2010;**5**(6):1019-1032

[36] Chen W, Zu Y, Huang Q, Chen F, Wang G, Lan W, et al. Study on metabonomic characteristics of human lung cancer using high resolution magic-angle spinning ^{1}H NMR spectroscopy and multivariate data analysis. Magnetic Resonance in Medicine. 2011;**66**(6): 1531-1540

[37] Mirnezami R, Jimenez B, Li JV, Kinross JM, Veselkov K, Goldin RD, et al. Rapid diagnosis and staging of colorectal cancer via high-resolution magic angle spinning nuclear magnetic resonance (HR-MAS NMR) spectroscopy of intact tissue biopsies. Annals of Surgery. 2014;**259**(6):1138-1149

[38] Wang H, Zhang H, Deng P, Liu C, Li D, Jie H, et al. Tissue metabolic profiling of human gastric cancer assessed by (1)H NMR. BMC Cancer. 2016;**16**:371

[39] Craig A, Cloarec O, Holmes E, Nicholson JK, Lindon JC. Scaling and normalization effects in NMR spectroscopic metabonomic data sets. Analytical Chemistry. 2006;**78**(7): 2262-2267

[40] Louis E, Bervoets L, Reekmans G, De Jonge E, Mesotten L, Thomeer M, et al. Phenotyping human blood plasma by ^{1}H-NMR: A robust protocol based on metabolite spiking and its evaluation in breast cancer. Metabolomics. 2014;**11**(1):225-236

[41] Louis R, Louis E, Stinkens K, Mesotten L, De Jonge E, Thomeer M, et al. Metabolic phenotyping of blood plasma by proton nuclear magnetic resonance to discriminate between colorectal cancer, breast cancer and lung cancer. Metabolomics (Los Angel). 2016;**6**(3):187

[42] Wiklund S, Johansson E, Sjostrom L, Mellerowicz E, Edlund U, Shockcor J, et al. Visualization of GC/TOF-MS-based metabolomics data for identification of biochemically interesting compounds using OPLS class models. Analytical Chemistry. 2008;**80**(1):115-122

[43] DeBerardinis RJ, Lum JJ, Hatzivassiliou G, Thompson CB. The biology of cancer: Metabolic reprogramming fuels cell growth and proliferation. Cell Metabolism. 2008;**7**(1):11-20

[44] Marien E, Meister M, Muley T, Fieuws S, Bordel S, Derua R, et al. Non-small cell lung cancer is characterized by dramatic changes in phospholipid profiles. International Journal of Cancer. 2015;**137**(7):1539-1548

[45] Vincent EE, Sergushichev A, Griss T, Gingras MC, Samborska B, Ntimbane T, et al. Mitochondrial phosphoenolpyruvate carboxykinase regulates metabolic adaptation and enables glucose-independent tumor growth. Molecular Cell. 2015;**60**(2):195-207

[46] Leithner K, Hrzenjak A, Trotzmuller M, Moustafa T, Kofeler HC, Wohlkoenig C, et al. PCK2 activation mediates an adaptive response to glucose depletion in lung cancer. Oncogene. 2015;**34**(8):1044-1050

[47] Louis E, Cantrelle FX, Mesotten L, Reekmans G, Bervoets L, Vanhove K, et al. Metabolic phenotyping of human plasma by ^{1}H-NMR at high and medium magnetic field strengths: A case study for lung cancer. Magnetic Resonance in Chemistry. 2017;**55**(8):706-713

[48] Bertram HC, Malmendal A, Petersen BO, Madsen JC, Pedersen H, Nielsen NC, et al. Effect of magnetic field strength on NMR-based metabonomic human urine data. Comparative study of 250, 400, 500, and 800 MHz. Analytical Chemistry. 2007;**79**(18):7110-7115

[49] Nicholson JK, Holmes E, Kinross JM, Darzi AW, Takats Z, Lindon JC. Metabolic phenotyping in clinical and surgical environments. Nature. 2012;**491**(7424):384-392

[50] Ocak S, Sos ML, Thomas RK, Massion PP. High-throughput molecular analysis in lung cancer: Insights into biology and potential clinical applications. The European Respiratory Journal. 2009;**34**(2):489-506

[51] Wender R, Fontham ET, Barrera E Jr, Colditz GA, Church TR, Ettinger DS, et al. American cancer society lung cancer screening guidelines. CA: A Cancer Journal for Clinicians. 2013;**63**(2):107-117

[52] Aberle DR, Adams AM, Berg CD, Black WC, Clapp JD, Fagerstrom RM, et al. Reduced lung-cancer mortality with low-dose computed tomographic screening. The New England Journal of Medicine. 2011;**365**:395-409

[53] Bach PB, Mirkin JN, Oliver TK, Azzoli CG, Berry DA, Brawley OW, et al. Benefits and harms of CT screening for lung cancer: A systematic review. Journal of the American Medical Association. 2012;**307**(22):2418-2429

[54] Wood DE, Eapen GA, Ettinger DS, Hou L, Jackman D, Kazerooni E, et al. Lung cancer screening. Journal of the National Comprehensive Cancer Network. 2012;**10**(2):240-265

[55] Spitz MR, Etzel CJ, Dong Q, Amos CI, Wei Q, Wu X, et al. An expanded risk prediction model for lung cancer. Cancer Prevention Research (Philadelphia, Pa.). 2008;**1**(4):250-254

[56] Atwater T, Massion PP. Biomarkers of risk to develop lung cancer in the new screening era. Annals of Translational Medicine. 2016;**4**(8):158

[57] Burotto M, Thomas A, Subramaniam D, Giaccone G, Rajan A. Biomarkers in early-stage non-small-cell lung cancer: Current concepts and future directions. Journal of Thoracic Oncology. 2014;**9**(11):1609-1617

[58] Clayton TA, Lindon JC, Cloarec O, Antti H, Charuel C, Hanton G, et al. Pharmaco-metabonomic phenotyping and personalized drug treatment. Nature. 2006;**440**(7087): 1073-1077

[59] Puchades-Carrasco L, Pineda-Lucena A. Metabolomics applications in precision medicine: An oncological perspective. Current Topics in Medicinal Chemistry. 2017;**17**(24): 2740-2751

[60] Everett JR. From metabonomics to pharmacometabonomics: The role of metabolic profiling in personalized medicine. Frontiers in Pharmacology. 2016;**7**:297

[61] Beger RD, Dunn W, Schmidt MA, Gross SS, Kirwan JA, Cascante M, et al. Metabolomics enables precision medicine: "A white paper, community perspective". Metabolomics. 2016;**12**(10):149

10

Noncoding RNAs in Lung Cancer Angiogenesis

Ioana Berindan-Neagoe, Cornelia Braicu,
Diana Gulei, Ciprian Tomuleasa and
George Adrian Calin

Abstract

Lung cancer is the major death-related cancer in both men and women, due to late diagnostic and limited treatment efficacy. The angiogenic process that is responsible for the support of tumor progression and metastasis represents one of the main hallmarks of cancer. The role of VEGF signaling in angiogenesis is well-established, and we summarize the role of semaphorins and their related receptors or hypoxia-related factors role as prone of tumor microenvironment in angiogenic mechanisms. Newly, noncoding RNA transcripts (ncRNA) were identified to have vital functions in miscellaneous biological processes, including lung cancer angiogenesis. Therefore, due to their capacity to regulate almost all molecular pathways related with altered key genes, including those involved in angiogenesis and its microenvironment, ncRNAs can serve as diagnosis and prognosis markers or therapeutic targets. We intend to summarize the latest progress in the field of ncRNAs in lung cancer and their relation with hypoxia related factors and angiogenic genes, with a particular focus on ncRNAs relation to semaphorins.

Keywords: noncoding RNAs, angiogenesis, lung cancer, semaphorins, therapy

1. Introduction

1.1. Noncoding RNAs (ncRNAs)—definition, biogenesis and classification

The noncoding RNAs evolved in the last few years as important regulators of numerous physiological and pathological processes with increased attention regarding cancer diagnosis, prognosis, and therapeutics [1]. The concept known as "dark matter" defined by the lack of function and lack of genetic information is now long gone, being replaced by the regulatory ncRNAs involved in cancer development and progression [1]. The transcription of the noncoding regions produces RNA sequences that can vary in size, short, mid-size, and long noncoding RNAs, and are able to influence the expression of tumor suppressor or tumor promoting coding genes, activity that further classifies this class of RNAs into oncogenic or tumor suppressor sequences [2].

The noncoding niche is rapidly expanding as new sequences are discovered and characterized. The ncRNAs, as their name underline, are RNAs that do not codify for proteins but new molecular concepts are revealed regarding the interplay between these types of RNA sequences and protein coding genes [3]. ncRNAs are also known as regulatory RNAs.

One of the most studied ncRNAs class is represented by microRNAs (miRNAs) that are small single-stranded nucleotide sequences (18–22 nucleotide length) capable of gene regulation through sequence complementarity [2], being involved in all hallmarks of cancer [4]. The biogenesis mechanism is presented in **Figure 1**. The discovery of miRNAs has enabled new

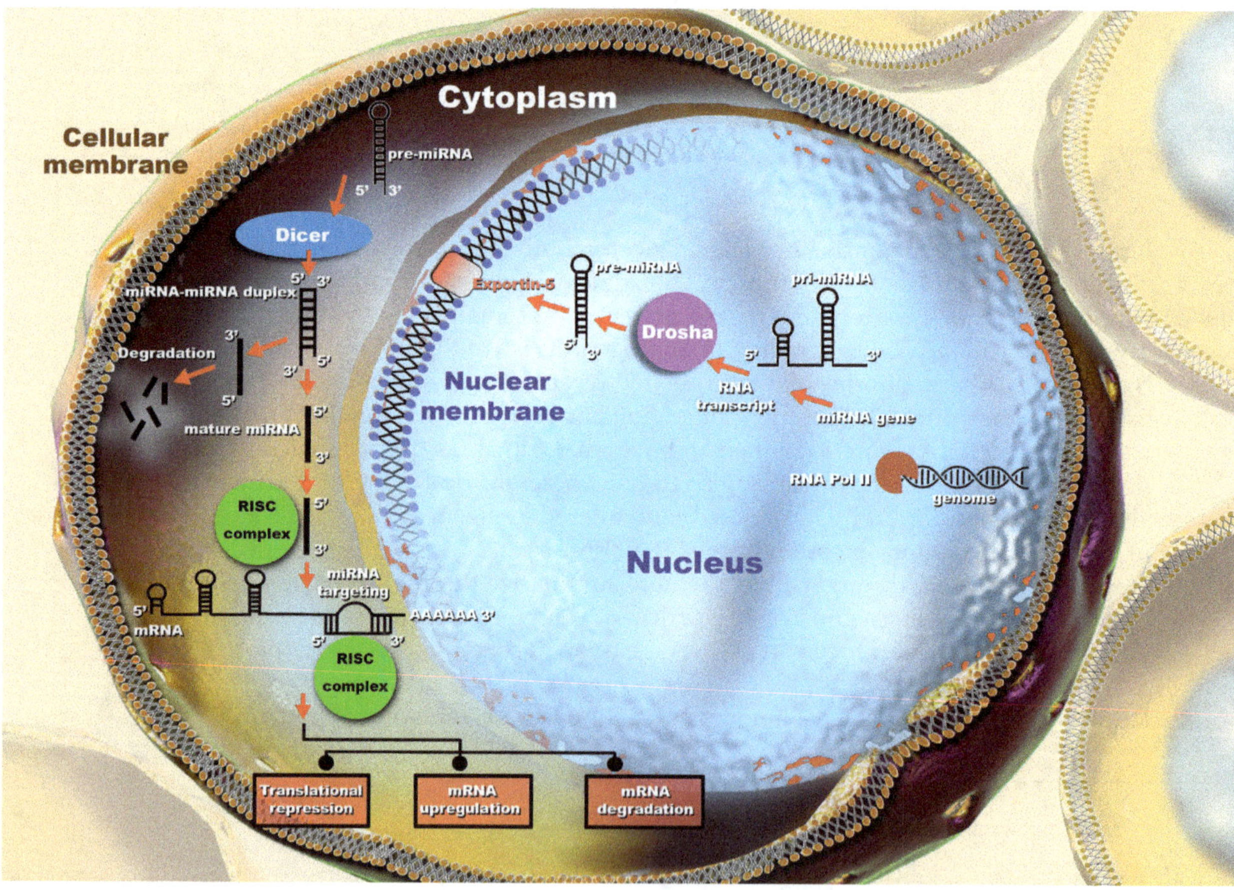

Figure 1. miRNA biogenesis mechanism. microRNAs are situated in the genome of the host as individual transcriptional units but also as clusters of a number of distinct microRNAs. For the first step, RNA polymerase II transcribes the target sequence resulting in a primary transcript named pri-miRNAs. This unprocessed sequence is then subjected to the activity of RNase III-type enzyme Drosha that transforms the pri-miRNA sequence into a transcript of approximatively 70 nt, pre-miRNA. This precursor is then transferred in the cytoplasm via Exportin-5, followed by another miRNA manipulation step governed by the RNase III protein Dicer, resulting in a double stranded RNA called miRNA-miRNA duplex. The less stable strand is further captured by the RISC complex, association that facilitates specific gene regulation through complementary interactions.

noninvasive diagnosis methods and also has conducted towards the development of more targeted therapeutics alternatives in a large number of cancers and other pathological states [4, 5]. Despite numerous discoveries in the ncRNA field, the two main noncoding fronts in cancer are still represented by microRNAs and the more recent characterized long noncoding RNAs (lncRNAs) [6]. As the technology advances, these last sequences are increasingly mentioned in pathological contexts, where differential expression levels are associated with malignant states and other diseases [6]. Despite the associations between lncRNAs expression patterns and different types of cancers, there are still many unknowns regarding the complex mechanism of action.

MiRNAs revolution has stimulated the investigation of other types of small ncRNAs such as small interfering RNAs (siRNAs), and Piwi-interacting RNAs (piRNAs) [3, 7, 8]. These last two types of molecules are similar to miRNAs in length and function, where siRNAs mediate posttranscriptional inhibitory processes and piRNAs act particularly on transposable elements and are capable of forming complexes with Piwi proteins [7, 8]. piRNAs transcribed from kiwi clusters together with Piwi proteins are capable of transposon modulation through interruption of the specific transcript that will be no longer able to exercise their specific activity. Other types of ncRNAs, circularRNA (ciRNA) are formed through base pairing of intronic repeats that ends up with a complete circular fragment that is able to act as a miRNA sponge through complementary interactions [3, 9].

Supplementing the complex regulatory networks of miRNAs, ciRNAs have recently emerged as new cancer modeling tools through miRNA targeting, escaping from the initial characterization as transcriptional "noise" [9, 10]. These types of transcripts are ubiquitous present in eukaryotic cells and competitively bind microRNAs sequences, functioning like an inhibitory sponge; process that could attribute a significant therapeutic potential to these circular fragments [9, 10, 11, 12]. In this sense, specific microRNAs are eliminated from the regulatory networks, influencing the expression scheme of target genes. Competitive endogenous RNA (ceRNA) describes a new mechanism of gene regulation, being involved in physiological and pathological processes [13].

The traditional concept that RNA molecules are just intermediary sequences between DNA and proteins is now replaced with more advanced molecular data, where short- and long-noncoding sequences play a key role in normal development and disease progression [14]. SiRNAs and miRNAs are similar in length, approximatively 22 nucleotides, and are both processed by Dicer through cleavage. SiRNAs are derived from complementary dsRNA duplexes, where miRNAs originate from imperfect RNA hairpins from short introns or long transcripts [15–18]. Both small noncoding types of sequences associate with Argonaute proteins in order to manipulate gene expression (generally through 3'UTRs) [19], although siRNAs are also involved in viral defense and transposon regulation. piRNAs are the longest fragments from the small RNAs group, having approximatively 26–30 in length. This class associates with PIWI-clade Argonaute proteins in order to guide transposon activity and chromatin status [15, 17]. Long noncoding RNA group consist in all RNA sequences that are not responsible for protein generation and their length exceed

200 nucleotides, being further grouped in concordance with their genomic localization: intronic, intergenic, sense, and antisense ncRNAs to host gene locus [6, 20]. Biogenesis of lncRNAs is very similar with the processing activity of mRNAs molecule, being transcribed by RNA Pol II and also being subjected to the same epigenetic modifications and splicing signals. The functional roles of lncRNAs are more extended than in the case of small ncRNAs, a significant part being still incompletely understood. Briefly, this type of sequences is not so well conserved as miRNAs and also can control gene activity at different levels in a more complex scheme [2, 6, 16].

2. Lung cancer—molecular classification and survival rates

Lung cancer occupies the first place regarding the mortality rates from the oncological field, being characterized by an aggressive profile that ends with numerous deadly metastatic sites. One of the main reasons for the high mortality rates consists in the late diagnosis [21]. According to the characteristics of the cancer cells, this malignancy presents itself in two major forms, one being *small-cell lung cancer* (SCLC), and the other being named *non-small-cell lung cancer* (NSCLC) according to the histological classification and another rare subtype, *lung carcinoid tumor* (*LCT*) [22, 23]. NSCLC ranks as the number one diagnosed type of lung cancer in the oncological field, being further divided into three histologic types: *squamous cell carcinoma, large-cell carcinoma, and adenocarcinoma. Adenocarcinomas* represent the most common subtype of NSCLC, with an incidence of 35–40% from all lung cancer cases, being the most lethal type of cancer in male population, and the second in women. This type of pulmonary malignancy frequently presents distant metastases and pleural effusions. Between a quarter and 30% of all lung cancer cases belong to the squamous cell carcinoma category. These particular tumors are mostly located in the central areas of the lungs, and were shown to be connected to tobacco smoking [24]. Lung carcinoid tumors are very rare and represent about 5% of the lung cancers which grows very slowly and are rarely associated with metastasis [25]. Despite the frequency drop, pulmonary tumors remain the major cause of death and morbidity around the world, being very aggressive and refractory to standard oncologic therapy [26], due to the late diagnostic [27].

Environmental and occupational exposure to different agents and an individual's susceptibility for these agents were associated with a risk of lung cancer in approximately 9–15% of cases. The cigarette smoke is the primary risk factor for the development of lung cancer and is estimated to be responsible for approximately 90% of all lung cancers [24], followed by asbestos [28], and radon [27]. More than 300 harmful substances with 40 known potent carcinogens were discovered in tobacco smoke.

The classical therapeutic strategies like surgery and chemotherapy or radiation fail to accomplish their purpose in advanced pathological states. In the case of patients diagnosed early in the disease, the chances of survival are more promising, being observed a partial response to drugs based on platinum. However, even in this case, the final outcome is not necessary a positive one due to acquisition of treatment resistance. According to National Cancer Institute, survival rates for early stages of NSCLC are extremely low compared to other types of cancer, where the rate for the late stages of the same malignancy can reach even 1%: the 5 years survival rate for stage IA is approximately 49%, 45% for stage IB, 30% for stage IIA and 31% for IIB. The next stages, IIIA and IIIB, are associated with even more dramatically numbers, 14% and 5% respectively (**Figure 2**). For the case of metastatic lung cancer, where the tumor has spread within different body sites, the survival rates are extremely low (1%) [29, 30]. Therefore, a critical part of lung cancer management is represented by the discovery of specific molecular carcinogenic pathways in order to precisely target key molecules that are responsible for tumor development and avoid treatment resistance. ncRNAs study represents an important research direction for achieving these goals.

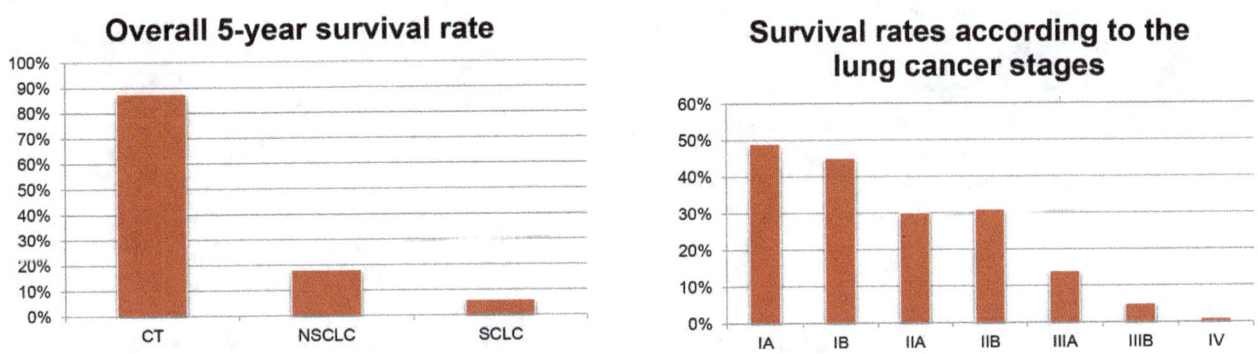

Figure 2. The overall survival rates associated with different lung cancer subtypes (NSCLC, SCLC) and the 5-year survival rate based on lung cancer stages.

3. Angiogenesis—beyond hallmarks of lung cancer

Nowadays, the cancer hallmarks are at the center of carcinogenesis: prolonged proliferation signals, escaping of growth inhibitors, apoptosis inhibition, indefinite replicative potential, vascular network development (angiogenesis) and activation of cell invasion, and thus metastasis (**Figure 3**) [31]. Although all of these hallmarks represent key elements without which tumorigenesis could not more or less advance, angiogenesis surpasses this listing of malignant processes: without the ability to receive oxygen and nutrients and evacuate waste products, the spreading of the tumor is naturally restricted. Moreover, the vessel network is one of the invasion routes used by transformed mesenchymal cell in order to evade from the original carcinogenic site and invade other tissues [31]. All these features stand at the base of the therapeutic concept, where angiogenesis is one of the main signaling pathway targeted in the treatment of cancer patients, including individuals with lung cancer. Inhibition of this malignant progression pathway through exogenous administration of targeted agents in the form of ncRNAs/anti-ncRNAs will enable the proper management of tumor spreading and will serve as a feasible therapeutic strategy for lung cancer [33].

The most promising proangiogenic target in lung cancer is VEGF (vascular endothelial growth factor), more precisely the interaction of VEGF with the transmembrane receptors or receptors downstream the signaling pathways. However, prolonged exposure to VEGF/VEGFR inhibitors may force tumor cells to find alternative pathways for vascular

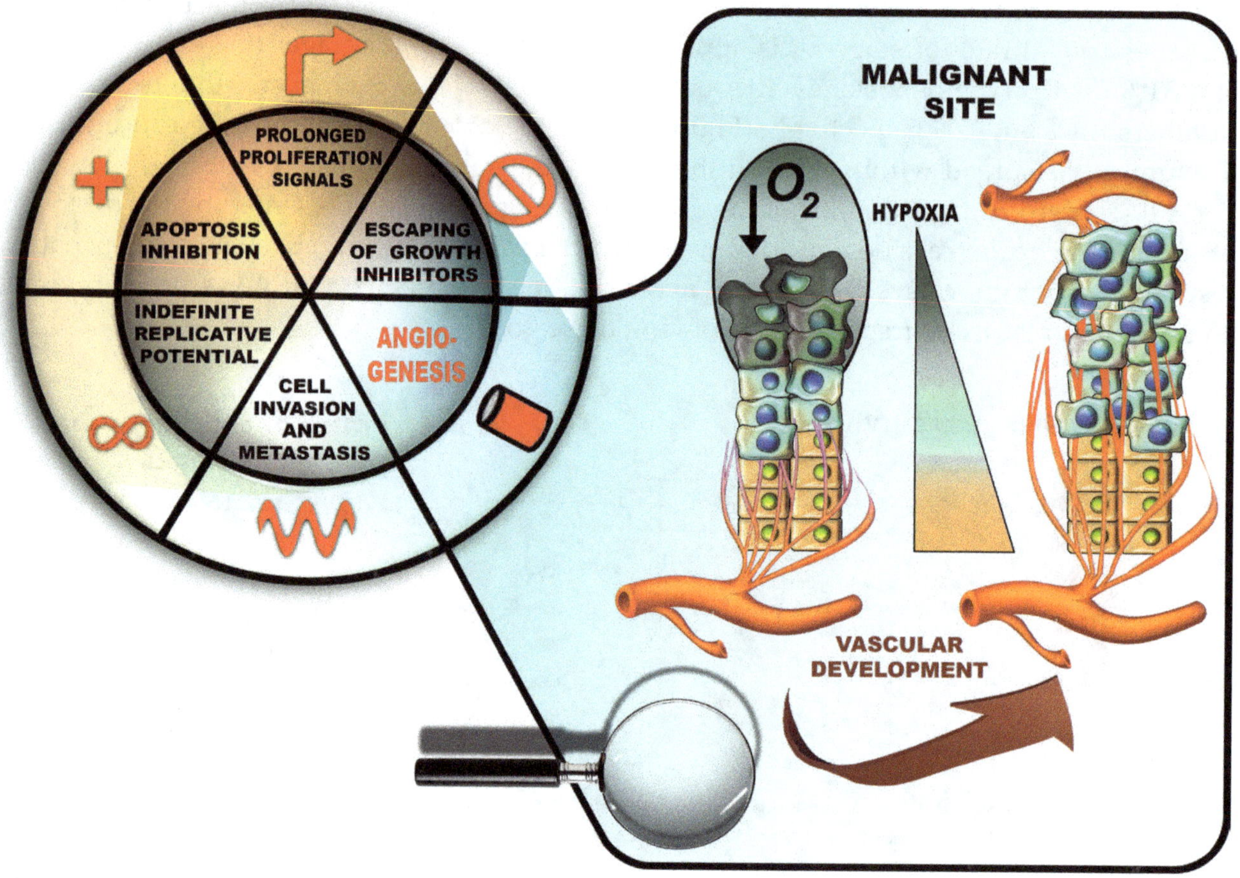

Figure 3. Lung cancer hallmarks with focus on angiogenesis.

development [34]. Additionally, some other angiogenic pathways have been explored with the same purpose, where FGFRs (fibroblast growth factor receptors), angiopoietin, PDGFRs (platelet-derived growth factor receptors), and, in the last few years, semaphorins and the related receptors captured the attention [32, 34]. The metastatic cascade, a multievent process that leads to the spreading of the tumor cells to numerous sites in the organism and causes death, represents the main challenge in cancer treatment and angiogenesis plays a major role in this progression [35].

3.1. Implication of ncRNAs in regulation of lung cancer angiogenesis

As a result of the limited success of the classical antiangiogenic therapies targeting VEGF and its related receptors [35, 36], researchers have deepened their knowledge by analyzing the expression of ncRNAs sequences in this pathology (**Figure 4**) [37, 38]. The mechanism of lung cancer angiogenesis is far from being completely deciphered and implicit the process of therapeutic inhibition via ncRNAs remains to be further investigated. Targeting ncRNAs will enable a more precise treatment and will avoid compensatory mechanisms retrieved in lung cancer [2, 37, 38].

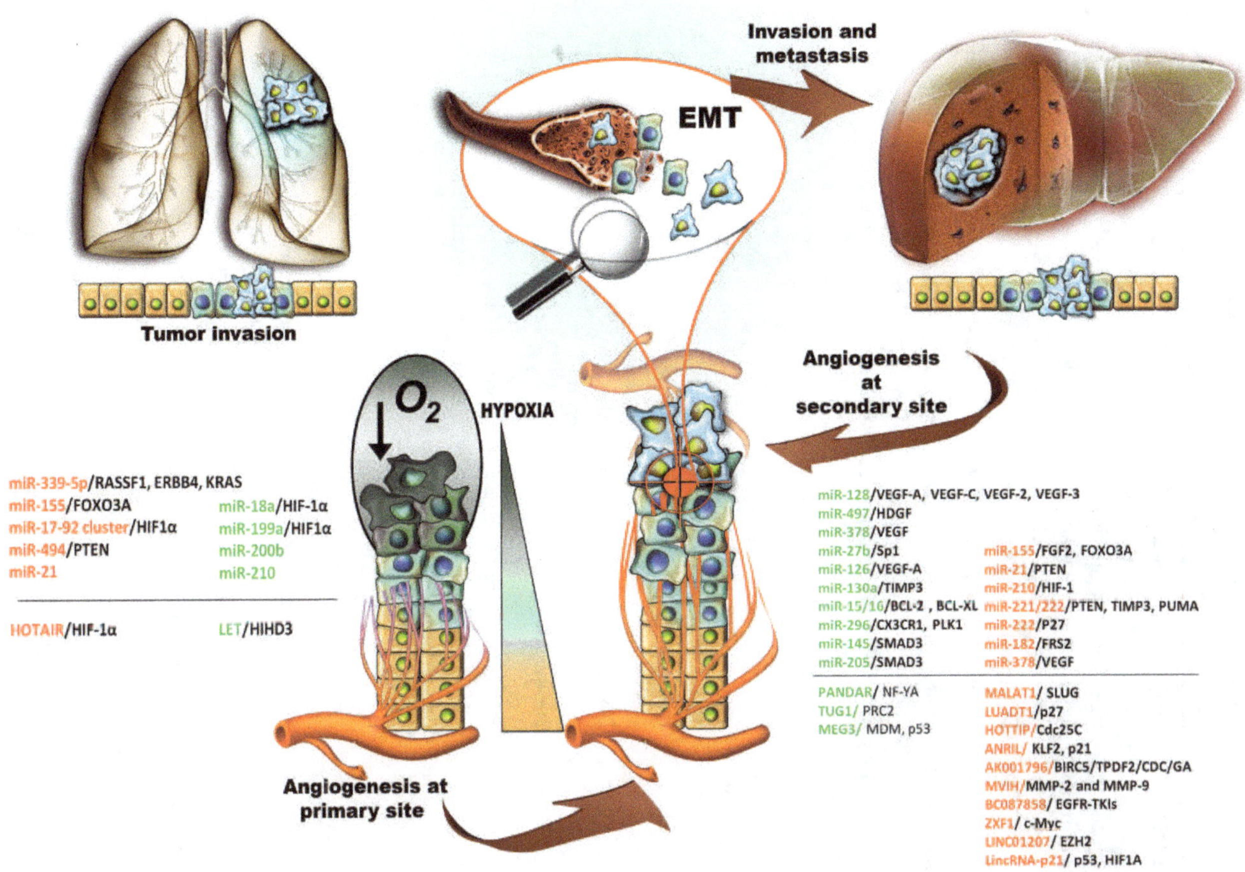

Figure 4. Evolution of vascular network within lung cancer. Malignant cells lacking nutrients and oxygen enter in hypoxic stress, state that promotes the signaling pathways related to angiogenesis in order to sustain cell proliferation. The same process is present at the metastatic sites, where mesenchymal cells that went through epithelial to mesenchymal transition are establishing new malignant formations. The complex malignant scheme is strictly regulated by noncoding RNAs (miRNAs and lncRNAs). Red - overexpressed ncRNAs; Green- downregulated ncRNAs.

3.2. miRNAs related to lung cancer angiogenesis

Among all types of ncRNAs, miRNAs molecules are the most intensive studied in what regards novel cancer therapies. Although the majority of the studies are concentrated on oncogenic miRNA inhibition via exogenous delivery of complementary (antisense) sequences through different vectors, it seems that another therapeutic alternative consists in miRNA replacement. This last type of targeted treatment may be even more effective due to the fact that the predominant pathological model consists more in dowregulated tumor suppressor sequences than overexpressed oncogenic genes [5, 21, 39].

Until this moment, several miRNA patterns involved in different lung cancer processes such as cell proliferation, resistance to therapy, invasion, metastasis, and angiogenesis have been identified. We will focus on some important miRNAs that presented the most aberrant expression related to lung cancer angiogenesis (**Tables 1** and **2**).

No.	Name	Location	Length (nucleotides)	Expression level	Target gene	Activity	Possible role in lung cancer angiogenesis	Clinical potential	References
1	miR-27b	9q22.32	22	▼	Sp1	Possible key miRNA regarding the development of lung cancer; ectopic expression reduced the cell growth and invasion	Sp1, a target gene of miR-27b, was associated with the angiogenic phenotype in gastric cancer, with key roles in the manipulation of this process; patients with high levels of Sp1 presented a more vascularized phenotype	Therapeutic target	[40, 41]
2	miR-126	9q34.3	22	▼	VEGF-A	Low expression of this miRNA is associated with high vascular density in NSCLC; this data were also observed in vitro	Due to direct targeting of miR-126 on VEGF-A, overexpression of this miRNA could be suitable for anti-angiogenic therapies	Therapeutic target and also prognosis tool	[42]
3	miR-130a	11q12.1	21	▼	MET	miR-130a downregulates the expression levels of two oncogenic miRNAs, miR-221 and miR-222; MET suppression	MET represents a key factor for vascular development and miR-221/222 cluster could also play an important role in angiogenesis due to the direct down regulation of TIMP3, an inhibitor of MET; miR-130 is able to reduce the levels of both this systems	Important therapeutic potential	[43, 44]
4	miR-15/16	13q14.3	–	▼	BCL-2 and BCL-XL	MiR-15/16 cluster was found as downregulated in NSCLCs; miR-15 directly targets BCL-2 and BCL-XL	BCL-2 has a suppressive action on VEGF and TP in lung cancer, both strongly implicated in angiogenesis development	Contradictory results; further studies needed	[45–47]
5	miR-378	5q32	21	▼	VEGF	Inhibition of lung cancer angiogenesis through VEGF targeting	Regulator of a central element in lung cancer angiogenesis	*In vivo* demonstrated therapeutic target	[48, 49]
6	miR-296	20q13.32	21	▼	CX3CR1, PLK1	Tumor suppressor role in lung cancer development targeting chemosensitivity and cell viability	MIR-296 has been associated with angiogenesis	Potential therapeutic target	[50–52]

No.	Name	Location	Length (nucleotides)	Expression level	Target gene	Activity	Possible role in lung cancer angiogenesis	Clinical potential	References
7	miR-128	2q21.3	23	▼	VEGF-A, VEGF-C, VEGF-2, VEGF-3	*In vitro* and *in vivo* overexpression of miR-128 led to significant suppression of angiogenesis due to down regulation of the target genes; furthermore miR-128 expression is correlated with the development stages of lung cancer	Current data shows that miR-128 could be used effectively as therapeutic target or prognostic tool	Therapeutic target for enhanced expression and prognosis tool	[53]
8	miR-497	17p13.1	20	▼	HDGF	Ectopic expression of this sequence in an animal model demonstrated positive effects through inhibition of cell proliferation and angiogenesis	Experimental data shows that miR-497 could be used with success as an antiangiogenic agent for lung cancer	Therapeutic target	[54]
9	let-7b	22q13.31	2[illegible]	▼	RAS	Lung cancer tumors tissue revealed a downregulated pattern and was associated with increased vascular density	The collected data suggest a possible role for miR-7b as antiangiogenic tool in the moment of ectopic expression	Prognosis and therapeutic tool	[55]
10	miR-145	5q32	22	▼	SMAD3	Implicated in EMT and invasion	Enhancement of this miR expression could serve as a therapeutic strategy for lung cancer	Possible therapeutic target	[56]
11	miR-205	1q32.2	20	▼	VEGF	Implicated in EMT and invasion	Enhancement of this miR expression could serve as a therapeutic strategy for lung cancer	Possible therapeutic target	[57]

Table 1. The main tumor suppressor altered miRNAs implicated in lung cancer angiogenesis.

No	Name	Location	Length (nucleotides)	Expression level	Target gene	Activity	Possible role in lung cancer angiogenesis	Clinical potential	References
1	miR-221 miR-222	Xp11.3	23	▲	PTEN, TIMP3	Highly expressed in lung cancer cells; promotes invasion and migration	miR-221/222 cluster could have a role in angiogenesis promotion through down regulation of TIMP3, an inhibitor of MET, an angiogenesis promoter	Therapeutic target and patients stratification toll	[58]
					PUMA	Co-modulation of the two miRNAs on PUMA promotes cell proliferation and inhibits apoptosis			[59]
2	miR-222	Xp11.3	23	▲	P27	Increased miR-221/222 expression promotes H460 cells viability and proliferation	Considering the possible in vivo role of p27, where the overexpression of this gene impaired angiogenesis, miR-222 that inhibits the expression of p27 could become a potent therapeutic target regarding antiangiogenic strategies	Therapeutic target for inhibition	[60, 61]
3	miR-210	11p15.5	22	▲		Significantly up-regulated in lung cancer tissues and associated with angiogenic potential in other types of cancers	Due to the regulation by HIF-1 involved in hypoxia (event that triggers angiogenesis development), miR-210 could also become a therapeutic target	Still limited data	[62, 63]
4	miR-155	21q21.3	22	▲/▼	FGF2	MIR-155 expression is correlated with FGF2 levels, an important molecule for lung cancer angiogenesis. Also, mimR-155 was correlated with VEGF-A in the N+ subgroup of NSCLC	Several studies have investigated the role of this miR in angiogenesis	Prognosis and therapeutic tool	[64, 65]
					FOXO3A, SOCS1, SOCS6, and PTEN	Hypoxia promotes miR-155 increased expression concomitant with the downregulation of FOXO3A target			[65, 66]

No	Name	Location	Length (nucleotides)	Expression level	Target gene	Activity	Possible role in lung cancer angiogenesis	Clinical potential	References
5	miR-21	17q23.1	21	▲	PTEN, SOCS1, and, SOCS6	After antiangiogenic therapy this miR was observed as downregulated	Possible role in lung cancer angiogenesis observed after the post-antiangiogenic down regulation	Possible therapeutic target	[66]
6	miR-182	7q32.2	23	▲	FRS2	miR-182 directly targets FRS2 in lung cancer, gene that represents a key molecule for NSLC progression and antigenesis	N/A	Therapeutic and diagnosis tool	[67]
7	miR-106a	Xq26.2	22	▲	–	Augmented expression of miR-106 in NSCLC was reported in several studies	Previously associated with hypoxia progression in colon and breast cancer that could enable a possible role in lung cancer hypoxia/ angiogenesis	Possible therapeutic target	[67–69]

Table 2. The main oncogenic miRNAs involved in lung cancer angiogenesis.

3.3. LncRNAs related to lung cancer angiogenesis

The number of lncRNAs has significantly increased due to the progresses offered by sequencing methods in genomic research. Long noncoding transcripts act as gene regulators via a wide range of mechanism [70], those related to lung cancer being summarized in **Table 3**. The first long noncoding sequence associated with lung cancer was MALAT1 that through increased expression and gene targeting (caspase-8, caspase-3, BCL-XL, BCL-2, and BAX) promotes the proliferation and invasiveness of cancer cells. Recently it was emphasized to target SLUG gene via a competitively "sponging" miR-204 [71]. Following this initial lncRNA, a significant list of lncRNA was associated with lung cancer progression or inhibition through modulation of key mechanisms involved in the hallmarks of lung pathology. The regulatory process is complex, lncRNAs being able to escort chromatin modifying enzymes to target loci within the genome, to bind the promoter of genes and modify the transcription process, to be processed into miRNAs and further act as short noncoding transcripts, and finally to modify the stability of specific mRNAs through direct binding [70].

Recent evidences suggested the role of PANDAR in lung cancer cell proliferation through p53/PANDAR/NF-YA/Bcl-2 axis [72]. Another lncRNA positively regulated by p53 is TUG1, whose downregulation is associated with increased cell proliferation and poor survival rate in lung cancer patients [73]. Also, considering the antiangiogenetic role of the p53 gene and the positive correlation between the two sequences, there is a possible role for TUG1 in angiogenesis suppression, however further investigations are necessary. HOTTIP is a long noncoding transcript that is associated with tumor growth [74], process that involves the formation of new blood vessel network, fact that could transform HOTTIP into a new target for antiangiogenetic therapies. MVIH is associated with microvascular invasion in HCC, being upregulated in this type of cancer with an increased oncogenic potential. Further studies have investigated the possible role of the same lncRNA in lung cancer and the results were increasingly similar with the previous pathology, MVIH representing a biomarker for poor prognosis and associated tumor cell proliferation [75]. There are also other lncRNAs with tumor suppressor or tumor promoting roles in lung cancer malignancies, like MEG3 (tumor suppressor), ANRIL, and AK001796 (oncogenic role) that are involved in cell proliferation and cell viability, processes that go hand in hand with the angiogenetic transformation [76–78]. lnRNA BC087858 is overexpressed in NSCLC and was demonstrated to be connected with drug resistance via EGFR-TKIs axis [80]. MEG3 was proved to be downregulated in tumoral tissue, and directly related with high tumoral stage. Preclinical studies demonstrated a reduced proliferation rate in the case of MEG3 overexpression, by targeting MDM2 and p53 proteins. MEG3 is presented not only as prognostic marker but also as important therapeutic target [76]. ANRIL is overexpressed in lung cancer tissue, being correlated with tumor-node-metastasis stages and tumor size, but until now there are not presented data with a direct connection with angiogenesis [78].

3.4. Ultraconserved regions (UCRs)

Ultraconserved regions (UCRs) are genome sequences longer than 200 bp and, as the name suggests, are conserved within humans, rats, and mouse, preserving their nucleotide

lncRNA	Target gene	Biological role	Reference
TUG1	PRC2	Tumor suppressor lncRNA regulated by p53, gene that promotes the expression of TUG1	[73]
MEG3	MDM and p53	Tumor suppressor role through cell proliferation reduction and increased survival. P53 expression is frequently correlated with the expression of the MEG3, with possible cumulative role in angiogenesis suppression	[76]
MALAT1	SLUG	Promoter of EMT and metastasis, via miR-204	[71]
PANDAR	NF-YA	Inhibits tumor cell proliferation in the moment of overexpression through p53/PANDAR/NF-YA/Bcl-2 axis	[72]
LUADT1	p27	Oncogenic role through promotion of cell proliferation; knockdown of the target gene significantly contribute to the reduced tumor size by inhibition of cell expansion	[79]
HOTTIP	Cdc25C	Promotes tumor growth and is overexpressed in lung cancers	[74]
ANRIL	KLF2 and p21	Oncogenic role; knockdown of this lncRNA reduced proliferation and increased apoptosis	[78]
MEG3	MDM and p53	Tumor suppressor role exercised through cell proliferation reduction and increased survival. P53 expression is frequently correlated with the expression of the MEG3, with possible cumulative role in angiogenesis suppression	[76]
AK001796	BIRC5/TPDF2/CDC/GA	Oncogenic role; involved in maintaining the tumor cell viability through complex mechanisms	[77]
MVIH	MMP-2 and MMP-9	Overexpressed in lung malignancies, being associated with increased cell proliferation and poor prognosis, previously recognized as angiogenesis promoter in HCCs	[75]
BC087858	EGFR-TKIs	Promotes cells invasion and induces drug resistance to EGFR-TKIs by activating PI3K/AKT and MEK/ERK pathways and EMT via up-regulating ZEB1 and Snail	[80]
ZXF1	c-Myc	LncRNA ZXF1overexpression was connected with a relatively poor prognosis; Knockdown by siRNA has no effect on cell proliferation, but decreased the migration and invasion of lung cancer cells	[81, 82]
LINC01207	EZH2	Cancer initiation and progression	[83]
LincRNA-p21	p53 and HIF1A	Regulation of TP53-dependent apoptosis and Warburg effect and angiogenesis	[84]

Table 3. The main lncRNAs involved in lung cancer angiogenesis and possible therapeutic targets for inhibiting lung cancers.

succession during the evolution [85, 86]. Until this moment there are a number of 481 conserved sequences, a part of them being situated at sensitive sites regarding cancer susceptibility and are further transcribed (T-UCR) into pathological expression patterns. Considering this recent discovery, it has been postulated that the differential expression pattern could serve as stratification tool in the oncology domain, being able to differentiate between human cancers and possible between molecular subtypes of carcinomas [85, 86].

The exact mechanism that leads to aberrant expression of T-UCR is not fully deciphered, although it is thought that the primary regulation models are represented by miRNAs interactions and epigenetic modifications in CpG islands hypermethylation [85].

Calin et. al. were the first to discover the T-UCR spectrum in malignant cells compared with healthy ones and found significant differences between the two states [85]. So far, molecular analysis have revealed different T-UCR signatures in a number of carcinomas, including prostate, hepatocellular, and colorectal cancer, as well as in chronic lymphocytic leukemia and neuroblastoma. Presently was observed upregulation of several T-UCRs and demonstrated by multiple investigations to be related with increased risks for tumour occurrence and a high metastatic rate. Therefore, the main investigation area is focused on integration of synthetic antisense oligonucleotides (ASOs) to inhibit T-UCR functions [85]. In lung cancer, an important number of T-UCRs need to be characterized and then used for developing novel therapies. In spite of the interest on the T-UCR, there are only few investigations on T-UCR therapy.

4. ncRNAs related to hypoxia in lung cancer

Hypoxia is a preangiogenetic process driven by specific gene modifications, alterations that are able to induce the installation of the mesenchymal phenotype through epithelial to mesenchymal transition (EMT), acquisition of drug and radiation resistance, and propagation of lung cancer stem cells [87, 88]. Compared to other cancers, lung malignancy is severely sustained by the installation of hypoxia through complex interactions between specific molecules (HIF1α and miRNAs or other ncRNAs, as displayed in **Tables 4** and **5**) and establishment of noncoding regulatory networks related to connection with the cell cycle regulation, apoptosis or autophagy [88].

In terms of lung cancer hypoxia, miRNAs play a pivotal role through the ability to orchestrate extensive signaling networks involved in this carcinogenic step. MiR-200 family has been extensively characterized in numerous malignant scenarios and miR-200b member seems to have a role that could be exploited in the context of the clinical area regarding hypoxia induced EMT where cells acquire motility characteristic and are able to invade secondary sites within the organism promoting lung cancer metastasis [89]. Reinforced expression of the tumor suppressor miRNAs inhibited EMT through regulation of key genes involved in this pathway [88]. Another possible therapeutic target is represented by miR-21, that is elevated in NSCLC-derived cells grown under hypoxic conditions [90]. Hypoxic conditions also triggered miR-155 overexpression and downregulation of FOXO3A target gene, and protects lung cancer cells to irradiation, elucidating a possible course of treatment through inhibition of miR-155 combined with radiotherapy [65].

Type of miRNA	Expression level	Name	Target gene	miRNA role in lung cancer hypoxia	Possible clinical role of miRNAs in lung cancer	References
Tumor suppressor miRNAs	▼	miR-200b	–	Hypoxia-induced EMT in lung cancer, influencing the activity of key genes involved in mesenchymal transition miR-200 mimic blocks hypoxia-induced EMT	Novel therapeutic strategy via Nobiletin delivery	[89]
	▼	miR-210	–	Regulate cellular response under hypoxic conditions High levels connected with a positive outcome in NSCLC patients	Biomarker for prognosis and patient stratification	[63, 91]
	▼	miR-18a	HIF-1α	Connected with lung metastasis of breast cancer cells ability to decrease the hypoxic stress *in vitro* and reduce cell invasiveness	Possible prognosis factor of lung metastasis in breast cancer	[92]
	▼	miR-199a	HIF1α	Inhibition of cancer cell hypoxia induced proliferation in NSCLC cells	Possible prognosis factor	[93]
Oncogenic miRNAs	▲	miR-21	–	NSCLC derived cell lines grown under hypoxic condition showed an elevated miR-21 expression; modulates radiation resistance via hypoxic mechanism	Possible therapeutic and prognosis role	[87, 90]
	▲	miR-339	RASSF1, ERBB4, KRAS	Activity correlated with the process of response to hypoxia	Possible target for therapeutic strategies	[94]
	▲	miR-155	FOXO3A	Correlates with poor prognosis and protects hypoxic lung cancer cells to irradiation and conversely	Therapeutic potential for radio sensitization of hypoxic lung cancer cells	[65]
	▲	miR-17-92 cluster	HIF1α	Downregulation of HIF1α does not affect the cellular adaptation to hypoxia	Possible prognosis factor	[95]
	▲	miR-494	PTEN	Promotes angiogenesis through direct targeting of PTEN and activation of Akt/eNOS pathway; expression is induced during hypoxia	Possible prognosis and therapeutic tool	[96]

Table 4. Tumor suppressor and oncogenic miRNAs involved in lung cancer hypoxia with possible roles in diagnosis, prognosis, and therapy.

Type of lncRNA	Expression level	Name	Target gene	lncRNA role in lung cancer hypoxia	Possible clinical role of lncRNAs in lung cancer	References
Tumor supressor lncRNAs	▼	lncRNA-LET (Low expression in tumor)	HIHD3; hypoxia-induced histone deacetylase 3	Squamous-cell lung carcinomas downregulated by HIHD3 promotes hypoxia-induced cancer cell invasion	New methods for therapeutic intervention	[97]
	▼	GAS5-AS1	–	Downregulation of GAS5-AS1 contributes to hypoxia tumor metastasis in non-small cell lung cancer	Prognosis and therapeutic marker	[98]
	▼	LincRNA-p21	TP53 and HIF-1α	Target angiogenic mechanisms	Prognosis marker	[84]
Oncogenic lncRNAs	▲	HOTAIR (HOX transcript antisense intergenic RNA)	HIF-1α	HOTAIR is upregulated in hypoxic conditions and is a direct target of HIF-1α; Promotion of cancer cell proliferation and ability to migrate and invade other sites	Novel therapeutic target	[99, 100]
	▲	H19	HIF-1α	Possess oncogenic properties triggered by hypoxic stress Correlates with p53 tumor suppressor status	Prognosis/ Diagnosis marker	[101]

Table 5. LncRNAs involved in lung cancer hypoxia with possible roles in diagnosis, prognosis, and therapy.

Hypoxia management has led to reduced angiogenesis and thus obtuse the malignant cell proliferation and survival due to deprivation of nutrients and oxygen via various molecules including the noncoding transcripts represented by miRNAs and lncRNAs. Multiple targeting through ncRNAs that are able to influence the fate of the hypoxic microenvironment will bring new insights into the pathogenesis of lung cancer, permitting the development of new clinical tools for cancer management, improving the concerning survival rate of this pathology. The list of miRNAs and lncRNAs implicated in the vascular invasion of the pulmonary malignancy is presented in **Tables 4** and **5**.

LncRNAs have recently emerged as important prognosis and therapeutic tolls in different malignancies and even for specific carcinogenic processes as lung cancer hypoxia. One of the main studied lncRNAs is HOTAIR, pathological expressed in numerous malignant scenarios, being associated with tumor promoting roles and a negative outcome in oncological patients. It was demonstrated that this lncRNA is a direct target for HIF-1α that act as an enhancer of expression and contribute together to the securitization of hypoxia followed by cell proliferation, migration, and metastasis. This information could transform HOTAIR in a possible therapeutic target under hypoxic conditions for NSCLC, that is limited in what regards the therapeutic options [99, 100]. Another newly discovered lncRNAs in lung cancer hypoxia that is lncRNA-LET targeted by HIHDR. The interaction between these two molecules ends with reduction of histone acetylation at the promoter region of the noncoding transcripts and thus decreased expression. Moreover, the downregulation process secures the expression of nuclear factor 90 proteins, a key element for cell migration induced by hypoxia. This data suggest that lncRNA-LET can be used as a clinical tool against cancer promotion [97].

LincRNA-p21 impacts prognosis in resected nonsmall-cell lung cancer patients through angiogenesis regulation. LincRNA-p21 was proved to be activated by TP53 and HIF1A [84]. It was proved to target the apoptosis pathway via regulation by p53 and the Warburg effect. LincRNA-p21 is downregulated in tumor tissue, and has effect on the lung cancer patients via angiogenesis regulation [84].

Other important ncRNA structures with a significant role in the development of novel molecular therapies are represented by PIWI-interacting RNAs (piRNAs). piRNAs are recognized to be involved in transposon silencing and gene expression during development and the complete role on the somatic cells remains to be deciphered [8]. In a recent paper were emphases a different piRNASs expression profiles between normal bronchial epithelial cells and lung cancer cells. The most downregulated piRNAs in lung cancer cells was piRNA-like-163 (piR-L-163) having as direct target the phosphorylated ERM (p-ERM) [102]. S100A4-small interfering RNA (S100A4-siRNA) was proved to activate the apoptosis and increase the radiosensitivity of A549 lung cells. S100A4 may promote A549 cell proliferation but also invasion, and metastasis by regulating the expression of E-cadherin and p53 protein [103].

5. ncRNAs targeting semaphorines and its related receptors in lung cancer

Semaphorins are guidance molecules which were characterized initially as directing elements for axon outgrowth; however advances in genomic and translational medicine revealed a more complex role for these proteins, being involved in cell migration, vascular network, and tissue development [32, 104]. Considering their vital role in physiological processes is not surprising that these guidance proteins are also involved in similar pathological processes especially from the oncologic area, where they exercise the same functions, but in a negative manner [32]. Therefore, semaphorins are implicated in carcinogenic establishment, metastasis, and especially angiogenesis in numerous cancers, including lung cancer. Regarding their role in angiogenesis, the family of semaphorins is divided into two main pathological classes: tumor suppressors inhibiting the angiogenic process and oncogenes through promotion of vascular invasion. Therefore, loss of expression in the case of antiangiogenic semaphorins and/or increased expression pattern for the procarcinogenic ones translates into sustaining of the malignant cells [106]. Immediately after the establishment of their newly discovered role, *in vitro* and *in vivo* studies confirmed the ability of semaphorins to serve as therapeutic targets in the form of suppression or enhancement [32]. Despite the fact that their role in pulmonary malignant processes is quite extensively studied, little is known about the ncRNAs regulatory action on the expression pattern of semaphorins. Deciphering the regulatory noncoding sequence panel for these proteins will enable a more advanced and specific molecular management of lung cancer, especially in angiogenesis that has a vital role regarding the maintenance of tumor cells integrity and proliferation.

The process of angiogenesis, can also occur through semaphorin receptors, neuropilins, and plexins (**Figure 5**). In the case of neuropilins, we encounter a multiple ligation system, this membrane proteins being able to bind both class-3 semaphorins, VEGF and growth factors. Also, this type of receptors that are essential to proper vascular development during organism development are generally mutated in lung cancer. On the other hand, *in vivo* suppression of neuropilins led to improper vascular network.

Among the first studies that elucidated the role of neuropilins in vascular development is the research where the authors observed that overexpressing of *Nrp1* was lethal for embryos due to extensive vascular defects like overdevelopment of blood vessel network and deformed hearts [107]. This discovery paved the way for further research in the area of cancer management with focus on targeted therapy. Therefore, it has been proven that a combined form of therapy represented by neuropilins inhibitors (semaphorin, anti-NRP, soluble NRP - B domain, and VEGF mimetics) administrated concomitant with anti-VEGF signaling molecules (kinase inhibitors, anti-VEGF, anti-VEGFR-2, and soluble VEGFR for VEGF) is more efficient than the classical antiangiogenic therapeutic strategy targeted towards VEGF alone [104]. Research studies demonstrated a role for NRP1 and NRP2 in lung cancer progression and angiogenesis where these two molecules were observed as normally expressed in bronchial basal cells, and as it progressed in the severity of the cell lesions, the level of neuropilins increased significantly, concomitant with VEGF expression [104]. NRP1 has been previously associated with cancer angiogenesis: overexpression of NRP1 in AT2.1 cells (*in vitro* model of prostate cancer) resulted in advanced vascular density, cell proliferation, and also inhibited apoptosis [108]; rat estrogen-induced pituitary tumors presented increased levels of NRP1, level that was also correlated in a positive manner with the aggressiveness of angiogenesis development [109].

The competitive binding of class-3 semaphorins and VEGF that in physiological conditions leads to the proper development of the vascular platform is changed during malignant scenarios where proangiogenic VEGF takes the lead due to mutations in the structure of the binding domain that decreases the complementarity with semaphorins or enhances the expression of receptors. Therefore, an alternative therapeutic pathway could be represented by the

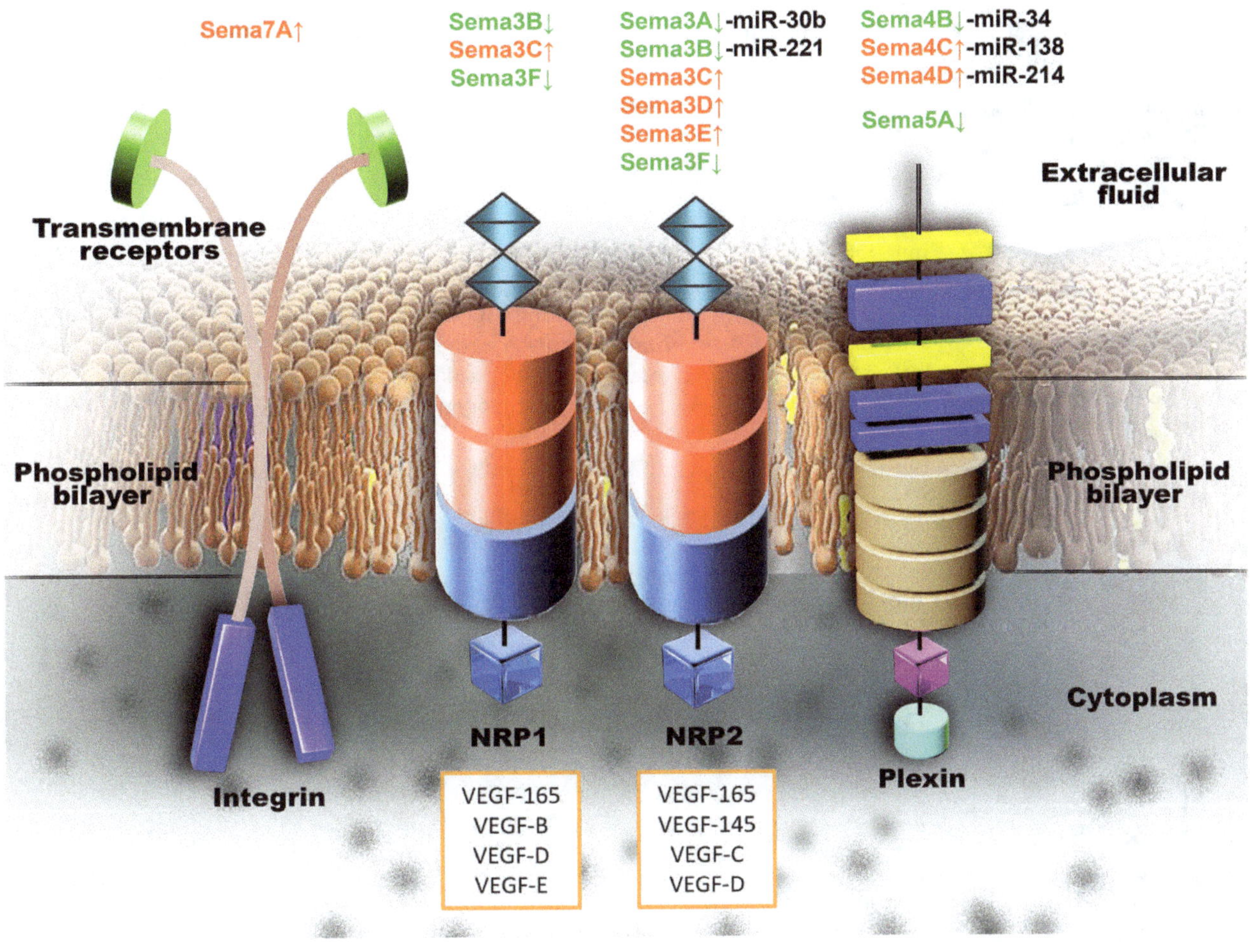

Figure 5. Semaphorin receptors and ncRNAs regulation. Green – downregulated genes; Red – overexpressed genes.

modulation of neuropilins (NRPs) expression. Furthermore, the specific malignant expression is most likely influenced by other molecules such as miRNAs and lncRNAs (**Table 6**).

Lung cancer therapies focused on semaphorins and their receptors are still an insufficiently explored domain that could hold great promises regarding the inhibition of cancer spreading. Considering the competitive binding between class-3 semaphorins and VEGF in vascular development, antiangiogenic strategies as antibodies for VEGF or NRP inhibition, soluble NRP or NRP blocking peptides have been tested with effective results [104, 106]. A more recent treatment compromising both VEGF and SEMA3A inhibitors have been applied *in vitro* and *in vivo* for colon cancer [105]. Another type of action could be represented by the induced internalization of the neuropilins through administration of dextran sulfate and fucoidan that significantly decreased the number of endothelial surface receptors, including VEGFR [131]. Although anti-VEGF molecules are well-known as efficient angiogenesis inhibitors, combining the modulation of VEGF/VEGFR with SEMA/NRP may hold significant clinical usage. Moreover, extension of the molecular insight regarding noncoding RNAs regulation of semaphorins and their receptor could improve even more the inhibition of angiogenesis if we take in consideration the ability of noncoding RNAs to regulate waste singling networks that involve more than one target gene.

Semaphorin	Regulatory miRNAs	Predicted targeting miRNAs	Role in lung cancer	Potential clinical role in lung cancer	Ref.
Semaphorin 3A (SEMA 3A)	miR-30b	miR-95-3p miR-589-5p	NSCLC-anticarcinogenic activity; low expression of SEMA 3A correlates with lymph node metastasis	Biomarker for prognosis	[104, 110]
Semaphorin 3B (SEMA 3B)	miR-221	miR-155-5p miR-107 miR-187-5p miR-18a-3p miR-708 miR-3074-5p miR-106b-3p miR-340-3p miR-3074-5p	Cell proliferation and invasion Small-cell lung cancer-tumor suppressor role via induction of apoptosis and inhibition of angiogenesis	Marker for cancer progression	[111, 112]
Semaphorin 3C (SEMA 3C)	–	miR-4746-5p miR-500a-5p miR-187-5p miR-301a-5p miR-21-3p miR-106a-3p miR-4677-3p miR-3074-5p let-7g-3p miR-183-3p miR-29a-3p miR-519a-5p miR-200c-5p miR-4668-3p miR-16-2-3p miR-193a-3p miR-4326 miR-4417 miR-3664-3p miR-155-5p miR-590-5p miR-616-3p miR-3182 miR-103a-2-5p miR-501-5p miR-362-3p miR-330-5p miR-30e-5p	A549 lung cancer cells -p65-SEMA3C (cleaved SEMA3C) – protumorigenic activities	Novel antitumorigenic drug	[113]
Semaphorin 3D (SEMA 3D)	–	miR-484 miR-15b-3p miR-16-2-3pmiR-32-3p miR-32-5p miR-33a-5p miR-33b-3p miR-340-5p miR-4668-3p miR-345-5p miR-629-5p miR-18a-5p miR-1306-5p	Proangiogenic and metastatic role	Prediction of response and survival	[114, 115]

Semaphorin	Regulatory miRNAs	Predicted targeting miRNAs	Role in lung cancer	Potential clinical role in lung cancer	Ref.
		let-7a-3p miR-183-3p miR-21-3p miR-21-5p miR-4742-5p miR-425-5p miR-200a-5p miR-301a-5p miR-3619-3p miR-589-5p miR-3614-3p miR-141-5p miR-106a-3p miR-93-3p			
Semaphorin 3E (SEMA 3E)	–	miR-340-5p miR-1306-5p miR-15b-3p let-7d-5p miR-1307-3p miR-629-5p miR-629-3p miR-4677-3p let-7g-3p miR-301a-5p miR-15b-5p miR-19a-3p miR-16-2-3p miR-105-3p miR-18a-5p miR-1306-5p miR-19a-3p miR-1307-5p miR-505-5p	*In vivo* promotion of lung metastasis and tumor progression	Possible target for therapeutic strategies	[116]
Semaphoring 3F (SEMA 3F)	–	miR-29c-3p miR-191-3p miR-29b-1-5p miR-18a-5p miR-20a-5p miR-29b-2-5p miR-200c-5p let-7g-3p let-7a-3p let-7d-5p miR-7-5p miR-3619-3p miR-590-5p miR-29b-2-5p miR-30e-5p miR-676-3p miR-135b-3p miR-30c-1-3p miR-140-3p miR-135b-3p miR-140-3p	Role in TGF-beta1-induced EMT Antitumor role; Downregulated in lung cancer Targets HIF-1 and VEGF	Possible prognosis biomarker and therapeutic target	[117, 118]

Semaphorin	Regulatory miRNAs	Predicted targeting miRNAs	Role in lung cancer	Potential clinical role in lung cancer	Ref.
Semaphorin 4B (SEMA 4B)	miR-34	miR-34	NSCLC—inhibition of invasion and growth—prevention of metastasis-direct target of hypoxia-inducible factor 1 (HIF-1) miR-34/p53 axis	Novel therapeutic target for inhibition of metastasis and growth -Novel therapeutic target through inhibition of HIF-1	[119–121]
Semaphorin 4C (SEMA 4C)	miR-138	miR-138	NSCLC-cell proliferation and EMT	New target or prognosis marker for lung cancer treatment	[122]
Semaphorin 4D (SEMA 4D)	miR-214	miR-199b-3p miR-127-3p miR-185-5p miR-421 miR-500a-5p miR-22-3p miR-500a-5p miR-22-3p miR-505-5p let-7g-3p miR-1269a miR-18a-5p miR-3614-3p miR-331-3p miR-18a-5p miR-18a-3p	Highly expressed in lung cancer; promotion of angiogenesis; NSCLC-*in vitro* inhibition of cell proliferation, migration, and invasion	Possible early prognosis tool and therapeutic target	[124–126]
Semaphorin 5A (SEMA 5A)	-	miR-3677-3p miR-3200-3p miR-32-5p miR-29b-1-5p miR-183-3p miR-345-5p miR-454-5p miR-3614-3p miR-18a-3p miR-500a-5p miR-106b-3p miR-27b-5p let-7g-3p miR-660-5p miR-135b-3p miR-1306-5p miR-29a-3p miR-29b-2-5p miR-425-3p miR-365a-5p miR-3136-3p miR-93-3p miR-4787-3p miR-19a-3p	NSCLC-tumor suppressor role; low levels associated with poor survival rate	New biomarker for NSCLC	[127]

Semaphorin	Regulatory miRNAs	Predicted targeting miRNAs	Role in lung cancer	Potential clinical role in lung cancer	Ref.
Semaphorin 6A (SEMA 6A)	miR-27a/b	miR-1307-3p miR-940 miR-3187-3p miR-33a-5p miR-425-3p miR-99b-5p miR-99b-3p miR-183-3p miR-3176 miR-760 miR-345-5p miR-4461	Endothelial cell repulsion	New therapeutic target through manipulation of miR-27a/b expression	[128, 129]
Semaphorin 7A (SEMA 7A)	–	22_40957679_40957783 (novel miRNA)	Promotion of tumor microenvironment and metastasis through regulation of prototypic chitinase-like protein (Chi3l1)	Possible role as therapeutic target	[130]

Table 6. Semaphorin and the targeting miRNAs with implication in lung cancer.

6. ncRNAs therapies targeting lung cancer angiogenesis

Once considered the "trash" of the genome, the noncoding RNA sequences are now emerging as important therapeutic targets (**Table 7**). Due to the complex regulatory network involving ncRNAs and also because of the personalized pathological expression pattern among cancer types, subtypes and malignant stages, ncRNAs are subjected to numerous preclinical studies regarding their silencing or induced expression [2]. A lipid-based delivery vehicle for tumor suppressor miR-34 was developed in order to enhance the expression of the specific molecule in a mouse model of non-small-cell lung cancer [132]. This approach has demonstrated to be efficient in both locally and systemically administration, being observed a reinforced miR expression concomitant with downregulation of the specific targets. Moreover, the intravenous delivery of miR-34 mimic did not produce an immune reaction in mice, but unfortunately this was not the case in humans. Very recently, MRX34, the miR-34 mimic, was stopped to be administrated in a cancer clinical trial due to major immune reactions [133].

Another therapeutic alternative that is currently on the scientific spotlight consist in the manipulation of the ciRNAs that can function as microRNA sponges, modulating their oncogenic or tumor suppressor activity [136]. Despite the fact that there is a number of research studies focused on this type of noncoding RNAs, relatively little is known about the regulatory mechanism of circRNAs in cancer development. Future perspectives imply ciRNAs-based therapy that can stand as "super-sponges" and modulate the activity of extended regulatory miRNA networks, influencing at a superior level the carcinoma progression [136].

miRNAs	Lung cancer subtype	Experimental model	Therapeutic approach	Delivery system	Target gene	Obtained results	References
miR-128	NSCLC	NSCLC cells	Ectopic miR-128 overexpression		VEGF-C	Inhibition of VEGF-C expression concomitant with angiogenesis restriction	[53]
		HUVECs and NSCLC cells			VEGF-A, VEGFR-2 and VEGFR-3	Low expression of the target genes that are critical factors for angiogenesis	
		Nude mice (A549 cells)	*In vivo* replacement therapy			Inhibition of lymphangiogenesis	
miR-497	NSCLC	NSCLC cells	Over expression of the miRNA		VEGF-A	Decreases in the levels of VEGF-A protein with no significant changes for the VEGF-A mRNA; inhibition of cell invasion	[123]
			miRNA inhibition			Increased levels of VEGF-A protein with no significant changes for the VEGF-A mRNA; increased cell invasion	
		NSCLC cells SCID mouse xenograft model	Ectopic expression of the miRNA sequence		HDGF	Restoration of the miR-497 levels reduced tumor development and angiogenesis in both *in vitro* and *in vivo* experimental models	[54]
miR-378	NSCLC	Swiss nude immunodeficient murine model (NCI-H292-Luc cells overexpressing miR-378—subcutaneous xenografts)	Overexpression of miR-378	Lentiviral vectors particles (pEZX-MR03 backbone)	HMOX1	mir-378 over expression models presented tumors with decreased vascularisation compared to the models with HMOX1 induced over expression; increased oxygen partial pressure; increased MUC5AC, Ang-1,MMP12 levels and decreased TNF-α and IL-1β levels - all essential genes for angiogenesis	[48]
miR-126		A549, Y-90 and SPC-A1 cells	Overexpression of miR-126	mir-126 expression vector (LV-miR-126)	VEGF-A	Dowregulation of VEGF-A gene correlated with inhibited cell growth	[42]
		Tumor xenograft model (A549 infected with LV-miR-126)	mir-126 expression vector (LV-miR-126)				

miRNAs	Lung cancer subtype	Experimental model	Therapeutic approach	Delivery system	Target gene	Obtained results	References
miR-222	NSCLC	H460 cells	Inhibition of miR-222 expression	miR-222 inhibitor	p27 (*in vivo* over expression of p27 impaired angiogenesis)	Inhibition of oncogenic miR expression resulted in decreased cell viability and proliferation	[60, 61]
miR-27b	NSCLC	HEK293 cells	Cotransfection of miR-27b mimics and WT Sp1 in order to express both miRNA and target gene	psiCHECK-2 vector	Sp1	Expression of miR-27b resulted in suppression of cell growth and reduced invasion	[128]
miR-130a	NSCLC	A549,CALU-1, H1299 and A459 cells	Transfection with miR-130a in order to increase the endogenous levels of this sequence	pre-miR 130a	MET	Strong reduction of MET (angiogenesis promoter) mRNA and protein levels; down regulation of miR-221 and miR-222, that are able to inhibit TIMP3 expression, molecule that in turn inhibits MET	[44]
miR-210	Adenocarcinoma	A549 cells	Knocked down of miR-210 in hypoxic parameters	antimiR-210	SDHD (positive-regulatory loop between miR-210 and HIF-1α)	Decreased cell survival and alteration of mitochondrial phenotype	[63]
miR-155	Adenocarcinoma	A549 and H460 cells	Inhibition of miR-155 levels in cells preserved in hypoxic conditions	Synthetic antimiR-155	FOXO3A (associated with roles in angiogenesis)	miR-155 inhibition exercise a positive role through radiosensitization of the cells	[65, 134]
miR-21	NSCLC	A549	*In vitro* inhibition of miR-21	miR-21-sponge	PDCD4 (associated with angiogenesis development)	Inhibition of miR-21 ameliorates cell proliferation, migration, and invasion through PDCD4 modulation; knockdown of PDCD4 has been demonstrated to stimulate angiogenesis through positive regulation of Ang-2 (negative prognostic factor in lung cancer)	[66, 135]

Table 7. Some relevant miRNAs tested on cell culture and animal models as potential therapeutic agents in lung cancer.

The discovery of lncRNAs as regulators of cancer development has naturally conducted towards potential therapeutic alternatives using these long fragments as direct targets. The expression pattern of these sequences has been also investigated in lung cancer and the list of oncogenic and tumor suppressor pathological expressed lncRNAs is continuously growing. Administration of siRNA, shRNA, and miRNAs or antisense oligonucleotides in order to inhibit oncogenic lncRNAs is currently under investigation [137]. HOTAIR has been on the spotlight of artificial knockdown via siRNA delivery with great rates of success in lung cancer and also breast and pancreatic malignancies [100].

Moreover, the same approaches have been shown to be effective for the reverse of cisplatin resistance through reduced expression of p21 [138]. Downregulation of MALAT1 through shRNA delivery is also a potent therapeutic approach for lung cancer as it was shown reduced cell viability after this type of treatment [71]. MALAT1 has been also inhibited by exogenous antisense oligonucleotides, approach that induced reduced cancer progression through cell cycle arrest [151]. Considering that in lung cancer there are also downregulated tumor suppressor lncRNAs, the replacement therapy could also stand as an effective therapeutic approach for this type of carcinoma, but nonetheless the scientific information are quite limited regarding this area.

The discovery that miRNA sequences can act as key regulators in cancer pathways through aberrant expression has led to the idea that these fragments could serve as potent therapeutic targets [139]. In this sense, several strategies have been implemented until now: inhibition strategies—inhibitory antisense oligonucleotides and delivery vectors (miRNA sponges) and enhancement strategies—miRNA replacement therapy (**Figure 6**) [139, 140].

For the case of therapeutics that follow an antagonistic pattern, the activity of tumor promoting miRNAs that are hazardous expressed is inhibited via administration of single stranded oligonucleotides complementary with the specific molecule or with the target binding site on the mRNA molecule; in either situation, the interaction between miRNAs and mRNA molecules is blocked and the downstream pathological pathway is strongly affected [140].

Delivery of anti-miRNA oligonucleotides (AMOs) in the context of preclinical studies is still a problematic area considering the necessity of target administration, prolonged stability, and increased pharmacokinetic properties [140]. In this means, there is an urgent need for efficient delivery vectors/vehicles that are able to fulfill the reminded request in order to accomplish the treatment purpose. The majority of the freely administrated oligonucleotides is retrieved in the liver and kidneys and then eliminated through the urine. Also, the necessary dose of synthetic sequences is usually very high and the chance for off-target delivery is also increasing. Establishment of an effective delivery system will break the grounds of miRNAs therapeutics and also other noncoding treatment strategies [139]. The current strategy for *in vivo* administration implies conjugation-based methods, where miRNA sequences are conjugated with different molecules like cholesterol [141] and α-tocopherol [142]. Although these studies have demonstrated promising results, the efficiency of miRNA targeting is still limited. Another type of delivery method consists in liposome-mediated delivery of siRNAs, where the first attempt [143] was to inhibit the replication of hepatitis B virus (HBV) in an animal model through administration of siRNAs integrated in as polyethylene glycol (PEG)–lipid conjugate (SNALP). Since then, different liposome-based vehicles have been tested and the results are encouraging considering that the administration dose is significantly decreased

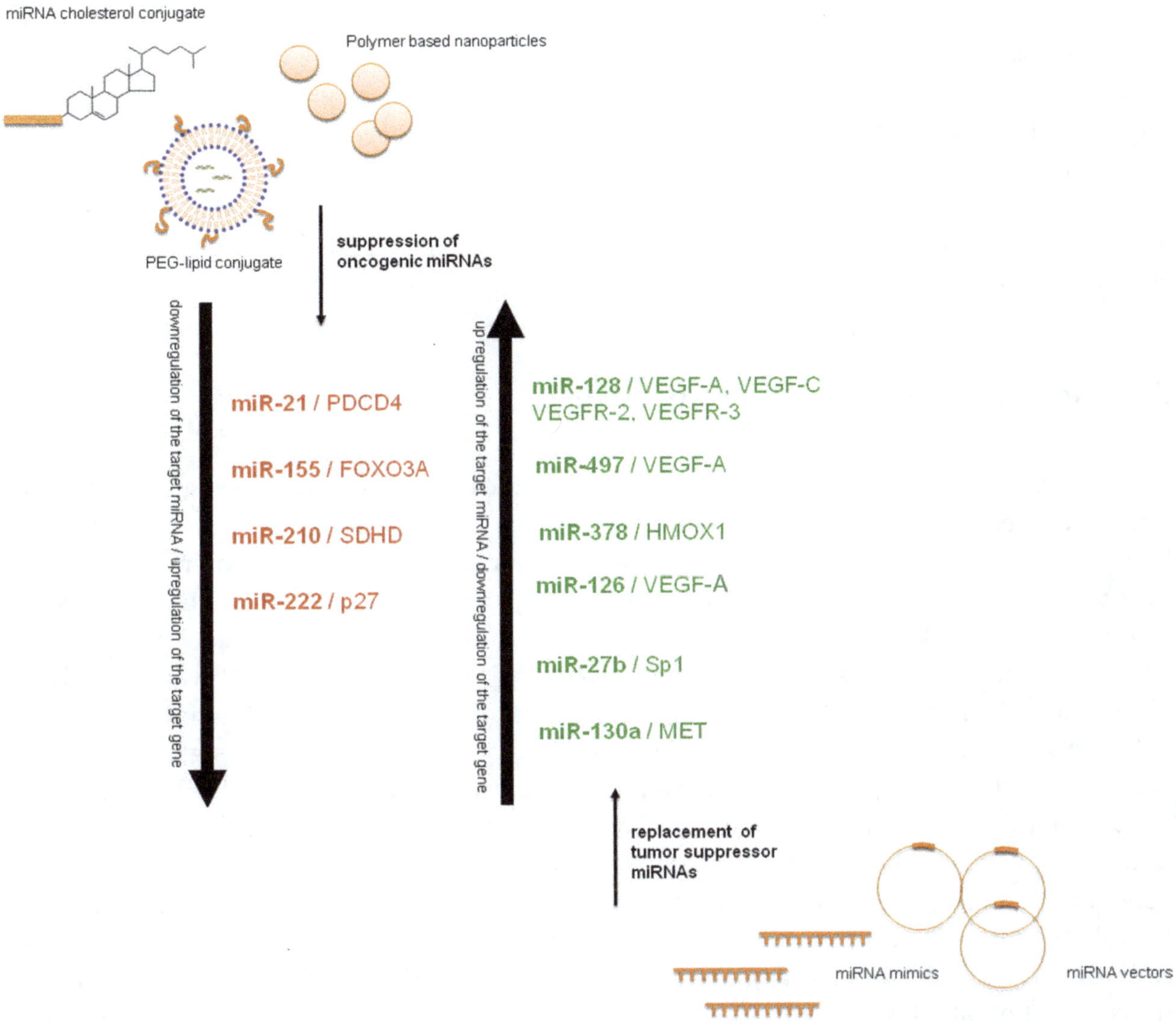

Figure 6. MicroRNAs have emerged as important regulators of lung cancer angiogenesis and also as key therapeutic targets regarding inhibition or enhancement strategies. MiRNAs sequences that are marked with green composed the tumor suppressor group that have been tested in the context of replacement therapies; the genes marked with the same color represent the target genes that have been downregulated after therapeutic modulation of miRNAs. Inversely, miRNAs sequences marked with red are oncogenic ones proposed for inhibition in what regards antiangiogenic programs; the genes marked with the same color also represent the target genes, but in this case their expression has been augmented.

comparing to the naked oligonucleotides [144–147]. Progresses in the area of material science produced a promising *in vivo* delivery system in the form of polymer-based nanoparticles that are more flexible than liposomes and also can be produced in a more homogenous manner regarding their size and form [139]. In respect of siRNAs and anti-miRs delivery, the size of the vehicle is very important in order to permit the passing through cellular compartments, where nanoparticles can fulfill this request having a size between 10 and 100 nm [139]. Moreover, in order to avoid the stimulation of the immune system, cyclodextrin–PEG conjugated nanoparticles have been developed and tested for the inhibition of EWS–FLI1 in an *in vivo* model of Ewing's sarcoma [148]. Attracting strategies for targeted therapies consist in the conjugation of siRNAs or anti-miR sequences with specific antibodies able to conduct the small fragments towards distinctive cells expressing the desired antigen [147, 149, 150].

MiRNA replacement therapy is more limited regarding the current attempts and results, although it seems to emerge as a more efficient form of treatment considering that the majority of pathological expressed miRNAs consist in downregulated or inhibited tumor suppressor sequences [140]. Even if the success of this therapeutic strategy could be greater than miRNA inhibition workflows, the requirements for the structure and composition of the replacement fragment are much more stringent considering the necessity of RISC uptake. Furthermore, the impediments regarding the delivery system for these oligonucleotides are the same as in the case of inhibitory antisense attempts.

7. Conclusions and future perspectives

Lung cancer remains the most deadly disease from the oncological field, being an aggressive form of cancer that is usually diagnosed in late stages with minimal therapeutic alternatives. Even in the case of early discovery, the classical treatments have failed numerous times due to compensatory mechanisms developed within the tumor environment leading to the same negative outcome. Therefore, we face a crisis situation where we need to develop new therapeutic tools for lung cancer management able to target key elements/pathways, but avoid in the same time the possibility of alternative carcinogenic pathways activation. One of the hallmarks of cancer is represented by angiogenesis, process that is in the sight of researchers for some time, but the classical inhibition of central molecules like VEGF has failed to deliver long-lasting results. Therefore, ncRNAs have emerged as potential lifesaving agents due to the capacity of extensive modulation, where the same ncRNA is able to target multiple genes and regulate their function. Also the same microRNA, or more recently discovered, the lncRNA can be encounter in different consecutive processes in pulmonary carcinogenesis, as in the case of hypoxia and angiogenesis. Development of novel therapeutic tools able to transform the pathological expression of ncRNAs, mainly through silencing of upregulated patterns, will enable a more extensive, and in the same time, specific approach that will probably excludes the installation of compensatory mechanism and significantly contribute to a better outcome in lung cancer patients. The concept of noncoding RNAs as therapeutic targets in the clinical context is now more feasible than ever, being supported by numerous preclinical studies. One of the main approaches should involve manipulation of miRNAs that are actively implicated in the regulation of VEGF genes expression, genes that hold a key role in the vascular development process. Even more, a heterogeneous approach that implies the administration of different miRNA sequences able to target multiple genes and naturally multiple pathological pathways within the angiogenic process will represent a more extended form of therapy that could modify extensive regulatory networks. This type of targeting will also minimize the compensatory mechanisms that are usually encountered after the implementation of classical therapeutic strategies due to concomitant regulation of multiple signaling pathways. Additionally, some other approaches may be used for the inhibition of angiogenesis. For example, semaphorins are now emerging as important regulators of vascular density in malignancies, with possible roles as prognostic tools or even therapeutic targets. Inhibition of procarcinogenic semaphorins would represent a novel course of action regarding cancer treatment considering their central role in vascular density. Moreover, the receptors associated with semaphorins contain binding sites for both semaphorins and VEGF molecules, engaging the competitive binding between these types of molecules. Managing the expression of VEGF via miRNA therapy concomitant with the levels of neuropilins (semaphorins receptors) will enable a more dramatic approach that could have more drastic results for cancer development.

Current therapeutic programs are promoting the effectiveness of specific sequence inhibition or enhancement through administration of antisense oligonucleotides or supplementation of the same sequence through exogenous enhancement. Development of chemically modified oligonucleotides under the form of medication for individuals diagnosed with cancer is now at the close horizon. Administration of synthetic oligonucleotides for noncoding RNAs inhibition or upregulation will enhance the effect of the current therapeutic strategies by modulation of specific gene expression able to influence the carcinogenic process or even reverse the malignant installation. In this sense, it is now clearly understood that the major strategy towards cancer treatment is focused on taking advantage of the key roles of noncoding sequences regarding the modulation of entire aberrant regulatory networks through manipulation of central molecules.

Acknowledgments

This work was supported by the POC-P_37_796 grant, entitled "Clinical and economical impact of personalized targeted anti-microRNA therapies in reconverting lung cancer chemoresistance"-CANTEMIR.

Author details

Ioana Berindan-Neagoe[1,2,3]*, Cornelia Braicu[1], Diana Gulei[2], Ciprian Tomuleasa[1,4] and George Adrian Calin[5]

*Address all correspondence to: ioana.neagoe@umfcluj.ro

1 Research Center for Functional Genomics, Biomedicine and Translational Medicine, "Iuliu Hatieganu", University of Medicine and Pharmacy Iuliu-Hatieganu, Cluj-Napoca, Romania

2 Medfuture—Research Center for Advanced Medicine, University of Medicine and Pharmacy Iuliu-Hatieganu, Cluj-Napoca, Romania

3 Department of Functional Genomics and Experimental Pathology, The Oncological Institute "Prof. Dr. Ion Chiricuta", Cluj-Napoca, Romania

4 Department of Hematology, The Oncological Institute "Prof. Dr. Ion Chiricuta", Cluj-Napoca, Romania

5 Department of Experimental Therapeutics, The University of Texas M.D. Anderson Cancer Center, Houston, TX, USA

References

[1] Mattick, J.S. and I.V. Makunin, *Non-coding RNA*. Hum Mol Genet, 2006. **15 Spec No 1**: pp. R17–29.

[2] Braicu, C., et al., *NCRNA combined therapy as future treatment option for cancer*. Curr Pharm Des, 2014. **20**(42): pp. 6565–74.

[3] Choudhuri, S., *Small noncoding RNAs: biogenesis, function, and emerging significance in toxicology*. J Biochem Mol Toxicol, 2010. **24**(3): pp. 195–216.

[4] Berindan-Neagoe, I., et al., *MicroRNAome genome: a treasure for cancer diagnosis and therapy*. CA Cancer J Clin, 2014. **64**(5): pp. 311–36.

[5] Berindan-Neagoe, I. and G.A. Calin, *Molecular pathways: microRNAs, cancer cells, and microenvironment*. Clin Cancer Res, 2014. **20**(24): pp. 6247–53.

[6] Kung, J.T., D. Colognori, and J.T. Lee, *Long noncoding RNAs: past, present, and future*. Genetics, 2013. **193**(3): pp. 651–69.

[7] Liu, Y. *MicroRNAs and PIWI-interacting RNAs in oncology*. Oncol Lett, 2016. **12**(4): pp. 2289–2292.

[8] Ng, K.W., C. Anderson, E.A. Marshall, B.C. Minatel, K.S. Enfield, H.L. Saprunoff, W.L. Lam, and V.D. Martinez, *Piwi-interacting RNAs in cancer: emerging functions and clinical utility*. Mol Cancer, 2016. **15**: p. 5.

[9] Hansen, T.B., J. Kjems, and C.K. Damgaard, *Circular RNA and miR-7 in cancer*. Cancer Res, 2013. **73**(18): pp. 5609–12.

[10] Peng, L., X.Q. Yuan, and G.C. Li, *The emerging landscape of circular RNA ciRS-7 in cancer (Review)*. Oncol Rep, 2015. **33**(6): pp. 2669–74.

[11] Ebbesen, K.K., T.B. Hansen, and J. Kjems, *Insights into circular RNA biology*. RNA Biol, 2016 Dec 16:0. [Epub ahead of print]

[12] Hansen, T.B., et al., *Natural RNA circles function as efficient microRNA sponges*. Nature, 2013. **495**(7441): pp. 384–8.

[13] Shao, T., et al., *Identification of module biomarkers from the dysregulated ceRNA-ceRNA interaction network in lung adenocarcinoma*. Mol Biosyst, 2015. **11**(11): pp. 3048–58.

[14] Taft, R.J., et al., *Non-coding RNAs: regulators of disease*. J Pathol, 2010. **220**(2): pp. 126–39.

[15] Malone, C.D. and G.J. Hannon, *Small RNAs as guardians of the genome*. Cell, 2009. **136**(4): pp. 656–68.

[16] Carthew, R.W. and E.J. Sontheimer, *Origins and mechanisms of miRNAs and siRNAs*. Cell, 2009. **136**(4): pp. 642–55.

[17] Ghildiyal, M. and P.D. Zamore, *Small silencing RNAs: an expanding universe*. Nat Rev Genet, 2009. **10**(2): pp. 94–108.

[18] Sobecka, A., W. Barczak, and W.M. Suchorska. *RNA interference in head and neck oncology*. Oncol Lett., 2016. **12**(5): pp. 3035–3040.

[19] Meister, G. *Argonaute proteins: functional insights and emerging roles*. Nat Rev Genet, 2013. 14(7): pp. 447–59.

[20] Tordonato, C., P.P. Di Fiore, and F. Nicassio, *The role of non-coding RNAs in the regulation of stem cells and progenitors in the normal mammary gland and in breast tumors*. Front Genet, 2015. **6**: p. 72.

[21] Kilgoz, H.O., et al., *KRAS and the reality of personalized medicine in non-small cell lung cancer*. Mol Med, 2016. **22**.

[22] Nicholson, S.A., et al., *Small cell lung carcinoma (SCLC): a clinicopathologic study of 100 cases with surgical specimens*. Am J Surg Pathol, 2002. **26**(9): pp. 1184–97.

[23] Nicholson, A.G., et al., *The international association for the study of lung cancer lung cancer staging project: proposals for the revision of the clinical and pathologic staging of small cell lung cancer in the forthcoming eighth edition of the TNM classification for lung cancer*. J Thorac Oncol, 2016. **11**(3): pp. 300–11.

[24] Cheng, T.D., et al., *The international epidemiology of lung cancer: latest trends, disparities, and tumor characteristics*. J Thorac Oncol, 2016. 11(10):1653–71.

[25] Okereke, I.C., et al., *Outcomes after surgical resection of pulmonary carcinoid tumors*. J Cardiothorac Surg, 2016. **11**: p. 35.

[26] Govindan, R., et al., *Changing epidemiology of small-cell lung cancer in the United States over the last 30 years: analysis of the surveillance, epidemiologic, and end results database*. J Clin Oncol, 2006. **24**(28): pp. 4539–44.

[27] Urman, A. and H.D. Hosgood, *Curbing the burden of lung cancer*. Front Med, 2016. **10**(2): pp. 228–32.

[28] Landrigan, P.J., *Comments on the 2014 Helsinki Consensus Report on Asbestos*. Ann Glob Health, 2016. **82**(1): pp. 217–20.

[29] http://www.cancer.org/cancer/lungcancer-non-smallcell/detailedguide/non-small-cell-lung-cancer-survival-rates, accessed, august 2016

[30] http://globocan.iarc.fr/old/FactSheets/cancers/lung-new.asp, accessed, august 2016

[31] Hanahan, D. and R.A. Weinberg, *Hallmarks of cancer: the next generation*. Cell, 2011. **144**(5): pp. 646–74.

[32] Neufeld, G., N. Shraga-Heled, T. Lange, N. Guttmann-Raviv, Y. Herzog, and O. Kessler, *Semaphorins in cancer*. Front Biosci, 2005. **10**: pp. 751–60.

[33] Piperdi, B., A. Merla, and R. Perez-Soler, *Targeting angiogenesis in squamous non-small cell lung cancer*. Drugs, 2014. **74**(4): pp. 403–13.

[34] Cabebe, E. and H. Wakelee, *Role of anti-angiogenesis agents in treating NSCLC: focus on bevacizumab and VEGFR tyrosine kinase inhibitors*. Curr Treat Options Oncol, 2007. **8**(1): pp. 15–27.

[35] Lee, S.M., et al., *Anti-angiogenic therapy using thalidomide combined with chemotherapy in small cell lung cancer: a randomized, double-blind, placebo-controlled trial*. J Natl Cancer Inst, 2009. **101**(15): pp. 1049–57.

[36] Arnedos, M., et al., *Personalized treatments of cancer patients: a reality in daily practice, a costly dream or a shared vision of the future from the oncology community?* Cancer Treat Rev, 2014. **40**(10): pp. 1192–8.

[37] Li, H. and X. Lv, *Functional annotation of noncoding variants and prioritization of cancer-associated lncRNAs in lung cancer*. Oncol Lett, 2016. **12**(1): pp. 222–230.

[38] Stenvang, J., M. Lindow, and S. Kauppinen, *Targeting of microRNAs for therapeutics*. Biochem Soc Trans, 2008. **36**(Pt 6): pp. 1197–200.

[39] Zhang, B., X. Pan, G.P. Cobb and T.A. Anderson, *microRNAs as oncogenes and tumor suppressors*. Dev Biol, 2007 Feb 1. **302**(1): pp. 1–12.

[40] Wang, L., et al., *Altered expression of transcription factor Sp1 critically impacts the angiogenic phenotype of human gastric cancer*. Clin Exp Metastasis, 2005. **22**(3): pp. 205–13.

[41] Safe S. *MicroRNA-Specificity Protein (Sp) Transcription factor interactions and significance in carcinogenesis*. Curr Pharmacol Rep, 2015. **1**(2): pp. 73–78.

[42] Liu, B., et al., *MiR-126 restoration down-regulate VEGF and inhibit the growth of lung cancer cell lines in vitro and in vivo*. Lung Cancer, 2009. **66**(2): pp. 169–75.

[43] Zhou, Y.M., J. Liu, and W. Sun, *MiR-130a overcomes gefitinib resistance by targeting met in non-small cell lung cancer cell lines*. Asian Pac J Cancer Prev, 2014. **15**(3): pp. 1391–6.

[44] Acunzo, M., et al., *miR-130a targets MET and induces TRAIL-sensitivity in NSCLC by down-regulating miR-221 and 222*. Oncogene, 2012. **31**(5): pp. 634–42.

[45] Sun, C.Y., X.M. She, Y. Qin, Z.B. Chu, L. Chen, L.S. Ai, L. Zhang, and Y. Hu. *miR-15a and miR-16 affect the angiogenesis of multiple myeloma by targeting VEGF*. Carcinogenesis, 2013. **34**(2): pp. 426–35.

[46] Tafsiri, E., et al., *Expression of miRNAs in non-small-cell lung carcinomas and their association with clinicopathological features*. Tumour Biol, 2015. **36**(3): pp. 1603–12.

[47] Koukourakis, M.I., et al., *bcl-2 and c-erbB-2 proteins are involved in the regulation of VEGF and of thymidine phosphorylase angiogenic activity in non-small-cell lung cancer*. Clin Exp Metastasis, 1999. **17**(7): pp. 545–54.

[48] Skrzypek, K., et al., *Interplay between heme oxygenase-1 and miR-378 affects non-small cell lung carcinoma growth, vascularization, and metastasis*. Antioxid Redox Signal, 2013. **19**(7): pp. 644–60.

[49] Chen, L.T., et al., *MicroRNA-378 is associated with non-small cell lung cancer brain metastasis by promoting cell migration, invasion and tumor angiogenesis*. Med Oncol, 2012. **29**(3): pp. 1673–80.

[50] Luo, W., et al., *miRNA-296-3p modulates chemosensitivity of lung cancer cells by targeting CX3CR1*. Am J Transl Res, 2016. **8**(4): pp. 1848–56.

[51] Xu, C., et al., *miR-296-5p suppresses cell viability by directly targeting PLK1 in non-small cell lung cancer*. Oncol Rep, 2016. **35**(1): pp. 497–503.

[52] Suarez, Y. and W.C. Sessa, *MicroRNAs as novel regulators of angiogenesis*. Circ Res, 2009. **104**(4): pp. 442–54.

[53] Hu, J., et al., *microRNA-128 plays a critical role in human non-small cell lung cancer tumourigenesis, angiogenesis and lymphangiogenesis by directly targeting vascular endothelial growth factor-C*. Eur J Cancer, 2014. **50**(13): pp. 2336–50.

[54] Zhao, W.Y., et al., *Downregulation of miR-497 promotes tumor growth and angiogenesis by targeting HDGF in non-small cell lung cancer*. Biochem Biophys Res Commun, 2013. **435**(3): pp. 466–71.

[55] Xia, X.M., W.Y. Jin, R.Z. Shi, Y.F. Zhang, and J. Chen. *Clinical significance and the correlation of expression between Let-7 and K-ras in non-small cell lung cancer*. Oncol Lett, 2010. **1**(6): pp. 1045–1047.

[56] Hu, H., et al., *MiR-145 and miR-203 represses TGF-beta-induced epithelial-mesenchymal transition and invasion by inhibiting SMAD3 in non-small cell lung cancer cells*. Lung Cancer, 2016. **97**: pp. 87–94.

[57] Li, J., et al., *The role of miR-205 in the VEGF-mediated promotion of human ovarian cancer cell invasion*. Gynecol Oncol. 2015. **137**: pp. 125–133.

[58] Garofalo, M., et al., *miR-221&222 regulate TRAIL resistance and enhance tumorigenicity through PTEN and TIMP3 downregulation*. Cancer Cell, 2009. **16**(6): pp. 498–509.

[59] Zhang, C., et al., *PUMA is a novel target of miR-221/222 in human epithelial cancers*. Int J Oncol, 2010. **37**(6): pp. 1621–6.

[60] Zhong, C., et al., *MicroRNA-222 promotes human non-small cell lung cancer H460 growth by targeting p27*. Int J Clin Exp Med, 2015. **8**(4): pp. 5534–40.

[61] Goukassian, D., et al., *Overexpression of p27(Kip1) by doxycycline-regulated adenoviral vectors inhibits endothelial cell proliferation and migration and impairs angiogenesis*. FASEB J, 2001. **15**(11): pp. 1877–85.

[62] Devlin, C., et al., *miR-210: More than a silent player in hypoxia*. IUBMB Life, 2011. **63**(2): pp. 94–100.

[63] Puissegur, M.P., et al., *miR-210 is overexpressed in late stages of lung cancer and mediates mitochondrial alterations associated with modulation of HIF-1 activity*. Cell Death Differ, 2011. **18**(3): pp. 465–78.

[64] Donnem, T., et al., *Prognostic impact of MiR-155 in non-small cell lung cancer evaluated by in situ hybridization*. J Transl Med, 2011. **9**: p. 6.

[65] Babar, I.A., et al., *Inhibition of hypoxia-induced miR-155 radiosensitizes hypoxic lung cancer cells*. Cancer Biol Ther, 2011. **12**(10): pp. 908–14.

[66] Xue, X., Y. Liu, Y. Wang, M. Meng, K. Wang, X. Zang, et al. MiR-21 and MiR-155 promote non-small cell lung cancer progression by downregulating SOCS1, SOCS6, and PTEN. Oncotarget, 2016.

[67] Yanaihara, N., et al., *Unique microRNA molecular profiles in lung cancer diagnosis and prognosis*. Cancer Cell, 2006. **9**(3): pp. 189–98.

[68] Donnem, T., et al., *MicroRNA signatures in tumor tissue related to angiogenesis in non-small cell lung cancer*. PLoS One, 2012. **7**(1): pp. e29671.

[69] Patnaik, S.K., et al., *Evaluation of microRNA expression profiles that may predict recurrence of localized stage I non-small cell lung cancer after surgical resection*. Cancer Res, 2010. **70**(1): pp. 36–45.

[70] Sang, H., et al., *Long non-coding RNA functions in lung cancer*. Tumour Biol, 2015. **36**(6): pp. 4027–37.

[71] Li, J., et al., *LncRNA MALAT1 exerts oncogenic functions in lung adenocarcinoma by targeting miR-204*. Am J Cancer Res, 2016. **6**(5): pp. 1099–107.

[72] Han, L., et al., *Low expression of long noncoding RNA PANDAR predicts a poor prognosis of non-small cell lung cancer and affects cell apoptosis by regulating Bcl-2*. Cell Death Dis, 2015. **6**: p. e1665.

[73] Zhang, E.B., et al., *P53-regulated long non-coding RNA TUG1 affects cell proliferation in human non-small cell lung cancer, partly through epigenetically regulating HOXB7 expression*. Cell Death Dis, 2014. **5**: p. e1243

[74] Deng, H.P., et al., *Long non-coding RNA HOTTIP promotes tumor growth and inhibits cell apoptosis in lung cancer*. Cell Mol Biol (Noisy-le-grand), 2015. **61**(4): pp. 34–40.

[75] Nie, F.Q., et al., *Long non-coding RNA MVIH indicates a poor prognosis for non-small cell lung cancer and promotes cell proliferation and invasion*. Tumour Biol, 2014. **35**(8): pp. 7587–94.

[76] Lu, K.H., et al., *Long non-coding RNA MEG3 inhibits NSCLC cells proliferation and induces apoptosis by affecting p53 expression*. BMC Cancer, 2013. **13**: pp. 461.

[77] Yang, Q., et al., *A novel long noncoding RNA AK001796 acts as an oncogene and is involved in cell growth inhibition by resveratrol in lung cancer*. Toxicol Appl Pharmacol, 2015. **285**(2): pp. 79–88.

[78] Nie, F.Q., et al., *Long noncoding RNA ANRIL promotes non-small cell lung cancer cell proliferation and inhibits apoptosis by silencing KLF2 and P21 expression*. Mol Cancer Ther, 2015. **14**(1): pp. 268–77.

[79] Qiu, M., et al., *A novel lncRNA, LUADT1, promotes lung adenocarcinoma proliferation via the epigenetic suppression of p27*. Cell Death Dis, 2015. **6**: pp. e1858.

[80] Pan, H., et al., *Long non-coding RNA BC087858 induces non-T790M mutation acquired resistance to EGFR-TKIs by activating PI3K/AKT and MEK/ERK pathways and EMT in non-small-cell lung cancer*. Oncotarget, 2016. **7**(31): pp. 49948–60.

[81] Zhang, L., et al., *Enhanced expression of long non-coding RNA ZXF1 promoted the invasion and metastasis in lung adenocarcinoma*. Biomed Pharmacother, 2014. **68**(4): pp. 401–7.

[82] Yang, Z.T., et al., *Overexpression of Long Non-Coding RNA ZXF2 Promotes Lung Adenocarcinoma Progression Through c-Myc Pathway*. Cell Physiol Biochem, 2015. **35**(6): pp. 2360–70.

[83] Wang, G., H. Chen, and J. Liu, *The long noncoding RNA LINC01207 promotes proliferation of lung adenocarcinoma*. Am J Cancer Res, 2015. **5**(10): pp. 3162–73.

[84] Castellano, J.J., et al., *LincRNA-p21 impacts prognosis in resected non-small-cell lung cancer patients through angiogenesis regulation*. J Thorac Oncol, 2016. **11**(12):2173–82

[85] Calin, G.A., et al., *Ultraconserved regions encoding ncRNAs are altered in human leukemias and carcinomas*. Cancer Cell. **12**(3): pp. 215–229.

[86] Peng, J.C., J. Shen, and Z.H. Ran, *Transcribed ultraconserved region in human cancers*. RNA Biol, 2013. **10**(12): pp. 1771–7

[87] Jiang, S., et al., *MicroRNA-21 modulates radiation resistance through upregulation of hypoxia-inducible factor-1alpha-promoted glycolysis in non-small cell lung cancer cells*. Mol Med Rep, 2016. **13**(5): pp. 4101–7.

[88] Kenneth, Niall S. and S. Rocha, *Regulation of gene expression by hypoxia*. Biochem J, 2008. **414**(1): pp. 19–29.

[89] Gao, X.J., et al., *Nobiletin inhibited hypoxia induced epithelial-mesenchymal transition of lung cancer cells by inactivating of Notch-1 signaling and switching on miR-200b*. Pharmazie, 2015. **70**(4): pp. 256–62.

[90] Haigl, B., et al., *Expression of microRNA-21 in non-small cell lung cancer tissue increases with disease progression and is likely caused by growth conditional changes during malignant transformation*. Int J Oncol, 2014. **44**(4): pp. 1325–34.

[91] Eilertsen, M., et al., *Positive prognostic impact of miR-210 in non-small cell lung cancer*. Lung Cancer, 2014. **83**(2): pp. 272–8.

[92] Krutilina, R., et al., *MicroRNA-18a inhibits hypoxia-inducible factor 1alpha activity and lung metastasis in basal breast cancers*. Breast Cancer Res, 2014. **16**(4): p. R78.

[93] Ding, G., et al., *MiR-199a suppresses the hypoxia-induced proliferation of non-small cell lung cancer cells through targeting HIF1alpha*. Mol Cell Biochem, 2013. **384**(1–2): pp. 173–80.

[94] Guo, W.G., et al., *Bioinformatics analyses combined microarray identify the desregulated microRNAs in lung cancer*. Eur Rev Med Pharmacol Sci, 2013. **17**(11): pp. 1509–16.

[95] Taguchi, A., et al., *Identification of hypoxia-inducible factor-1 alpha as a novel target for miR-17-92 microRNA cluster*. Cancer Res, 2008. **68**(14): pp. 5540–5.

[96] Mao, G., et al., *Tumor-derived microRNA-494 promotes angiogenesis in non-small cell lung cancer*. Angiogenesis, 2015. **18**(3): pp. 373–82.

[97] Yang, F., et al., *Repression of the long noncoding RNA-LET by histone deacetylase 3 contributes to hypoxia-mediated metastasis*. Mol Cell, 2013. **49**(6): pp. 1083–96.

[98] Wu, Y., et al., *Downregulation of the long noncoding RNA GAS5-AS1 contributes to tumor metastasis in non-small cell lung cancer*. Sci Rep, 2016, **6**: p. 31093.

[99] Zhou, C., et al., *Long noncoding RNA HOTAIR, a hypoxia-inducible factor-1alpha activated driver of malignancy, enhances hypoxic cancer cell proliferation, migration, and invasion in non-small cell lung cancer*. Tumour Biol, 2015. **36**(12): pp. 9179–88.

[100] Yao, Y., J. Li, and L. Wang, *Large intervening non-coding RNA HOTAIR is an indicator of poor prognosis and a therapeutic target in human cancers*. Int J Mol Sci, 2014. **15**(10): pp. 18985–99.

[101] Matouk, I.J., et al., *The oncofetal H19 RNA connection: hypoxia, p53 and cancer*. Biochim Biophys Acta, 2010. **1803**(4): pp. 443–51.

[102] Mei, Y., et al., *A piRNA-like small RNA interacts with and modulates p-ERM proteins in human somatic cells*. Nat Commun, 2015. **6**: p. 7316.

[103] Qi, R., T. Qiao, and X. Zhuang, *Small interfering RNA targeting S100A4 sensitizes non-small-cell lung cancer cells (A549) to radiation treatment*. Onco Targets Ther, 2016. **9**: pp. 3753–62.

[104] Geretti, E. and M. Klagsbrun, *Neuropilins: novel targets for anti-angiogenesis therapies*. Cell Adh Migr, 2007. **1**(2): pp. 56–61.

[105] Nguyen, Q.D., et al., *Inhibition of vascular endothelial growth factor (VEGF)-165 and semaphorin 3A-mediated cellular invasion and tumor growth by the VEGF signaling inhibitor ZD4190 in human colon cancer cells and xenografts*. Mol Cancer Ther, 2006. **5**(8): pp. 2070–7.

[106] Geretti, E., A. Shimizu, and M. Klagsbrun, *Neuropilin structure governs VEGF and semaphorin binding and regulates angiogenesis*. Angiogenesis, 2008. **11**(1): pp. 31–9.

[107] Kitsukawa, T., et al., *Overexpression of a membrane protein, neuropilin, in chimeric mice causes anomalies in the cardiovascular system, nervous system and limbs*. Development, 1995. **121**(12): pp. 4309–18.

[108] Miao, H.Q., et al., *Neuropilin-1 expression by tumor cells promotes tumor angiogenesis and progression*. FASEB J, 2000. **14**(15): pp. 2532–9.

[109] Banerjee, S.K., et al., *Overexpression of vascular endothelial growth factor164 and its co-receptor neuropilin-1 in estrogen-induced rat pituitary tumors and GH3 rat pituitary tumor cells*. Int J Oncol, 2000. **16**(2): pp. 253–60.

[110] Han, F., et al., *MicroRNA-30b promotes axon outgrowth of retinal ganglion cells by inhibiting Semaphorin3A expression*. Brain Res, 2015. **1611**: pp. 65–73.

[111] Loginov, V.I., et al., *Tumor suppressor function of the SEMA3B gene in human lung and renal cancers*. PLoS One, 2015. **10**(5): pp. e0123369.

[112] Cai, G., S. Qiao, and K. Chen, *Suppression of miR-221 inhibits glioma cells proliferation and invasion via targeting SEMA3B*. Biol Res, 2015. **48**: p. 37.

[113] Mumblat, Y., et al., *Full-length semaphorin-3C is an inhibitor of tumor lymphangiogenesis and metastasis*. Cancer Res, 2015. **75**(11): pp. 2177–86.

[114] Meert, A.P., et al., *[Difficulties and limitations in conducting translational research in thoracic oncology. A practical example]*. Rev Mal Respir, 2016. **33**(7): pp. 594–9.

[115] Foley, K., et al., *Semaphorin 3D autocrine signaling mediates the metastatic role of annexin A2 in pancreatic cancer*. Sci Signal, 2015. **8**(388): p. ra77.

[116] Christensen, C., et al., *Proteolytic processing converts the repelling signal Sema3E into an inducer of invasive growth and lung metastasis*. Cancer Res, 2005. **65**(14): pp. 6167–77.

[117] Nasarre, P., et al., *Neuropilin-2 Is upregulated in lung cancer cells during TGF-beta1-induced epithelial-mesenchymal transition*. Cancer Res, 2013. **73**(23): pp. 7111–21.

[118] Clarhaut, J., et al., *ZEB-1, a repressor of the semaphorin 3F tumor suppressor gene in lung cancer cells*. Neoplasia, 2009. **11**(2): pp. 157–66.

[119] Jian, H., et al., *SEMA4B inhibits growth of non-small cell lung cancer in vitro and in vivo*. Cell Signal, 2015. **27**(6): pp. 1208–13.

[120] Jian, H., B. Liu, and J. Zhang, *Hypoxia and hypoxia-inducible factor 1 repress SEMA4B expression to promote non-small cell lung cancer invasion*. Tumour Biol, 2014. **35**(5): pp. 4949–55.

[121] Jian, H., et al., *SEMA4b inhibits MMP9 to prevent metastasis of non-small cell lung cancer*. Tumour Biol, 2014. **35**(11): pp. 11051–6.

[122] Li, J., Q. Wang, R. Wen, J. Liang, X. Zhong, W. Yang, et al. *MiR-138 inhibits cell proliferation and reverses epithelial-mesenchymal transition in non-small cell lung cancer cells by targeting GIT1 and SEMA4C*. J Cell Mol Med, 2015. **19**(12): pp. 2793–805.

[123] Gu, A., J. Lu, W. Wang, C. Shi, B. Han, M. Yao. *Role of miR-497 in VEGF-A-mediated cancer cell growth and invasion in non-small cell lung cancer*. Int J Biochem Cell Biol, 2016. **70**: pp. 118–25.

[124] Ruan, S.S., et al., *Expression and clinical significance of Semaphorin4D in non-small cell lung cancer and its impact on malignant behaviors of A549 lung cancer cells*. J Huazhong Univ Sci Technolog Med Sci, 2014. **34**(4): pp. 491–6.

[125] Liu, Y., et al., *MiR-214 suppressed ovarian cancer and negatively regulated semaphorin 4D*. Tumour Biol, 2016. **37**(6): pp. 8239–48.

[126] Fazzari, P., et al., *Plexin-B1 plays a redundant role during mouse development and in tumour angiogenesis*. BMC Dev Biol, 2007. **7**: p. 55.

[127] Lu, T.P., et al., *Identification of a novel biomarker, SEMA5A, for non-small cell lung carcinoma in nonsmoking women*. Cancer Epidemiol Biomarkers Prev, 2010. **19**(10): pp. 2590–7.

[128] Veliceasa, D., et al., *Therapeutic manipulation of angiogenesis with miR-27b*. Vasc Cell, 2015. **7**: p. 6.

[129] Urbich, C., et al., *MicroRNA-27a/b controls endothelial cell repulsion and angiogenesis by targeting semaphorin 6A*. Blood, 2012. **119**(6): pp. 1607–16.

[130] Ma, B., et al., *Role of chitinase 3-like-1 and semaphorin 7a in pulmonary melanoma metastasis*. Cancer Res, 2015. **75**(3): pp. 487–96.

[131] Narazaki, M., M. Segarra, and G. Tosato, *Sulfated polysaccharides identified as inducers of neuropilin-1 internalization and functional inhibition of VEGF165 and semaphorin3A*. Blood, 2008. **111**(8): pp. 4126-36.

[132] Wiggins, J.F., et al., *Development of a lung cancer therapeutic based on the tumor suppressor microRNA-34*. Cancer Res, 2010. **70**(14): pp. 5923–30.

[133] AUSTIN, Texas, BUSINESS WIRE - *Mirna Therapeutics*, Inc. (Nasdaq:MIRN) September 20, 2016

[134] Potente, M., et al., *Involvement of Foxo transcription factors in angiogenesis and postnatal neovascularization*. J Clin Invest, 2005. **115**(9): pp. 2382–92.

[135] Krug, S., et al., *Knock-down of Pdcd4 stimulates angiogenesis via up-regulation of angiopoietin-2*. Biochim Biophys Acta, 2012. **1823**(4): pp. 789–99.

[136] Wang, F., A.J. Nazarali, and S. Ji, *Circular RNAs as potential biomarkers for cancer diagnosis and therapy*. Am J Cancer Res, 2016. **6**(6): pp. 1167–76.

[137] Ricciuti, B., et al., *Long noncoding RNAs: new insights into non-small cell lung cancer biology, diagnosis and therapy*. Med Oncol, 2016. **33**(2): p. 18.

[138] Liu, Z., M. Sun, K. Lu, J. Liu, M. Zhang, W. Wu, et al. *The long noncoding RNA HOTAIR contributes to cisplatin resistance of human lung adenocarcinoma cells via downregualtion of p21(WAF1/CIP1) expression*. PLoS One, 2013. **8**(10): p. e77293.

[139] Li, Z. and T.M. Rana. *Therapeutic targeting of microRNAs: current status and future challenges*. Nat Rev Drug Discov, 2014. **13**(8): pp. 622–38.

[140] Roberts, T.C. and M.J. Wood. *Therapeutic targeting of non-coding RNAs*. Essays Biochem, 2013. **54**: pp. 127–45.

[141] Krutzfeldt, J., N. Rajewsky, R. Braich, K.G. Rajeev, T. Tuschl, M. Manoharan, et al. *Silencing of microRNAs in vivo with 'antagomirs'*. Nature, 2005. **438**(7068): pp. 685–9.

[142] Bagga, S., J. Bracht, S. Hunter, K. Massirer, J. Holtz, R. Eachus, et al. *Regulation by let-7 and lin-4 miRNAs results in target mRNA degradation*. Cell, 2005. **122**(4): pp. 553–63.

[143] Morrissey, D.V., J.A. Lockridge, L. Shaw, K. Blanchard, K. Jensen, W. Breen, et al. *Potent and persistent in vivo anti-HBV activity of chemically modified siRNAs*. Nat Biotechnol, 2005. **23**(8): pp. 1002–7.

[144] Akinc, A., et al., *A combinatorial library of lipid-like materials for delivery of RNAi therapeutics*. Nat Biotechnol, 2008. **26**(5): pp. 561–9.

[145] Peer, D., et al., *Systemic leukocyte-directed siRNA delivery revealing cyclin D1 as an anti-inflammatory target*. Science, 2008. **319**(5863): pp. 627–30.

[146] Palliser, D., et al., *An siRNA-based microbicide protects mice from lethal herpes simplex virus 2 infection*. Nature, 2006. **439**(7072): pp. 89–94.

[147] Kumar, P., et al., *A single siRNA suppresses fatal encephalitis induced by two different flaviviruses*. PLoS Med, 2006. **3**(4): pp. e96.

[148] Hu-Lieskovan, S., et al., *Sequence-specific knockdown of EWS-FLI1 by targeted, nonviral delivery of small interfering RNA inhibits tumor growth in a murine model of metastatic Ewing's sarcoma*. Cancer Res, 2005. **65**(19): pp. 8984–92.

[149] Song, E., et al., *Antibody mediated in vivo delivery of small interfering RNAs via cell-surface receptors*. Nat Biotechnol, 2005. **23**(6): pp. 709–17.

[150] Yao, Y.D., et al., *Targeted delivery of PLK1-siRNA by ScFv suppresses Her2+ breast cancer growth and metastasis*. Sci Transl Med, 2012. **4**(130): p. 130ra48.

[151] Gutschner, T., et al., *The noncoding RNA MALAT1 is a critical regulator of the metastasis phenotype of lung cancer cells*. Cancer Res, 2013. **73**(3): pp. 1180–9.

11

Paraneoplastic Syndromes in Lung Cancer

Dilaver Tas

Abstract

In recent years, the incidence of lung cancer (LC) has been increasing throughout the world and is the most common type of cancer in all regions of the world, occurring more frequently in men than in women. Paraneoplastic syndromes (PNS) refer to clinical conditions that develop in relation to tumors, without physical effects of the primary or metastatic tumors. The development of PNS is not associated with the size of the primary tumor or the extent of metastases. It is usually seen in small-cell lung cancer (SCLC) as well as other types of lung cancer. PNS developed in almost 1 in 10 patients with lung cancer and it may be an indicator for the diagnosis of lung cancer and it can be seen during later stages of cancer or at the time of cancer recurrence. Accordingly, the identification of these syndromes can be helpful in the early diagnosis of occult cancers, allowing timely treatment. PNS decreases the quality of life of the patients with cancer and thus requires specific treatment. Moreover, these conditions can be used as a marker of cancer activity and can predict prognosis. In this section, a detailed description of PNS is provided.

Keywords: lung cancer, small-cell lung cancer, non-small-cell lung cancer, paraneoplastic syndromes

1. Introduction

1.1. Definition

The term "paraneoplastic syndrome (PNS)" refers to tumor-related symptoms and findings that are independent of the direct, local extent or physical effects of metastases. PNS develops in response to the effects of hormones and cytokines released from cancer cells, or due to the immunologic response of cancer cells [1, 2]. In this regard, there is no single mechanism underlying the development of PNS, and potential mechanisms have not yet been clearly understood. On the other hand, several tumor-secreted proteins that may be associated with the development of PNS have been defined in the recent years. Generally, the ectopic production of peptide hormones with hormonal activity and immunological mechanisms can be seen in patients with PNS.

The diagnosis and treatment of PNS are complementary parts of lung cancer (LC) management. PNS may involve several organs and systems, and so may therefore result in neurological, dermatological, hematological, nephrological, rheumatologic, metabolic, immunologic and constitutional signs and symptoms.

1.2. History

In 1865, Armand Trousseau, a French internal diseases specialist, stated that the identification of unexpected or migratory thrombophlebitis could indicate an occult visceral malignancy [3], and today, the development of superficial migratory thrombophlebitis related to visceral cancer is known as Trousseau syndrome. An Austrian dermatologist, Ferdinand von Hebra, underlined the significance of internal disease in the etiology of several skin manifestations such as urticaria, generalized pruritus, xanthoma, and pemphigus. In 1868, he further stated that skin pigmentation could be an indicator of cervical cancer [4, 5]. In 1890, a French physician named Auche defined peripheral nervous system involvement in patients with stomach, pancreas, and uterus cancer [6], while acanthosis nigricans associated with malignancy was reported separately by Pollitzer and Janovsky in 1890 [7]. Later, Brown identified the Cushing syndrome in a patient with small-cell lung cancer (SCLC) in 1928 [8], and in 1933, neuropathy development was reported in a patient with oat cell carcinoma (small-cell lung cancer) [9]. Guichard and Vignon used the term "paraneoplastic" for the first time in 1949 when they identified central and peripheral neuropathies in a patient with cervical cancer [10]. In 1957, Schwartz et al. reported hyponatremia in a patient with LC [11]. In 1967, Bartter and Schwartz defined the syndrome of inappropriate antidiuretic hormone secretion (SIADH) [12]. The relationship between the neurological PNS and LC was first suggested by Oppenheim at the end of the nineteenth century [9].

In the following years, etiologic and pathogenetic studies were carried out to evaluate the relationship between PNS and cancer including LC. Additionally, new PNS definitions and new developments have been made which are still ongoing.

1.3. Epidemiology

LC is currently the most common type of cancer throughout the world [13]. Due to the high incidence rate of LC and the relatively high frequency of PNS in SCLC cases, LC-related PNS is more common than other types of cancer [14–17]. However, it is difficult to estimate PNS frequency due to challenges in the identification of PNS and uncertainty in the differentiation of its symptoms because of the underlying disease. PNS can be seen in all age groups of patients with cancer. However, due to the nature of cancer, it is more common in middle-aged and older individuals. PNS develops in 1–7.4% of all patients with cancer, although it is estimated to develop in 20% of all patients with cancer [14]. The inclusion of generalized malignancy symptoms, such as cachexia and fever, increases PNS frequency up to 70% [18].

PNS can occur both in patients with SCLC and with non-small-cell lung cancer (NSCLC). SCLC has a neuroendocrine origin and PNS is more common in such cancer types. PNS is seen by 7–15% of all patients with LC. Systemic symptoms and findings of PNS develop in 50% of patients with SCLC and almost 10% of patients with NSCLC [19]. PNS develops secondary to LC and increases the severity of the disease. It is therefore crucial to recognize PNS in these patients.

Incidences of PNS will increase in the coming years thanks to the improvements in diagnosis and treatment of LC as well as in the diagnosis of PNS.

1.4. Pathophysiology

PNS may develop under the effects of substances released by the tumor or as a result of the cross-reactions between tissues and the antibodies produced against the tumor.

Studies investigating the pathogenesis of PNS offer some evidences that PNS develops based on different pathogenetic mechanisms, such as:

1. The production of special substances by tumor cells, leading specifically to the development of PNS. These substances may be hormones, growth factors, vasoactive peptides, cytokines, enzymes or other signaling molecules.
2. Abnormal immune response of the host organ to the neo-antigens produced by the tumor or to other tumor products [7, 18, 20].

Endocrinologic PNS generally develops due to the increased production of hormones or hormone precursors by malignant cells. The best example for this is paraneoplastic Cushing syndrome seen in patients with SCLC [21].

Paraneoplastic hypercalcemia is an example of PNS associated with cytokine production. Some cytokines (IL-1, 3, and 6, prostaglandins, TGF-α, TNF-α [lymphotoxin], and TNF-β [cachectin], etc.) that are synthesized by the malignant cells may result in hypercalcemia by activating osteoclasts [22].

Cancer cells are recognized by the immune cells and lead to the production of antibodies. As cancer cells are identical to normal cells in nature, the antigens on the cancer cells are similar to those of natural cells. Therefore, the formed antibodies may have a cross-reaction with normal tissues. This pathophysiological condition is most commonly seen in neurological PNS [23, 24].

The main mechanism underlying above-described pathological response in patients with LC and other types of cancer still presents an unanswered question. The most appropriate answer to that would be inappropriate gene expression (IGE). IGE may be described as the formation of an inappropriate gene programmed to produce tumoral proteins in cancer cells. This may lead to the development of new disorders that will negatively affect patient well-being. Thus, the quality of life of the patient is impaired and the severity of the disease increases [18].

Genetic studies that will be performed in the future to identify IGEs in cancer patients will allow the early detection of PNS, even before the clinical diagnosis, and more importantly, will be helpful to identify malignant formations.

2. Paraneoplastic syndromes

The diagnosis of PNS is relatively challenging, as lesions may develop in regions distant to the cancer and may not resemble a cancer-related disease, and the disorder has benign forms in general as well as malignant forms. PNS should be suspected in the presence of below characteristics: absence of a defined etiology for the associated syndrome; correlation between the time of diagnosis of the syndrome and that of cancer; clinical and histological remission after complete surgical or chemotherapy treatment and a worsening of symptoms due to tumor residue [25].

Although PNS may be associated with a lot of malignancies, they are associated most commonly with lung cancer, specifically SCLC. Humoral hypercalcemia and SIADH, which is seen in orderly squamous cell and SCLC, are the most common PNSs. Multiple paraneoplastic syndromes can be seen in patients with SCLC. In the literature, there have been patients with two or more paraneoplastic syndromes associated with SCLC, even though rarity. Paraneoplastic syndromes usually have a course parallel to the underlying malignancy. Treating the underlying tumor is the first choice and symptomatic therapy can be useful [2, 26–29].

2.1. Classification

Paraneoplastic symptoms in LC can be seen almost in all systems, which can be listed as follows:

- Endocrine paraneoplastic syndromes
- Neurologic paraneoplastic syndromes
- Dermatologic paraneoplastic syndromes
- Rheumatologic paraneoplastic syndromes
- Nephrological paraneoplastic syndromes
- Hematologic paraneoplastic syndromes
- Others

2.2. Endocrine paraneoplastic syndromes

Endocrinological PNS generally develops due to excessive synthesis of hormones or hormone precursors with low bioactivity, or the conversion of the precursors to more effective product(s) in the tumor tissue.

2.2.1. Ectopic Cushing syndrome

Secretion of ectopic adrenocorticotropic hormone (ACTH) from the tumor may result in Cushing syndrome, and high ACTH levels can be noted in almost 50% of patients with LC. Cushing syndrome may develop in 1–5% of patients with SCLC [30, 31], and of all the pulmonary neuroendocrine tumors, about 1–2% are accompanied by Cushing syndrome due to ectopic ACTH secretion, or the production of its precursor, proopiomelanocortin (POMC) [32].

Patients are typically admitted to clinics due to myopathy, centripetal obesity, facial plethora, hypertension, osteoporosis, hyperglycemia, hirsutism, and acne. The clinical symptoms have a rapid onset and are generally accompanied by hypokalemia and hyperglycemia.

Due to its rapid onset, patients generally are found to have electrolyte imbalances rather than having a cushingoid appearance, although typical cushingoid characteristics such as moon face and buffalo hump generally do not manifest, as hypercortisolism is an acute phenomenon and patients do not live long enough for the manifestation of morphological changes [33, 34].

Increased levels of free cortisol in the urine, elevated serum levels of ACTH or ACTH precursors, hypokalemia and hyperglycemia are helpful for the diagnosis of ectopic Cushing syndrome (ECS).

The prognosis of SCLC patients with Cushing syndrome is worse than in SCLC patients without Cushing syndrome [35].

Treatment essentially involves treating the primary tumor. In the presence of non-resectable tumors, medications that inhibit steroid biosynthesis (metyrapone, ketoconazole) can be used for the treatment of ECS. Aminoglutethimide can be used to prevent androgenic side effects and octreotide may be helpful in reducing ACTH release. A bilateral adrenalectomy may also be considered [31].

2.2.2. Inappropriate antidiuretic hormone syndrome

Inappropriate antidiuretic hormone syndrome (IADHS) develops as a result of free water retention and increased extracellular fluid volume due to the irregular release of the antidiuretic hormone (ADH). This initiates a process characterized by a progressive dilution of plasma sodium and sodium loss through the kidneys.

It is generally seen in patients with SCLC, accounts for around 75% of all cancer-related IADHS. It is seen in 7–16% of patients with SCLC but may also occur in patients with NSCLC [36, 37].

Antidiuretic hormone (ADH) levels are generally elevated in LC patients with IADHS and in addition, patients may also have increased levels of atrial natriuretic peptide [38].

IADHS symptoms rarely manifest when plasma sodium levels are higher than 125 mEq/L. Plasma sodium levels below 125 mEq/L may result in symptoms such as weakness, tiredness, nausea, headache, lethargy, and confusion, while levels below 120 mEq/L may lead to seizure and coma [39].

Based on the definition of Bartter and Schwartz, a diagnosis of IADHS can be made in the presence of following findings:

- Serum Na < 134 mEq/l
- Plasma osmolality <275 mOsm/kg

- Urine osmolality >500 mOsm/kg
- High urinary sodium concentration (>20mEq/l)
- Absence of clinical signs of volume depletion
- Presence of normal adrenal functions
- Presence of normal thyroid functions [1, 12]
- Presence of IADHS is a marker of poor prognosis [38]

If plasma sodium levels are higher than 130 mEq/L, fluid intake may be limited (500 mL/day) and/or patients may be given demeclocycline, which is a medication that blocks the response of renal tubules to ADH. A slow infusion of hypertonic saline solution and an IV furosemide infusion may be preferred in severe cases [31].

2.2.3. *Hypercalcemia*

Hypercalcemia develops in 6% of LC patients, and is most commonly seen in the presence of squamous cell carcinoma [40, 41]. In LC, hypercalcemia is caused by the production of parathyroid hormone-related protein (PTHrP) of the tumor and secretion of parathyroid hormone. Another mechanism leading to the development of hypercalcemia involves PTHrP increase as a result of granulocyte colony-stimulating factor signal. While increased 1.25$(OH)_2$ Vitamin D synthesis may result in hypercalcemia in some malignancies, this mechanism is not associated with hypercalcemia in LC [41].

Early symptoms of hypercalcemia include loss of appetite, nausea, vomiting, constipation, numbness, polyurea, polydypsia, and dehydration, while late symptoms include renal failure, nephrocalcinosis, confusion, and coma.

Elevated serum levels of ionized calcium, normal or decreased levels of parathyroid hormone and high PTHrP levels are diagnostic factors [9].

Treatment is essentially based on the treatment of the tumor-causing hypercalcemia. Symptomatic patients with high serum calcium levels should be treated with hydration and bisphosphonates, and any calcium supplements, thiazide diuretics, and lithium, all of which may alleviate hypercalcemia, should be discontinued [42].

2.2.4. *Other endocrine paraneoplastic syndromes*

In LC patients, hypoglycemia may occur due to ectopic insulin secretion and insulin-like growth factor (IGF) secretion.

Acromegaly may also occur as a result of ectopic growth hormone-releasing hormone (GHRH) or IGF secretion.

Moreover, carcinoid syndrome may develop in relation to the secretion of serotonin and similar vasoactive amines [41, 43].

2.3. Neurologic paraneoplastic syndromes

Neurologic PNS may develop by the involvement of central nervous system, peripheral nervous system or the neuromuscular junction and muscles. The majority of patients with neurologic PNS have SCLC (at a rate of 5%). In its pathogenesis, immune-system mediated reactions are seen in general. Immune cross-reactivity is seen between tumor cells and components of the nervous system [9, 29, 44].

International criteria have been determined to facilitate the diagnosis of paraneoplastic neurologic syndromes, defining "definite" and "possible" diagnoses. The definite diagnostic criteria are as follows:

- neurological symptoms that will develop cancer within 5 years and commonly accompanying with cancer (limbic encephalitis, cerebellar degenerations, etc.);
- nonclassical neurologic syndrome that improves after cancer treatment without concomitant immunotherapy;
- nonclassical neurologic syndrome with positive antibodies and a diagnosis of cancer within 5 years; and
- neurologic syndromes accompanied by "well-characterized" antibodies in the absence of a cancer diagnosis (anti-Hu, anti-CV2, anti-Ri, anti-Yo, anti-Tr, and anti-Ma2).

There are three categories of possible paraneoplastic neurologic syndrome diagnoses:

- presence of classical neurologic syndrome in the absence of cancer or antibodies, but a high risk of underlying tumor;
- presence of neurologic syndrome with non-classical antibodies in the absence of cancer; and
- presence of classical neurologic syndrome without antibodies or a malignancy [9, 45].

2.3.1. Encephalomyelitis

Paraneoplastic encephalomyelitis should be considered in the presence of neuronal loss and inflammation in multiple regions of the central nervous system, primarily in the hippocampus (limbic encephalitis), Purkinje cells of the cerebellum (cerebellar degeneration), brainstem (brainstem encephalitis) and medulla spinalis (myelitis). Dorsal root-ganglion (sensorial neuronopathy), as well as sympathetic and parasympathetic nerve and ganglions (orthostatic hypotension, gastrointestinal paresis, arrhythmia, erectile dysfunction) are known to be involved in the majority of the cases [46, 47].

It is thought to be developed with SCLC and due to the immune response that develops against the neural proteins expressed by the tumor. The most commonly identified antibody in paraneoplastic encephalomyelitis is the Hu (ANNA-1) antibody, although cases associated with CV2, amphiphysin, and Ri antibodies have also been reported.

While it may start with relatively milder and focal signs such as epilepsia partialis continua, nonconvulsive epileptic status or frontal-type ataxia, the findings rapidly progress within weeks or months and may result in death in general. Neurological outcomes may not be satisfying despite the treatment, as irreversible neuronal damage occurs in most of cases when the diagnosis is made. The worst neurological outcomes are seen in paraneoplastic encephalomyelitis accompanied by Anti-Hu antibodies [48].

In addition to cancer treatment, immunomodulation plays a key role in the treatment of encephalomyelitis, and corticosteroids, steroid-sparing agents (azathioprine, cyclophosphamide, etc.), rituximab, IVIG, and plasmapheresis can be used for treatment [44].

2.3.2. *Limbic encephalitis*

Paraneoplastic limbic encephalitis manifests with major findings such as short-term memory loss, behavior/mood changes and epileptic seizures, and confusion, irritability, depression, sleep problems, hallucinations and psychosis in addition to major findings [49]. Moreover, hyperthermia and endocrine disorders may also develop due to hypothalamic dysfunction. Antibodies produced against the Hu, Ma2, CV2 and amphiphysin antigens expressed by the tumor have been identified in patients with paraneoplastic limbic encephalitis. For the diagnosis, demonstration of epileptic activity in the electroencephalographic examination, demonstration of temporal lobe involvement in magnetic resonance imaging (MR2), and an investigation of the cerebrospinal fluid (CSF) and auto-antibody test are required. The neurologic response to treatment varies between patients with paraneoplastic limbic encephalitis, while 30–50% of patients may recover after the tumor treatment.

Just like in encephalomyelitis, immunomodulation plays a key role in treatment along with cancer-specific therapies, and corticosteroids, steroid-sparing agents (azathioprine, cyclophosphamide, etc.), rituximab, IVIG, and plasmapheresis can be used for treatment [44].

2.3.3. *Cerebellar degeneration*

Paraneoplastic cerebellar degeneration is one of the most common PNS. Depending on the widespread cerebellar Purkinje cell death, it may have an acute or subacute onset and courses with a rapidly progressing pancerebellar syndrome. The antibodies associated with cerebellar degeneration include anti-Yo, Tr, Hu, Ma2, and Ri [50]. However, the most well-defined and frequently seen paraneoplastic cerebellar degeneration is associated with the Yo antibodies. Before developing findings of neurologic deficit, patients may experience flu-like prodromal signs and may then develop an ataxic gait, dysarthria, dysphagia, diplopia, blurred vision, and transient opsoclonus. Patients initially have normal MR and CSF findings, however, inflammatory findings in CSF develop rapidly and an MR may demonstrate advanced cerebellar atrophy. Fast and effective treatment may prevent the progression of symptoms, but cerebellar degeneration is one of the most treatment-resistant PNS.

Like in limbic encephalitis, treatment may include the use of corticosteroids, steroid-sparing agents (azathioprine, cyclophosphamide, etc.), rituximab, IVIG, and plasmapheresis [44].

2.3.4. Lambert-Eaton myasthenic syndrome

Almost 60% of the Lambert-Eaton myasthenic syndrome (LEMS) cases have a paraneoplastic origin. SCLC is observed in the vast majority of cancer cases with LEMS, while other types of cancer are seen in a small number of cases [51]. LEMS develops in 3% of all SCLC cases, and LEMS develops as a result of the autoimmune response to the P/Q-type anti-voltage-gated calcium channels (VGCC) that exist on the pre-synaptic membrane of the neuromuscular junction, and 95% of the cases are found to be positive for this antibody. Of all cases with LEMS and SCLC, 64% are positive for SOX1 antibodies [41], and patients are generally admitted with proximal muscle weakness, reduced or absent deep tendon reflexes, and findings of autonomic function impairment. Tumor treatment is known to be a key factor to predict the neurological outcomes. In cases with SCLC, treatment 3,4-diaminopyridine, a potassium channel antagonist, may provide significant recovery, and azathioprine and prednisolone may also be used for the treatment [41, 51, 52].

2.3.5. Opsoclonus-myoclonus

This syndrome is associated with involuntary chaotic conjugated rapid eye movements and myoclonic discharges in the head, neck, face, trunk, and legs as well as potential cerebellar ataxia. In some adult cases, anti-Ri, anti-Hu, anti-amphiphysin, and P/Q-type VGCC antibodies may accompany cancer. Paraneoplastic opsoclonus and myoclonus respond well to treatment. Successful treatment can be achieved by the resection of the underlying tumor and elimination of circulating antibodies such as corticosteroids, intravenous immunoglobulin and plasmapheresis [41, 53].

2.3.6. Chronic gastrointestinal pseudo-obstruction

Chronic gastrointestinal pseudo-obstruction (CGP) is an autonomic neuropathy that is characterized by gastrointestinal dysmotility without a mechanical obstruction, leading to symptoms of abdominal pain, nausea and constipation [41].

While CGP generally occurs in patients with SCLC, it may also be noted in patients with NSCLC. Anti-Hu antibodies are frequently positive. In addition to cancer treatment, agent such as octreotide, prednisone, and azathioprine can be used for the treatment of CGP [41, 54].

2.3.7. Others

Neurological PNS has a variety of clinical manifestations. Other than above-described syndromes, patients may experience subacute sensory neuropathy involving the peripheral nervous system, acute sensory-motor neuropathy (Guillain-Barre Syndrome, brachial neuritis), neuropathy with vasculitis, myasthenia gravis involving the neuromuscular junction and muscles, acquired myotonia, and acute necrotizing myopathy [41].

2.4. Dermatologic paraneoplastic syndromes

Dermatologic paraneoplastic syndromes are generally seen before patients are diagnosed with cancer. It is not possible to differentiate them from their benign variants in terms of clinical appearance and histopathological findings, although dermatologic PNS that suddenly develop at an atypical localization during the late stages of life and progress rapidly may indicate an accompanying malignancy and it should be investigated [7, 9, 17, 55].

2.4.1. Acanthosis nigricans

Acanthosis nigricans are characterized by skin hyperpigmentation and hyperkeratosis. It is most frequently seen on skin folds such as the axilla, neck, and groins. It usually accompanies lung adenocarcinoma.

The pathogenesis of acanthosis nigricans has not been clarified yet, although one possible etiology is the interactions between increased levels of insulin with insulin-like growth factor receptors and their effect on keratinocytes and dermal fibroblasts [56].

Malignant acanthosis nigricans regresses with the treatment of underlying malignancies, and isotretinoin may be preferred in cases that fail to recover [57].

2.4.2. Polymyositis/dermatomyositis

Polymyositis/dermatomyositis (PM/DM) is a disease characterized by specific skin findings (skin rashes and heliotropic appearance) and inflammatory myopathy accompanying with proximal muscle weakness. Violet-colored edema in periorbital tissues and the eyelids (heliotrophy), periungual telangiectasia, dystrophic changes in the cuticula and macular, violet-colored erythema on the forehead, neck, upper trunk, back, deltoid region, and dorsum of the hand are specific findings of PM/DM [58].

In 15–30% cases of PM/DM, an underlying malignancy is the cause of PNS. Ovarian and breast cancer in women and lung cancer in men are the most common malignancies associated with dermatomyositis [59].

Up to 30% of patients with PM/DM have auto-antibodies against cytoplasmic and nuclear antigens [60].

The treatment of the underlying malignancies can help in the resolution of the findings. Glucocorticoids are the most important medication for the PM/DM treatment, and immunosuppressive agents (azathioprine, cyclophosphamide, etc.) can also be beneficial [44].

LC patients with PM/DM have poor prognosis [61].

2.4.3. Erythema gyratum repens

Erythema gyratum repens (EGR) refers to multiple, erythematosus, serpiginous, concentric-shaped lesions that can grow by almost 1 cm/day [62, 63], but no face, hand or foot involvement is observed.

Rather than benign pathological diseases, EGR generally appears in the presence of malignant diseases and a carcinoma can be detected in more than 80% of patients with EGR. The most common type of malignancy associated with EGR is a SCLC [7, 18].

The pathogenesis of the disease is unknown and its treatment is based primarily on the identification and treatment of the underlying malignancy.

2.4.4. Erythema annulare centrifugum

Erythema annulare centrifugum (EAC) is an eruption characterized by slowly progressing, annular or polycyclic erythematosus lesions.

EAC, caused by benign reasons, is thought to develop due to hypersensitivity reaction. The pathogenesis of a figured erythema developing due to cancer, and thus EAC, is not clearly known, but a suggested hypothesis is that the tumor causes chemical changes in the surrounding tissues, inducing an antigenic status in these tissues, and these antigens lead to inflammation on the skin by causing cross-reactions since they are similar to the skin proteins [63].

EAC regresses with the treatment of the underlying tumor.

2.4.5. Bazex syndrome (acrokeratosis paraneoplastica)

Bazex syndrome is characterized by hyperkeratosis of the acral regions. It appears as erythematosus, papulosquamous plaques on the nose and ears, and less frequently on the fingernails, hands, feet, knees, and elbows. The lesions are generally likened to psoriasis [64, 65]. Benign forms are less frequent than malignant PNS forms.

Its mechanism of development is still unclear, however, it regresses with tumor treatment. Like in most PNS cases, it may appear during LC recurrence.

2.4.6. Tripe palms

It is also known as palmoplantar keratoderma, pachydermatoglyphy, or palmar hyperkeratosis, and is generally seen with LC and 90% of the cases are associated with neoplasm. The most common types of tumors are lung and gastric cancers [41].

2.4.7. Others

Other cutaneous PNS seen in LC patients include paraneoplastic pemphigus, leukocytoclastic vasculitis, multicentric reticulohistiocytosis, sign of leser-trelat, pruritus, and finger clubbing.

2.5. Rheumatologic paraneoplastic syndromes

2.5.1. Hypertrophic osteoarthropathy

Hypertrophic osteoarthropathy (HO) is a syndrome characterized by finger clubbing and periostitis. Secondary HO, which is a PNS, is most frequently seen in LC, particularly in NSCLC [66]. It manifests with a clubbing of the fingers and toes, periostitis of the long bones and polyarthritis in some cases [67].

More than 70% of HO cases are associated with LC, and the incidence rate of HO among LC patients has been found to be 0.7% [41]. Periostitis is a well-known radiographic feature with a generally symmetric distribution, and periosteal reactions involving the long bones are present [67].

While theories have been suggested to explain the mechanisms of HO development, it is still unclear.

In addition to the cancer treatment, nonsteroidal anti-inflammatory drugs, bisphosphonates, and octreotide have been shown to be beneficial for the treatment of HO [41].

2.6. Hematologic paraneoplastic syndromes

Hematologic abnormalities such as anemia, leucocytosis, thrombocytosis, and eosinophilia are common in LC patients. However, not all of these are associated with a PNS. These conditions generally follow an asymptomatic course, and coagulopathies, granulocytosis, anemia, and thrombocytosis can be listed among hematologic PNS [9, 68].

2.6.1. Paraneoplastic coagulopathies

Patients with LC tend to develop thrombosis. Thrombotic risk in lung cancer patients is 20-fold higher than in the general population. Also the risk of thrombosis development in LC is higher than other types of cancer. Several studies have demonstrated that the incidence of cancer diagnosis increases during the first 6 months following venous thromboembolism and venous thrombosis. There are several mechanisms of coagulopathies in patients with LC. The main mechanisms include thrombocytosis, activation of clotting due to injury on the vascular walls, increase in the level and activation of clotting factors, and production of procoagulant factor secondary to tumor hypoxia [18, 29, 69].

Venous thrombosis and hypercoagulability are known as Trousseau syndrome, and while these are mobile in character, long-term anticoagulant treatment should be considered when they are detected.

2.6.2. Paraneoplastic granulocytosis

Granulocytosis, in the absence of infection or leukemia, is relatively common at the time of diagnosis or during the follow-up of patients with LC, and it is seen in 14.5% of patients with LC, and the majority of which are giant-cell lung carcinoma cases [2, 68, 70].

Granulocytosis develops due to the production of paraneoplastic hematopoietic growth factors and certain cytokines (IL-6) [70].

No specific treatment is required other than cancer treatment.

2.6.3. *Paraneoplastic anemia*

Anemia is seen in several types of cancer. It occurs as a PNS in cancer patients and is a normocytic normochromic anemia. This condition presents with low serum iron levels, normal or elevated ferritin level, normal iron stores, and low serum erythropoietin levels [2].

In LC, anemia as a PNS may also develop depending on autoimmunity, known as autoimmune hemolytic anemia, although antibodies with a specific association are unknown [71].

Anemia generally recovers after the cancer treatment, but patients may be given an erythrocyte suspension in cases of severe anemia.

2.6.4. *Paraneoplastic thrombocytosis*

Thrombocytosis frequency is 13–32% in LC patients. IL-6 is the cytokine that is known to play a role in the development of paraneoplastic thrombocytosis [41]. It requires no specific treatment.

2.7. Nephrological paraneoplastic syndromes

Nephrological PNS involves a group of disorders that develop as a result of glomerulopathy, which may cause electrolyte imbalance and urea-creatinine elevation, leading eventually to renal failure.

2.7.1. *Membranous nephropathy*

Membranous nephropathy, developing as a PNS, is most commonly seen in patients with LC, and primarily in patients with NSCLC [72]. Proteinuria leads to the development of hypoproteinemia, resulting in edema in different parts of the body, and acute renal failure and hypertension may also develop in nephrotic syndrome.

The pathophysiology of membranous nephropathy involves the immune response given by tumor-related antigens, and antigen deposits in renal glomeruli have been reported in some patients [25, 73].

2.7.2. *Others*

Paraneoplastic glomerulopathies seen in LC patients include minimal change disease, IgA nephropathy, focal segmental glomerulosclerosis, membranoproliferative glomerulonephritis, crescentic glomerulonephritis, and thrombotic microangiopathies [73].

Effective cancer treatment will be sufficient when paraneoplastic glomerulopathies including membranous nephropathy are detected. However, renal functions should still be monitored and appropriately managed [74].

2.8. Ophthalmologic paraneoplastic syndromes

Ophthalmologic PNS related to the retina or optic nerves can be seen in LC cases, and particularly in SCLC, and retinopathy and optic neuropathy may develop and result in visual dysfunctions. Paraneoplastic syndrome in these cases is caused by the development of immune reaction. The antigens associated with paraneoplastic retinopathy are recoverin and alpha-enolase, whereas collapsin response mediator protein 5 is the antigen associated with paraneoplastic optic neuropathy [75].

Treatment is based primarily on immunosuppressive therapies. However, visual functions may not improve despite immunosuppressive therapy and effective treatment of underlying cancer [76].

2.9. Others

2.9.1. Cachexia

Cachexia is frequently seen in LC patients, and develops as a result of a rather complex process. Roughly, cachexia develops due to the chronic course of systemic inflammation associated with anorexia as well as the loss of muscle and fat mass in cancer patients [77]. While there is no specific treatment for cachexia, the most appropriate approach is to focus on cancer treatment and to provide nutritional support.

2.9.2. Fever

The diagnosis of fever as a PNS is difficult. Several conditions may cause fever in LC patients, including infections (bacterial, viral, parasitic, etc.), drug-induced fever, and autoimmune conditions other than cancer (rheumatoid arthritis, vasculitis, etc.). While the etiology of paraneoplastic fever is not completely understood, it is believed to be mediated by cytokines [78].

In addition to LC treatment, antipyretic medications can be preferred for the treatment.

3. Conclusion

Over the last century, there has been a great deal of progress in the diagnosis and pathogenesis of PNS. PNS is more common in LC patients and its frequency is higher in SCLC than in other types of LC.

PNS may involve almost all systems and may appear before or after the diagnosis of cancer. The diagnosis of the lesions that appear before LC diagnosis can significantly affect the outcomes by allowing the early identification of LC and changing its prognosis through timely treatment. Similarly, recurrences and remissions of PNS provide important clues during cancer follow-up.

A clear understanding of the mechanisms leading to PNS development in LC patients and improvements in the diagnostic and treatment methods will significantly provide positive improvements in the cancer treatment.

Author details

Dilaver Tas

Address all correspondence to: dilavertas@gmail.com

Istanbul Research and Training Hospital, Baskent University, Istanbul, Turkey

References

[1] Yeung SCJ, Habra MA, Thosani SN. Lung cancer-induced paraneoplastic syndromes. Current Opinion in Pulmonary Medicine. 2011;**17**:260-268

[2] Bilynski BT, Dzhus MB, Litvinyak RI. The conceptual and clinical problems of paraneoplastic syndrome in oncology and internal medicine. Experimental Oncology. 2015;**37**(2):82-88

[3] Varki A. Trousseau's syndrome: Multiple definitions and multiple mechanisms. Blood. 2007 Sep 15;**110**(6):1723-1729

[4] Silva JA, Mesquita KC, Igreja ACSM, Lucas ICRN, Freitas AF, Oliveira SM, et al. Paraneoplastic cutaneous manifestations: Concepts and updates. Anais Brasileiros de Dermatologia. 2013;**88**(1):9-22

[5] Holubar K. Ferdinand von Hebra 1816-1880: On the occasion of the centenary of his death. International Journal of Dermatology. 1981;**20**(4):291-295

[6] Auche M. Desnevrites peripherique schezles cancereux. Revista Médica. 1890;**10**:785-807

[7] Chung VQ, Moschella L, Zembowicz A, Liu V. Clinical and pathologic findings of paraneoplastic dermatoses. Journal of the American Academy of Dermatology. 2006;**54**:745-762

[8] Zhang HY, Zhao J. Ectopic Cushing syndrome in small cell lung cancer: A case report and literature review. Thoracic Cancer. 2017;**8**(2):114-117

[9] Paraschiv B, Diaconu CC, Toma CL, Bogdan MA. Paraneoplastic syndromes: The way an early diagnosis of lung cancer. Pneumologia. 2015;**64**(2):14-19

[10] Guichard A, Vignon G. La Polyradiculonéurite cancéreus emétastatique. Journal de Médecine de Lyon. 1949;**30**:197-207

[11] Schwartz WB, Bennett W, Curelop S, Bartter FC. A syndrome of renal sodium loss and hyponatremia probably resulting from inappropriate secretion of antidiuretic hormone. The American Journal of Medicine. 1957 Oct;**23**(4):529-542

[12] Bartter FC, Schwartz WB. The syndrome of inappropriate secretion of antidiuretic hormone. The American Journal of Medicine. 1967;**42**:790-806

[13] Gaga M, Powell C, Schraufnagel D, Schonfeld N, Rabe K, Hill NS, et al. An official American Thoracic Society/European Respiratory Society statement. The role of the pulmonologist in the diagnosis and management of lung cancer. American Journal of Respiratory and Critical Care Medicine. 2013;**188**(4):503-507

[14] Chabner BA, Thompson EC. Paraneoplastic syndromes. Hematology and Oncology MSD Manual. [Internet] 2018. Available from: http://www.msdmanuals.com/professional/hematology-and-oncology/overview-of-cancer/paraneoplastic-syndromes [Accessed: 14/02/2018]

[15] Baijens LWJ, Manni JJ. Paraneoplastic syndromes in patients with primary malignancies of the head and neck. Four cases and a review of the literature. European Archives of Oto-Rhino-Laryngology. 2006;**263**:32-36

[16] Cabry R, Ballyamanda S, Kraft M, Hong E. Understanding paraneoplastic syndromes in athletes. American College of Sports Medicine. 2013;**12**(1):33-40

[17] Cosar-Alas R, Yurut-Caloglu V, Karagol H, Caloglu M, Yalçin O, Turgut B, et al. Paraneoplastic syndrome of non-small cell lung carcinoma: A case with pancytopenia, leukocytoclastic vasculitis, and hypertrophic osteoarthropathy. Lung Cancer. 2007;**56**:455-458

[18] Tarin D. Update on clinical and mechanistic aspects of paraneoplastic syndromes. Cancer Metastasis Reviews. 2013;**32**:707-721

[19] Richardson GE, Johnson BE. Paraneoplastic syndromes in lung cancer. Current Opinion in Oncology. 1992 Apr;**4**(2):323-333

[20] Darnell RE, Posner JB. Paraneoplastic Syndromes. Oxford: Oxford University Press; 2011. p. 496

[21] Becker KL, Silva OL. Paraneoplastic endocrine syndromes. In: Becker KL, editor. Principles and Practice of Endocrinology and Metabolism. 3rd ed. Philadelphia: Lippincott Williams & Wilkins; 2001. pp. 2004-2015

[22] Stewart AF. Clinical practice. Hypercalcemia associated with cancer. New England Journal of Medicine. 2005;**352**:373-379

[23] Dalmau J, Gultekin HS, Posner JB. Paraneoplastic neurologic syndromes: Pathogenesis and physiopathology. Brain Pathology. 1999;**9**:275-284

[24] de Beukelaar JW, Sillevis Smitt PA. Managing paraneoplastic neurological disorders. The Oncologist. 2006;**11**:292-305

[25] De Oliveira Filgueira PH, Vasconcelos LF, da Silva GB, Daher Ede F. Paraneoplastic syndromes and the kidney. Saudi Journal of Kidney Diseases and Transplantation. 2010 Mar;**21**(2):222-231

[26] Franco DL, Thomas L. Small cell lung cancer associated with multiple paraneoplastic syndromes. Biomédica. 2017;**37**:8-10

[27] Tantisattamo E, Ng RC. Dual paraneoplastic syndromes: Small cell lung carcinoma-related oncogenic osteomalacia and syndrome of inappropriate antidiuretic hormone secretion: Report of a case and review of the literature. Hawaii Medical Journal. 2011;**70**:139-143

[28] Akinosoglou K, Siagris D, Geropoulou E, Kosmopoulou O, Velissaris D, Kyriazopoulou V, et al. Hyperamylasaemia and dual paraneoplastic syndromes in small cell lung cancer. Annals of Clinical Biochemistry. 2013;**51**(1):101-105

[29] Kanaji N, Watanabe N, Kita N, Bandoh S, Tadokoro A, Ishii T, et al. Paraneoplastic syndromes associated with lung cancer. World Journal of Clinical Oncology. 2014; **5**(3):197-223

[30] Mayer S, Cypess AM, Kocher ON, Berman SM, Huberman MS, Hartzband PI, et al. Uncommon presentations of some common malignancies: Case 1. Sequential paraneoplastic endocrine syndromes in small-cell lung cancer. Journal of Clinical Oncology. 2005;**23**:1312-1314

[31] Mazzone PJ, Arroliga AC. Endocrine paraneoplastic syndromes in lung cancer. Current Opinion in Pulmonary Medicine. 2003;**9**:313-320

[32] Scanagatta P, Montresor E, Pergher S. Cushing's syndrome induced by bronchopulmonary carcinoid tumours: A review of 98 cases and our experience of two cases. Chirurgia Italiana. 2004;**56**:63-70

[33] Howlett TA, Rees LH, Besser GM. Cushing's syndrome. Clinics in Endocrinology and Metabolism. 1985;**14**:911-945

[34] Jeong C, Lee J, Ryu S, Lee HY, Shin AY, Kim JS, et al. A case of ectopic adrenocorticotropic hormone syndrome in small cell lung cancer. Tuberculosis and Respiratory Diseases. 2015;**78**(4):436-439

[35] Ilias I, Torpy DJ, Pacak K, Mullen N, Wesley RA, Nieman LK. Cushing's syndrome due to ectopic corticotropin secretion: Twenty years experience at the national institutes of health. The Journal of Clinical Endocrinology and Metabolism. 2005;**90**:4955-4962

[36] Iyer P, Ibrahim M, Siddiqui W, Dirweesh A. Syndrome of inappropriate secretion of anti-diuretic hormone (SIADH) as an initial presenting sign of non small cell lung cancer-case report and literature review. Respiratory Medicine Case Reports. 2017 Aug 11;**22**:164-167

[37] Vanhees SL, Paridaens R, Vansteenkiste JF. Syndrome of inappropriate antidiuretic hormone associated with chemotherapy-induced tumor lysis in small-cell lung cancer: Case report and literature review. Annals of Oncology. 2000;**11**(8):1061-1065

[38] Gross AJ, Steinberg SM, Reilly JG, Bliss DP, Brennan J, Le PT, et al. Atrial natriuretic factor and arginine vasopressin production in tumor cell lines from patients with lung cancer and their relationship to serum sodium. Cancer Research. 1993;**53**:67-74

[39] McClelland MT. Paraneoplastic syndromes related to lung cancer. Clinical Journal of Oncology Nursing. 2010;**14**(13):357-364

[40] Hiraki A, Ueoka H, Takata I, Gemba G, Bessho A, Segawa Y, et al. Hypercalcemia leukocytosis syndrome associated with lung cancer. Lung Cancer. 2004;**43**(3):301-307

[41] Thomas L, Kwok Y, Edelman MJ. Management of paraneoplastic syndromes in lung cancer. Current Treatment Options in Oncology. 2004;**5**:51-62

[42] Karmy-Jones R, Vallières E. Carcinoid crisis after biopsy of a bronchial carcinoid. The Annals of Thoracic Surgery. 1993;**56**:1403-1405

[43] Antoine JC, Camdessanche JP. Paraneoplastic neuropathies. Current Opinion in Neurology. 2017;**30**:513-520

[44] Pelosof LC, Gerber DE. Paraneoplastic syndromes: An approach to diagnosis and treatment. Mayo Clinic Proceedings. 2010;**85**(9):838-854

[45] Graus F, Delattre JY, Antoine JC, Dalmau J, Giometto B, Grisold W, et al. Recommended diagnostic criteria for paraneoplastic neurological syndromes. Journal of Neurology, Neurosurgery, and Psychiatry. 2004;**75**(8):1135-1140

[46] Antoine JC, Hannorat J, Vocanson J, Koenig F, Aguera M, Belin MF, et al. Posterior uveitis, paraneoplastic encephalomyelitis and auto-antibodies reacting with developmental protein of brain and retina. Journal of the Neurological Sciences. 1993;**117**(1-2):215-223

[47] Graus F, Keime-Guibert F, Rene R, Benyahia B, Ribalta T, Ascaso C, et al. Anti Hu-associated paraneoplastic encephalomyelitis: Analysis of 200 patients. Brain. 2001;**124**(Pt 6):1138-1148

[48] Oh SJ, Gurtekin Y, Dropcho EJ, King P, Claussen GC. Anti-Hu antibody neuropathy: A clinical, electrophysiological, and pathological study. Clinical Neurophysiology. 2005;**116**(1):28-34

[49] Gultekin SH, Rosenfeld MR, Voltz R, Eichen J, Posner JB, Dalmau J. Paraneoplastic limbic encephalitis: Neurological symptoms, immunological findings and tumour association in 50 patients. Brain. 2000;**123**(Pt 7):1481-1494

[50] Dalmau J, Rosenfeld MR. Paraneoplastic syndromes of the CNS. Lancet Neurology. 2008;**7**(4):327-340

[51] Honnorat J, Antoine JC. Paraneoplastic neurologic syndromes. Orphanet Journal of Rare Diseases. 2007;**2**:22

[52] Sabafer L, Titulaer M, Saiz A, Verschuuren J, Gure AO, Graus F. SOX1 antibodies are markers of paraneoplastic Lambert Eaton myasthenic syndrome. Neurology. 2008;**70**(12): 924-928

[53] Bataller I, Graus F, Saiz A, Vilchez JJ. Clinical outcome in adult onset idiopathic or paraneoplastic opsoclonus-myoclonus. Brain. 2001;**124**:437-443

[54] Weinkauf C, McPhillips S, Krouse R, Levine I. Autoimmune gastrointestinal paralysis: Failure of conventional treatment without immunomodulation. Case Reports in Surgery. 2014:4. Article ID 180654

[55] Boyce S, Harper J. Paraneoplastic dermatoses. Dermatologic Clinics. 2002;**20**:523-532

[56] Karakas Y, Esin E, Laçin S, Ceyhan K, Heper AO, Yalcin S. A case of acanthosis nigricans as a paraneoplastic syndrome with squamous cell lung cancer. OncoTargets and Therapy. 2016 Aug 3;**9**:4815-4820

[57] Sabir S, James WD, Schuchter LM. Cutaneous manifestations of cancer. Current Opinion in Oncology. 1999;**11**(2):139-144

[58] DiRollo D, Abeni D, Tracanna M, Capo A, Amerio P. Cancer risk in dermatomyositis: A systematic review of the literature. Giornale Italiano di Dermatologia e Venereologia. 2014 Oct;**149**(5):525-537

[59] Ahuja S, Makkar P, Gupta S, Vigoda I. Paraneoplastic syndrome and underlying breast cancer: A worsening rash despite initiation of chemotherapy. Journal of Community and Supportive Oncology. 2016 May;**14**(5):229-231

[60] Castro A, Barroso A, Parente B. Dermatomyositis as the first manifestation of a lung tumor. Revista Portuguesa de Pneumologia. 2013;**19**(4):179-183

[61] Wang J, Guo G, Chen G, Wu B, Lu L, Bao L. Meta-analysis of the association of dermatomyositis and polymyositis with cancer. British Journal of Dermatology. 2013;**169**:838-847

[62] Bakos N, Krasznai G, Begany A. Erythema gyratum repens an immunologic paraneoplastic disorders. Pathology and Oncology Research. 1997;**3**(1):59-61

[63] Tas D, Demirer E, Ayhan G, Citici NU, Okutan O. Cutaneous paraneoplastic syndrome in a patient with non small cell lung cancer: Case report. Acıbadem Üniversitesi Sağlık Bilimleri Dergisi. 2013;**4**(1):26-29

[64] Yavuz E, Yeşilova Y, Sula B. Paraneoplastic dermatoses. The Medical Bulletin of Haseki. 2010;**48**:61-67

[65] Zarzour JG, Singh S, Andea A, Cafardi JA. Acrakeratosis paraneoplastica (Bazex syndrome): Report of a case associated with small cell lung carcinoma and review of the literature. Radiology Case. 2011;**5**(7):1-6

[66] Carlson S, Rauchenstein J. Hypertrophic osteoarthropathy. The Journal of the American Osteopathic Association. December 2015;**115**:745

[67] Özen A, Saynak M, Kocak Z, Bayır-Angin G, Uregen B, Çosar-Alas R, et al. Hypertrophic osteoartropathy associated with lung cancer: A case report. Turk Onkoloji Dergisi. 2007;**22**(3):141-145

[68] Sreevatsa A, Babu SM, Babu GK, Suresh TM. Hyperleucocytosis, an unusual paraneoplastic manifestation of lung cancer: Case report and review of literature. Journal of Cancer Research and Therapeutics. 2015;**11**:669

[69] Viau M, Renaud MC, Gregoire J, Sebastienelli A, Plante M. Paraneoplastic syndromes associated with gynecological cancers: A systematic review. Gynecologic Oncology. 2017;**146**:661-671

[70] Le Roy A, Pasquier P, Savard D, Bugier S, Merat S, Pilo JE, et al. Paraneoplastic granulocytosis in an advanced lung cancer patient. Annales de Biologie Clinique. 2014;**72**(3):367-370

[71] Holbrechts S, Gorham J, Sideris S, Meert AP, Durieux V, Berghmans T, et al. Autoimmune paraneoplastic syndromes associated to lung cancer: A systematic review of literature. Lung Cancer. 2017;**106**:93-101

[72] Ohara G, Satoh H, Kurishima K, Ohtsuka M, Hizawa N. Paraneoplastic nephrotic syndrome in patients with lung cancer. Internal Medicine. 2009;**48**:1817-1820

[73] Bacchetta J, Juillard L, Cochat P, Droz JP. Paraneoplastic glomerular diseases and malignancies. Critical Reviews in Oncology/Hematology. 2009;**70**:39-58

[74] Aytekin A, Ozet A, Bilgetekin I, Ogut B, Ciltas A, Benekli M. A case of membranous glomerulopathy associated with lung cancer and review of the literature. Molecular and Clinical Oncology. 2017;**7**:241-243

[75] Gordon LK. Paraneoplastic syndromes in neuro-ophthalmology. Journal of Neuro-Ophthalmology. 2015;**35**:306-314

[76] Rahimy E, Sarraf D. Paraneoplastic and non-paraneoplastic retinopathy and optic neuropathy: Evaluation and management. Survey of Ophthalmology. 2013;**58**:430-458

[77] Schcolnik-Cabrera A, Chávez-Blanco A, Domínguez-Gómez G, Dueñas-González A. Understanding tumor anabolism and patient catabolism in cancer-associated cachexia. American Journal of Cancer Research. 2017 May 1;**7**(5):1107-1135

[78] Zell JA, Chang JC. Neoplastic fever: A neglected paraneoplastic syndrome. Supportive Care in Cancer. 2005;**13**(11):870-877

Permissions

All chapters in this book were first published in LCSDT, by InTech Open; hereby published with permission under the Creative Commons Attribution License or equivalent. Every chapter published in this book has been scrutinized by our experts. Their significance has been extensively debated. The topics covered herein carry significant findings which will fuel the growth of the discipline. They may even be implemented as practical applications or may be referred to as a beginning point for another development.

The contributors of this book come from diverse backgrounds, making this book a truly international effort. This book will bring forth new frontiers with its revolutionizing research information and detailed analysis of the nascent developments around the world.

We would like to thank all the contributing authors for lending their expertise to make the book truly unique. They have played a crucial role in the development of this book. Without their invaluable contributions this book wouldn't have been possible. They have made vital efforts to compile up to date information on the varied aspects of this subject to make this book a valuable addition to the collection of many professionals and students.

This book was conceptualized with the vision of imparting up-to-date information and advanced data in this field. To ensure the same, a matchless editorial board was set up. Every individual on the board went through rigorous rounds of assessment to prove their worth. After which they invested a large part of their time researching and compiling the most relevant data for our readers.

The editorial board has been involved in producing this book since its inception. They have spent rigorous hours researching and exploring the diverse topics which have resulted in the successful publishing of this book. They have passed on their knowledge of decades through this book. To expedite this challenging task, the publisher supported the team at every step. A small team of assistant editors was also appointed to further simplify the editing procedure and attain best results for the readers.

Apart from the editorial board, the designing team has also invested a significant amount of their time in understanding the subject and creating the most relevant covers. They scrutinized every image to scout for the most suitable representation of the subject and create an appropriate cover for the book.

The publishing team has been an ardent support to the editorial, designing and production team. Their endless efforts to recruit the best for this project, has resulted in the accomplishment of this book. They are a veteran in the field of academics and their pool of knowledge is as vast as their experience in printing. Their expertise and guidance has proved useful at every step. Their uncompromising quality standards have made this book an exceptional effort. Their encouragement from time to time has been an inspiration for everyone.

The publisher and the editorial board hope that this book will prove to be a valuable piece of knowledge for researchers, students, practitioners and scholars across the globe.

List of Contributors

Fiona Lim Mei Ying
Department of Oncology, Princess Margaret Hospital, Hong Kong

Vivek Kaushik, Juan Sebastian Yakisich, Yogesh Kulkarni, Neelam Azad and Anand Krishnan V. Iyer
Department of Pharmaceutical Sciences, School of Pharmacy, Hampton University, Hampton, VA, USA

Alexandru C. Grigorescu
Department of Medical Oncolog, Institute of Oncology Bucharest, Romania

Jelena Stojšić
Department of Thoracopulmonary Pathology, Service of Pathology, Clinical Centre of Serbia, Belgrade, Serbia

Li Zhang and Yanyan Pan
Department of Central Laboratory, Dalian Municipal Central Hospital, Dalian, Liaoning, China

Anine Crous and Heidi Abrahamse
University of Johannesburg, Gauteng, South Africa

Milic Medenica and Danilo Cosovic
Hospital for Lung Diseases - Brezovik, Niksic, Montenegro

Miras Medenica
Wrightington, Wigan and Leigh NHS Foundation Trust, UK

Metin Budak and Mustafa Yildiz
Biophysics Department, Faculty of Medicine, Trakya University, Edirne, Turkey

Elien Derveaux
Faculty of Medicine and Life Sciences, Hasselt University, Hasselt, Belgium

Evelyne Louis
Department of Respiratory Oncology, University Hospitals KU Leuven, Leuven, Belgium

Karolien Vanhove
Faculty of Medicine and Life Sciences, Hasselt University, Hasselt, Belgium
Department of Respiratory Medicine, Algemeen Ziekenhuis Vesalius, Tongeren, Belgium

Liene Bervoets
Department of Medical Microbiology, Maastricht Universitair Medisch Centrum, Maastricht, The Netherlands

Liesbet Mesotten
Faculty of Medicine and Life Sciences, Hasselt University, Hasselt, Belgium
Department of Nuclear Medicine, Ziekenhuis Oost-Limburg, Genk, Belgium

Michiel Thomeer
Faculty of Medicine and Life Sciences, Hasselt University, Hasselt, Belgium
Department of Respiratory Medicine, Ziekenhuis Oost-Limburg, Genk, Belgium

Peter Adriaensens
Applied and Analytical Chemistry, Institute for Materials Research, Hasselt University, Hasselt, Belgium

Ioana Berindan-Neagoe
Research Center for Functional Genomics, Biomedicine and Translational Medicine, "Iuliu Hatieganu", University of Medicine and Pharmacy Iuliu-Hatieganu, Cluj-Napoca, Romania
Medfuture—Research Center for Advanced Medicine, University of Medicine and Pharmacy Iuliu-Hatieganu, Cluj-Napoca, Romania
Department of Functional Genomics and Experimental Pathology, The Oncological Institute "Prof. Dr. Ion Chiricuta", Cluj-Napoca, Romania

Cornelia Braicu
Research Center for Functional Genomics, Biomedicine and Translational Medicine, "Iuliu Hatieganu", University of Medicine and Pharmacy Iuliu-Hatieganu, Cluj-Napoca, Romania

Diana Gulei
Medfuture—Research Center for Advanced Medicine, University of Medicine and Pharmacy Iuliu-Hatieganu, Cluj-Napoca, Romania

Ciprian Tomuleasa
Research Center for Functional Genomics, Biomedicine and Translational Medicine, "Iuliu Hatieganu", University of Medicine and Pharmacy Iuliu-Hatieganu, Cluj-Napoca, Romania
Department of Hematology, The Oncological Institute "Prof. Dr. Ion Chiricuta", Cluj-Napoca, Romania

George Adrian Calin
Department of Experimental Therapeutics, The University of Texas M.D. Anderson Cancer Center, Houston, TX, USA

Dilaver Tas
Istanbul Research and Training Hospital, Baskent University, Istanbul, Turkey

Index

www.ingramcontent.com/pod-product-compliance
Lightning Source LLC
LaVergne TN
LVHW080946210926
848485LV00004B/787